To
Lyanne
My Best,

8

Powerful Secrets to Anti-Aging

Dr. Paul Ling Tai

Health Secrets USA
in conjunction with
United Writers Press, Inc.
P.O. Box 326
Tucker, Georgia USA 30085-0326

ISBN-13: 978-1-934216-90-3
ISBN-10: 1-934216-90-9

Printed in Indonesia

Disclaimer

This publication is designed to provide scientific, authoritative and personal anecdotal information in regard to the subject matter covered. The reader understands that the author and publisher are not engaged in rendering professional services.

If you require medical, psychological or any other expert assistance, please seek the services of a professional.

The information, personal experiences, anecdotal stories, procedures and suggestions contained within this book are not intended to replace the services of a trained health care professional or to serve as a replacement for a professional medical doctor's advice and care. You should consult a health care professional regarding any of the information, ideas, personal experiences, anecdotal stories, procedures, supplements, drug therapies or any other information from this book.

The author and publisher hereby specifically disclaim any and all liability arising directly or indirectly from the use or application of any of the products, ideas, procedures, drug therapies, or suggestions contained in this book and any errors, omissions, and inaccuracies in the information contained herein.

The treatments and supplements included in this book are for identification purposes only and are not intended to recommend or endorse the product.

Important Warning

    This book is intended for readers and physicians to evaluate hormone deficiencies occurring in the human body; however, it is not intended for pregnant or nursing women, nor is it intended for children below the age of 18.

    Optimal and deficient values presented within this book do not necessarily correspond to the reference values found in local laboratories. The values and references used in this book are purely subjective and come from the author's own personal experiences and by other physicians who have shared their experiences.

    The reader should not base his or her assessment solely on the values given in this book. Hormonal imbalances are determined by laboratories, and corrective approaches are determined by a trained medical professional.

    Laboratory values within this book constitute only some of the information the reader should gather. Much more emphasis should be placed on clinical evaluation, signs and symptoms. Many other clinical and laboratory tests should be used before deciding on a diagnosis and/or treatment. A reader should always seek a physician's advice before deciding to institute any form of medical treatment.

CONTENTS

Acknowledgments   **ix**

Foreword   **xi**

Dr. Morris Westfried M.D., FAAD, FASDS
Prof. Dr. Helton Traber de Castilho, M.D., Ph.D., M.S.

Introduction: Luck of the Draw—Bad Genetics   xv

Secret I 1

Chapter 1: Hormones Explained   3
Hormones and receptor cells + Steroids and peptides + Women and hormones + Men and hormones + Secretion+ Anabolic and Catabolic

Chapter 2: Chronological vs. Biological age   17
Chronological age + Biological age + Hormone deficiencies + Biological signs of aging + Free radicals + Antioxidants

Chapter 3: Counting Your Hormones: Easy as 1, 2, 3   37
Hormonal testing and monitoring + Saliva testing+ Contaminations + Urine testing + Serum testing + Determining hormonal normalcy + Hormonal fluctuations + Direct measurements

Secret II 49

Chapter 4: Synthetic vs. Bioidentical hormones   51
Cells and cell receptors+ Phytohormones + Synthetic hormone composition + Potential side effects of synthetic hormones + Bioidentical hormones

Chapter 5: Hormone Delivery   58
Pros and Cons of: Injections + Dermal Patches + Gels and lotions + Pills, tablets and capsules + Sublingual sprays + New technology: Liposomes

Secret III 67

Chapter 6: DHEA   69
DHEA production and secretion + DHEA conversion + Bioidentical supplementation + DHEA-S + DHEA in men + DHEA in women + DHEA and cancer + DHEA and sugar+ DHEA deficiency and excess

Chapter 7: Pregnenolone   83
Pregnenolone production and secretion + Pregnenolone and other hormones+ Memory + Mood+ Stress+ Pregnenolone deficiency and excess

Secret IV...91

Chapter 8: HGH   93
HGH production and secretion + IGF-1 + Chondrocytes + Determining who should use HGH+ HGH deficiency+ HGH and memory loss+ Dendrites + Side effects +Secretagogues + Deer Antler + Growth Factors+ HGH deficiency and excess

Chapter 9: Testosterone   106
Testosterone explained + Testosterone secretion+ Testosterone in the ovaries + Testosterone in the testes + Andropause + Menopause+ Injections + Liposomes+ Testosterone deficiency and excess

Secret V...121

Chapter 10: Estrogen   122
Estrogen explained+ Menstrual cycles + FSH and LH + E1 + E2 + E3 + Postpartum + Perimenopause + Menopause + Estrogen in men + Synthetic versus Natural+ Estrogen deficiency and excess

Chapter 11: Progesterone 148
Progesterone explained + Progesterone secretion and production+ Estrogen and progesterone + PMS +Bones+ Heart + Brain + Synthetic versus Natural+ Progesterone deficiency and excess

Secret VI...167

Chapter 12: Melatonin   168
Melatonin explained + Melatonin secretion and production + Sleep + Jet lag + Dosage+ melatonin deficiency and excess

Chapter 13: Thyroid   178
Thyroid functions + T3 and T4 + Hypothyroid + Iodine + Hyperthyroid + Metabolism + Thyroid support diet plan + Self-assessment + Synthetic versus Natural + Anti-aging Health Secret+ thyroid deficiency and excess

Chapter 14: Adrenals 198

Adrenals explained + Adrenal gland production + Cortisol+ Hypoadrenal + Adrenals and stress+ cortisol deficiency and excess

Secret VII...198

Chapter 15: Hormones and our Skin 212

Anatomy+ winkles+ cellulite+ skin thickness+ bruising+ Vitamins+ Antioxidants

Chapter 16: Building your skin with natural ingredients 228

Puereria Mirifica + Ginseng + Coenzyme Q10+ Argania + Peptides + L-caffeine + L-Carnitine Caffeine + Paullinia Cupana

Chapter 17: Look younger in 30 days 237

Skin after a certain age + Cosmetic surgeries + Pleoliposomes + Experts on liposomes + Fat and water soluble moisturizers + Expiration dates + Cleansers+ Soap + pH levels+ Exfoliating + Exfoliants + Diamonds + Moisturizing + SPF +Anti-aging Health Secret

Secret VIII..255

Chapter 18: Dr. Tai's Asian Diet 256

Fattening food allergies+ overeating + abundance and scarcity + Green tea and water + glycemic index + metabolism + hormones + hypothyroid and weight gain + condoments + alcohol+ Max-Digestion + Calcium +Vitamin C + Dr. Tai's Diet Plan and additional suggestions

Chapter 19: Delayed food allergy/Food intolerance 268

Delayed food allergy/intolerance + obesity + weight loss + food detective + tested foods

Chapter 20: Extreme Anti-aging Technology 275

Xeno stem cell + live cell technology + cell therapy + freeze drying + embryonic cells + screening treatment + rare risks + oval cell therapy + injectable cell therapy

Chapter 21: Is there life after 50? 285

by Katherine Lee

Chapter 22: Conditions & Supplements   289
Acne + Adrenal fatigue+ Alzheimer's, memory loss and learning difficulties + Andropause + Arthritis, Fibromyalgia and muscle, joint pain + Cell division + Diabetes + Edema, water retention + Fibrocystic breasts, ovarian and uterine fibroids + Heart disease, cholesterol, Arrhythmia + High blood pressure + Menopause + Migraines, headaches + Obesity + Osteoporosis + Prostate inflammation + Sexual dysfunction, female and male + Stress + Wrinkles

Resources   313

References   317

Index   337

ACKNOWLEDGMENTS

Profound thanks go to Katherine M. Lee. Also, special thanks to Kristale Ivezaj for her dedicated work in compiling this book.

I am extremely grateful to the thousands of patients worldwide who have shared their experiences with me—they were my primary inspiration for the writing of this book. Also, my very heartfelt thanks to all the doctors who were willing to share their stories, secrets, trials and tribulations for the sake of those who continuously strive for improvement. Thank you!

—*Dr. Paul Ling Tai*

For centuries, a healthy life has been an elusive goal. Food such as kefir, an eastern European yogurt-like drink, have been credited with contributing to long life. In New York, fish wholesalers M. Slavin & Sons Ltd. proclaim, "Eat fish and live longer." Does any one food guarantee a long life, or is the answer a lifestyle?

Ayurvedic medicine has three diets for three different body types: "xata," "pita" and "kappa." Dr. Adama assigns diets associated with your health type, and a myriad of other diet books promote their version of "diet nirvana." Regional diets that are healthy include the Mediterranean diet (olive oil and vegetables); the traditional Japanese diet (seafood, sea vegetables and soy); and the French paradox, with its beneficial effect of wine despite a diet rich in saturated fat. There are elements of these diets that lower risk factors for heart disease. Diets incorporated in the American Heart Association include five or more servings of fruit and vegetables. However, diet is not the only answer to a long, healthy life. Why?

What we do does not change our genetic makeup. Our cells are preprogrammed for eventual wear and tear. As we age, our peak performance will slow. The hormone levels of youth will fall, and we will show signs of aging: thinner skin, easier bruising, receding gums, hair loss, etc. Perhaps we can slow this process with supplements.

Any health-food store is stocked with numerous individual and combination supplements that are supposed to help one condition or another. The diversity and variety can be daunting even for an expert: vitamin E, ginkgo biloba, beta carotene, etc. Some studies question their value, so what's the answer?

In *8 Powerful Secrets to Super-Charged Anti-aging: A Natural, Simple and Effective Program to Feel Stronger, Look Younger and Live Longer,* Dr. Paul Tai comprehensively approaches aging from the perspective of hormones. Eight key hormones—DHEA (dehydropeplandosterone), HGH (human growth hormone), progesterone, estrogen, melatonin, testosterone, pregnenolone, adrenal hormone (cortisol), and thyroid—are all fully discussed. His user-friendly approach discusses health issues and how bioidentical hormones can make you healthier and improve your life. This natural and simple approach addresses menopause, weight gain, loss of sex drive, lack of stamina and other signs of aging.

Aging is inevitable, but a robust life is achievable. Finally, there may be gold in the golden years. Instead of a life filled with pills and doctor visits, a healthful, happier life is in your future with Dr. Tai's book.

—*Dr. Morris Westfried, M.D., FAAD, FASDS*
Cosmetic Dermatologist Surgeon

"Transforming men and women to younger and more beautiful human beings is my passion in life."

I spent my whole life dedicated to sharpening my surgical skills and medical knowledge in pursuit of the Anti-Aging solution. As a teacher and post graduate professor of plastic surgery, I was able to help young doctors acquire similar skills, but more importantly to share and instill in them my anti-aging passion.

In my observations of human health conditions and diseases, even watching my own family members and friends age, I can clearly say that "growing old is anything but graceful."

There is nothing "Sexy" or "Glamorous" about sagging wrinkles, graying hair, increasing fat, loss of sex drive and feeling old and ugly, except in the make-believe world of Hollywood with their magical cameras, make-up artists, and trick photography where everyone looks beautiful.

Yes, I have nearly perfected plastic surgery of the human face and body, but Dr. Paul Ling Tai's book *8 Powerful Secrets to Anti Aging* approaches beauty, youth, and vitality from the inside out; they are every surgeon's hope and dream come true!

Dr. Tai's work is tremendously inspiring as he delivers simple and concise tools you need for looking and feeling younger. Dr. Tai teaches you powerful secrets in natural bio-identical hormones, nutritional supplements, the latest testing to discover and evaluate your true "Biological Age," and food poisons that may be the cause of all your pains, inflammations, and miseries.

This is a step-by-step approach to Anti-Aging for the layman as well as physicians or health workers. For the first time, we have a clear and loud answer to the eternal question, "Is there an Anti-Aging solution?"

The answer is a resounding YES! It is in this wonderful, easy to read and science-backed book of the *8 Powerful Secrets to Anti Aging*.

Good luck, good health, and enjoy!

—*Prof. Dr. Helton Traber de Castilho, M.D., PhD. MS.*
Associate Professor in Plastic Surgery Section
Sao Paulo Federal University
Visiting Professor, West Virginia University, Morgantown, WV
Fellow in Otorrinolaringoplasty, Sao Paulo University, 1984

My father: dead at 43
My mother: open-heart surgery, twice
Brother #1: dead at 45
Brother #2: open-heart surgery at 42
Brother #3: dead at 5

Dub, Dub, Dub—this is the sound your heart makes when it's beating. Death comes to one whose heart stops beating, and, in my family, hearts stop beating too soon. It's genetic. I have bad genes, and because I recognized this, I've labored intensively to develop natural health supplements that will minimize the risks I've inherited. So far, I've made it; I'm nearly 60 and I feel good. I'm healthy and I'm happy.

My father and brother, the two most important men in my life died of heart failure. The second eldest of my brothers has had open-heart surgery; my aging mother has had two. None of these people drank or smoked; they ate well and have taken good care of themselves. Again, it's genetic. Acknowledging this was my first step towards avoiding problems that are known to run in my family.

But the deaths of my family members didn't convince me to alter my lifestyle—I didn't begin until the day I realized I felt like the thousands of patients I'd treated. I had studied their conditions, examined patients and treated them, but I didn't really understand how they felt until I felt the very same way.

Then I went on a mission—a mission to change how I felt and therefore the lives of my patients.

In the upcoming chapters, you will find fun, practical summaries of the extensive medical research I've conducted through the years. This book is about what works and what doesn't in a practical, everyday sense; it is not intended for academic use. Every detail included in every single chapter was derived from reading and learning from all the wonderful doctors I came to respect and, of course, from my personal experiences as well. This book is the story of my life, your life, every person's life. It is the story of the complex organism we call the human body.

I learned all this not for a paycheck or in order to pass a med-school exam. I learned it to save my own life. I know from first-hand experience that it is possible for you to feel stronger, look younger, and ultimately live longer.

MY STORY
Made in China

At a very early age, I became aware of all the ills and sufferings around the world. My father, a chemist by profession, died at the young age of 43 when I was only a year old; I don't remember him. Shortly after, my younger brother died unexpectedly; he was only five years old.

A few years after my father's passing, my mother, a master acupuncturist and herbalist, married a Dutch import-export business tycoon. In the 1940s and 50s, my stepfather was well-respected, known in Shanghai for social and financial prominence.

A kind man, he took in my two brothers, my sister and myself and provided for the whole family before communism took over. Everything he had the government took away, which meant everything "we" had vanished into the hands of those who did not work for it. Communism overthrew capitalism and things started getting crazy in the city, which meant we needed to get out of China.

Being Chinese aristocrats had its blessings and its burdens. We were once respected, but during the shift in government we were cursed and spat on. Luckily, we had maintained strong ties with old friends; my mother had been close to the wife of a Brazilian ambassador. We took advantage of the connection and applied for visas. Months later, we received notice from the Chinese government that our whole family would be allowed to leave China, unharmed.

To be able to leave Red China in 1954 was like winning the lottery—especially since I had a brother and sister who were old enough to be in the "People's Army." (During that time, Chinese communists wanted every able-bodied teenager for its military. I was seven so I didn't have to worry about any of that.)

I followed my family around the world and into Brazil. Circumnavigating the world for 35 days meant sea sickness, poor nutrition (if one ate at all) and sleeping in a cramped room; on the ship, we were sardines floating above sardines, leaving behind a home of comfort and luxury—permanently.

Red Clay
"A new life in the jungles of Brazil"

Brazil was strange. We had never seen so many green trees. Birds and insects abounded, and the soil, the soil was not brown or black (as we knew it). It was RED! There was red soil everywhere; it covered our tiny home as it did our bodies.

I was uncomfortable, and so was my family. We were foreigners in every sense. We didn't speak the language nor did we understand the culture. With no money or friends we depended on the Brazilian embassy for hand-outs and they kindly provided us with a small closet-like place to live in and a few loaves of bread on occasion when they recalled we existed.

In those days, dinner was a rarity for us but my mother made the family sit together every evening. (She referred to these evening chats as "family meetings.") Occasionally, we had a few pieces of bread or a can of sardines to munch on while we discussed our situation. During one of those family meetings, my mother asked my siblings (who were all older than I) to help her go door-to-door and sell some of our family trinkets to raise some cash. They refused.

I assume they rebuked Mother's offer because persuading people to buy our trinkets was far too embarrassing an act for my "cool" teenage siblings. But I, the youngest and most eager to explore, volunteered. I was excited, because helping my mother meant spending all day with her.

Together, we sold tablecloths, handkerchiefs, chopsticks and small porcelain. In the back streets of Sao Paulo, I learned Portuguese…and a lot about people. It was there that I made an observation that would shape the rest of my life.

"People," I said to myself, "are naturally good. And just as they have helped us, I want to help them." (I still believe this is true.) If approached honestly and straightforwardly, most people will try to help you. And If anyone needed help at the time, it was us.

Rule of Incentive:
"If we didn't sell, we didn't eat."

Every morning, shortly before the sun rose, my mother and I would share a cup of coffee and a piece of bread before setting out into the city streets of Sao Paulo.

Almost rhetorically, she would ask, "Why do we only drink half of a cup of coffee and eat half a piece of bread?" I didn't know how to answer her, because, well, I was seven and hungry. She answered her own question by delicately explaining that by eating half a slice of bread and by drinking half a cup of coffee we had saved enough for an evening dinner if we did not sell anything that day. In other words, "no sales, no food." From then on, the thought of having dinner was all it took for me to sell passionately.

I became known as Sao Paulo's seven-year-old Chinese sales boy. My mother, a beautiful and sincere woman, towered over me as I led the way through the alleys and back ways of Brazil speaking broken Portuguese and selling trinkets door-to-door. She followed every step I took and every word I uttered with a gentle smile and a soft and subtle nod. That is how we survived.

America

And then one day, my mother surprised me with the announcement that I was to go to America! She was determined that I would go to the United States. I protested, but somehow I was unable to influence her. I didn't want to leave Brazil—I was 17 and had a home, friends, a girlfriend (my first)—a reasonably normal teenaged life. During my strongest protests, my mother acted as if I was invisible and continued packing for my trip. Everything seemed surreal; I didn't realize I was really leaving until I found myself at the airport terminal with my bag in hand.

Traditional Chinese families rarely, if ever, touch one another. Hugs and kisses are never to be shared so it is noteworthy that the first time I had physical contact with my mother was at the Sao Paulo Airport. She shook my hand as a gesture of saying goodbye and she placed a tightly-rolled, crisp American $100 bill in my shirt pocket. I read her eyes as they spoke to me. "Don't call me, I'll call you." Twelve years passed before I saw or spoke to my mother again. There were no telephone calls, letters or visitations.

Big hearts in a big country
"Thank you America!"

I became my own best friend, caretaker and confidante. Yet I was fortunate enough to find a gracious family in Oregon who sponsored me for eight months. It was there I learned to speak English and act like an American.

Many families along the way "adopted" me; they fed me when I was hungry and gave me shelter when I had nowhere to go. Even so, after I applied and was accepted to college, I hated the holiday season. Everyone else would leave for the holidays while I stayed behind. There were times when I slept in unheated sheds on campus and literally ate what I was able to kill…with my car.

Miracles in Michigan

I was blessed to have a hospital residency in Detroit, Michigan where I honed my skills as a surgeon and clinician. I did a rotation through all the hospital departments, but enjoyed the emergency room most. Wow! I loved the drama of the emergency room—the adrenaline, the blood and the glory.

Once I finished, after a few years of diligent work, I was able to build one of the most successful reconstructive surgical clinics in the U.S. My specialty? Foot, ankle, leg, bone, joint and tendon reconstruction.

My partner and I saw over 100 patients a day. I was busy—life was picking up for me. We performed dozens of surgeries daily, both at our outpatient surgical clinic as well as at a dedicated surgical department at the local hospital. With our own internal radiology and physiotherapy departments, along with an ambulatory surgical center, we had the most modern facilities around.

The patients that came to our offices and clinics complained of broken-down joints, and were ravaged with diseases like diabetes, arthritis, and deteriorated central and peripheral nervous systems. All I could do was patch, repair and send them on their way the best I knew how.

And then I turned 40. And suddenly, I began to understand and empathize with my patients and their underlying health problems. I discovered the source of virtually all of them.

It's called *aging*.

I lived through almost six decades before I "got it." I needed to drastically change my life-style by starting at the core. I began to treat myself, becoming both the physician and the patient, and I asked myself a question.

"Dr. Tai, what makes you, moves you, energizes you, and beautifies you?"

And the answer that came to me was "Hormones." I began to pay attention to hormones—and the lack of them—and I understood at last that it is the gradual depletion of hormones of all kinds over time that results in what we call aging. I knew then that if I could just discover a way to naturally replace the hormones, I could change my life and those of my patients. And I did.

Now I'm excited about my life and the improvement I've seen in others because of natural supplementation and I'm here to tell you that you no longer have to suffer the crippling pain of inflammation and watch yourself wither away in despair. I am confident in sharing with you my health secrets for powerful energy and a healthier, longer life. I know I have finally discovered the secrets because I feel it, just as I learned of my patients' maladies. The truth is I've never had it this good.

But, as I said, it wasn't always this way. Travel back in time with me and see what I mean.

Flashback: I'm 40.

I'm semi-retired and pursuing other interests besides medicine. However, there is a problem—I can't think. I can't remember. I am forgetful. I'm forgetting common words and names of restaurants, people, and places. Everyone looks at me funny. Even the waiter at the restaurant I frequent.

I love halibut. I'm known for ordering it, and yet I can't remember the name of it, so I refrain from ordering it. I'm frustrated and embarrassed.I realize that I'm slowly developing Alzheimer's.

My solution? I place mini-fluorescent colored post-it notes on the outer rim of my glasses to remind myself of meetings, important dates, interesting ideas and that my favorite fish is known as the "Halibut." I look ridiculous but it works—until I forget to wear my glasses.

I have always been a slender guy, but at 40, I'm not anymore. My waist feels like an extra large truck tire—I can't zip, button or buckle my pants. I have gone from weighing 150 pounds to 190—40 extra pounds! Officially, I have become a "fatso."

Fast forward: I'm 50.

I can't remember, I'm fat, and now I'm falling asleep on my wife. I hate myself, but I can't help it.

As I zoom down the freeway, I tend to doze off and have to psyche myself up to stay awake. I roll down my car window and poke my head out, holding my hands out against 70mph winds. I assume other drivers think I'm attempting suicide but all I am doing is trying to stay awake!!!

Stop. Play: I'm 59 goin' on 60.

My hormones are balanced, my diet has changed, and I've lost 35 pounds. I go to bed early and get up early. I get plenty of sleep and spontaneously beat the alarm clock. I've re-developed muscle on my arms and my back has straightened (no longer do I resemble the hunch-back of Notre Dame). There's a bounce in my step, similar to that of a tap dancer. And at night, I sleep like a baby.

You

I am excited to share this information, which I'm certain will enrich your life. You can truly enjoy the benefits of break-through anti-aging technology just as much as I have.

In conclusion, I'm grateful for my life. On a weekly basis, I travel globally to lecture, learn and discover. Thousands of doctors from various anti-aging societies worldwide congregate to study the latest natural medical techniques, medical supplements, and bio-hormone balance strategies so they too may implement them within their own practices.

Creating exciting products, natural formulations and new inventions requires a great deal of energy and a high level of commitment. I recently obtained my eighth U.S. patent, the youngest of my babies— a patent in the field of satiety (anti-obesity) for a formula that stops irrational food cravings and normalizes food allergies.

I am blessed by the Supreme Being, God; He has given me a mission to share my ideas and knowledge with you and my visions have turned into realities. Endless hours of grueling research, hard work and perseverance have turned this endless quest for natural health into *8 Powerful Secrets to Supercharged AntiAging.*

These eight secrets lie within these pages; read them…but most importantly, practice them daily. Chances are that you'll be *healthier*, feel *stronger*, look *younger* and ultimately live *longer*!

Have a blessed life!

SECRET 1

**"Age is mind over matter.
If you don't mind, it doesn't matter."
—Leroy "Satchel" Paige**

Chapter 1

Hormones Explained

What are hormones?

Simply put, hormones are natural compounds produced by the body's glands (adrenals, thyroid, ovaries, etc.). They're made from cholesterol and act as messengers or signals between the nervous system and vital organs such as the brain, heart and lungs. These little boot-camp soldiers maintain an orderly sequence of bodily functions so you can go about your daily activities without much difficulty (e.g. eating, drinking, visiting the loo, learning, remembering and getting physical—the desire to touch, have sex or fight).

By origin, the word hormone comes from the Greek word meaning "to urge on." Holding true to its meaning, in order for a person to live and be active, hormones are necessary. When hormones flow into our bloodstreams they work throughout the entire body, inside every cell, nerve and organ. The glands that produce hormones are called endocrine glands, hence the word endocrinology.

Endocrinology is the study of hormones—it's considered one of the most complex fields in medicine. The reason why experts in the field are so few in number is because there's so much that goes into explaining what a hormone is.

"The body is like an orchestra. All the woodwinds, strings, percussion, and brass instruments have to play at the right moment in order for the music to sound synchronized. The same applies for hormones. When a hormone starts to come on strong during the wrong time of the day, it will cause havoc with your body's regular activity. Like an exquisite symphony, harmony and balance of hormones at specific times is crucial."

Recap:
What are hormones?

Messenger compounds (made from cholesterol) produced by various glands to communicate internal instructions with the whole body's system.

Hormones are major parts of an extremely complex network of signals; they concentrate on specific tasks that prompt various kinds of biological responses, which is why they're referred to as "the movers" of the emotional and physical well-being. Virtually all of our organs are affected by hormones. Hundreds of them concentrate specifically on the task they were meant to complete. When one or more of the hormones are deficient, other hormones must work harder to do the work that must be done. By doing this, their strengths become their weaknesses. In essence, hormones define us. They affect our personality and DNA; they can fight for or against you. Hormones form your whole being. Be good to them, and they will be oh so good to you!

Hormones are your friends
Company you want around for life

Hormones help your body feel; they're like friends who attempt to finish your sentences and tell you things you'd prefer not know. Hormones can be activated in many different ways at different times of the day. You may not always be able to communicate the sensations you experience verbally, but if you pay close attention to the feelings you're experiencing, you may be able to distinguish which hormone caused a particular signal, and how you communicated the signal through response. Some hormones are higher in the morning (i.e. cortisol, more on this later), and some of them are higher in the evening (i.e. melatonin). Some hormones circulate when you are upset, pleased or anxious, and they can be initiated through each of the five senses. Subsequently, your senses become historians, in that they register information sent by nerves and shoot chemicals to your brain from your hormones. How these feelings are expressed is completely up to the individual.

Hormones can provoke particular body language, as you'll read in the upcoming chapters. An absence of certain hormones can cause tremors, twitching, irregular heart beats and an assortment of other internal disruptions that will make you act in ways you'll have trouble controlling.

To a large extent, you are what your hormones are because they regulate everything. If you're to remember anything from this book, remember that your hormones regulate all internal functions. They're the body's administration and government—they're the police officers and message carriers. Hormones try to avoid chaos, and as faithful soldiers they fight in your favor until their demise. Hormones are released in response to various sorts of environmental and internal conditions so that you can adjust to various situations and surroundings. For example, because of hormones, we have depth perception, which prevents us from falling down stairs. We take larger and longer steps when our hormones tell us we need to, and by the same token, we take smaller steps when necessary. If it weren't for our hormones, we'd be bruised and broken. It's our eyes that take the credit for keeping us moving in the right direction, when really it's our hormones that deserve the recognition.

Hormones and Receptor cells

Hormones circulate freely in the bloodstream, waiting to be recognized by receptor cells that will take them to their assigned destination—receptor cells that can only be activated by a specific type of hormone. As a key is to a lock, once activated, the cell knows when to start a specific function.

The body contains more than 100 trillion cells and hormones are the chief regulators of these trillion and some cells. They control the way the circulatory system works, which includes every heartbeat, breath and flexed muscle. By depositing and burning fat, hormones build strong bones and regulate metabolism, which controls body temperature and energy production. In addition, hormones define female and male characteristics associated with sexuality—where do you think the terms sexy and sex appeal come from?

Steroids and peptides

There are two types of hormones: Steroids and Peptides.

In general, steroids are sex hormones related to sexual maturation and fertility. Steroids are made from cholesterol either in the placenta (while we rest in mom's womb), or in our adrenal glands or gonads (testes or ovaries) after birth. From puberty to old age, steroids determine physical development and fertility cycles. If we're not synthesizing the correct steroidal hormones, we can supplement them via bioidentical hormones like estrogen and progesterone.

Peptides regulate other functions such as sleep and blood sugar levels. They're made from long strings of amino acids, sometimes referred to as protein hormones. Human growth hormone, for example, helps us burn fat and build up muscles. Another peptide hormone, insulin, converts sugar into cellular energy.

Gals and hormones

Hormones govern a woman's body by giving her a monthly menstrual cycle (allowing her to give birth) and lactating ability (for breast feeding). When and if a woman becomes pregnant, hormones set the time for her to deliver the baby. These very same hormones will give her body the ability to cope with stress, prevent fatigue and provide a sense of calm during times of anxiety. Hormones in a woman's body also help her relieve the stress that has potential to develop into depression.

Guys and hormones

In men, hormones define their masculinity. Men are hairy because of their hormones. Men can develop muscle quicker than women because of their hormones. Men have a stronger sex drive because of their… you guessed it, hormones. Undoubtedly, hormones affect both sexes' decision-making, memory and self-confidence, which in turn will affect personality, character traits and behavior.

Recap:
◊ **Hormone: A chemical substance (the messenger) produced in the body's endocrine glands that stimulates various effects. For example, when calcium is low, the thyroid administers calcitonin to regulate the minimal amounts of calcium in a person's body. The hormone calcitonin will now secrete itself into your blood. When your blood signals that it has enough of the calcium hormone, it transmits the rest into your bones.**
◊ **Hormones are projected from the endocrine glands.**
◊ **Hormones are smart little guys. They're messengers, historians and regulators.**
◊ **Hormones circulate freely throughout the bloodstream. Once their carpool partner cells pick them up, they head directly towards their destination.**
◊ **There are two types of hormones: steroids (sex hormones) and peptides (hormones that burn fat and transmit energy).**

Let's begin.

I hope I keyed you up about your hormones. I wanted to share the excitement with you over the importance of your hormones, particularly with regard to your physical responses and immunities. Like a climax in a movie, bedroom, or story, hormones have their peaks and valleys. The highest point for your hormones is around the age of 20 to 25. After that, they start to diminish—slowly, gradually and consistently. Because of this, the immune system is weakened. The person experiencing a hormonal deficiency is more likely to experience difficulty fighting disease and infection as compared to a person who has replenished and functioning hormones.

Where do hormones come from?
East, west, north, south

As members of the endocrine system, glands manufacture hormones. Hormones are released by the thyroid, parathyroid, adrenal and other glands, under the general direction of pituitary gland, "the father" (or master gland). Glands work together in unison just as a family would.

Come on in and meet the family...
This is...

Hypothalamus: Mom, whom we love and know for the commands, "Go ask your father" and "Don't tell your father." A central area on the underside of the brain that secretes hormones that stimulate or suppress the release of hormones to the pituitary gland.

Pituitary: Dad, who makes sure we have everything we need, all the time. Tough at times, he makes sure everything runs smoothly at home. The master gland secretes hormones that influence many other glands and organs, affecting growth and reproduction.

Pineal: The little brother that never wants to get up for school, a.k.a. "Sleepy." Secretes melatonin (promotes sleep), a hormone involved with daily biological rhythms.

Thyroid: The older sister that's always on the run. The family's chess club champion and theatrical diva. Located on the neck, regulates metabolism and blood calcium levels.

Adrenal: The cousin all your girlfriends want to date. He's "The Fonz." He's "Mr. Cool," both a lover and a fighter. Located above each kidney, the adrenal glands secrete cortisol to combat inflammation and respond to stress. Adrenal glands also produce aldosterone which helps maintain the body's water, salt and potassium balances. They also secrete epinephrine (adrenaline) and norepinephrine (noradrenaline) which are involved in the "fight or flight" response. Lastly, the adrenal glands produce testosterone and DHEA and a myriad of other hormones.

Ovaries: The aunt, a feminist. She applauds anything a woman does, and is known for throwing "first time period parties." Secretes "female" hormones like estrogen for development and maintenance of female characteristics. Also secretes progesterone to prepare the uterus for pregnancy. Most importantly the ovaries produce eggs for fertilization.

Uterus: Grandma, she can be spotted doing laps around the neighborhood at 5 a.m. Secretes hormones and proteins that are almost always in response to the cyclical hormonal changes in a woman.

Testes: The hyperactive uncle who's always giving everyone motivational speeches and pep talks. Produces testosterone and sperm.

Pancreas: The motor-mouth cousin, niece or daughter who's always complaining about her weight. She's either too thin or too big. Nevertheless, she's a sweetie and is filled with energy. Secretes insulin; controls the use of sugar in the body and other hormones involved with sugar metabolism.

Born to die
Hormones go buh-bye!

When you complain about how "old" you feel, this means you're hormone levels are decreasing. Next time a friend asks you how you're feeling, instead of saying not so great, tell him or her that your hormones are diminishing. This will probably evoke a humorous response, yet it will also alert them that when they're going through a similar experience, they could be having more than just a "bad day"; they could be feeling the effects of hormone loss.

> **Let's talk finances. If your anabolic activity represented your "health wealth," you'd be rich. If more anabolic activity occurs in your bank account, you'd be at a surplus. If catabolic activity increased, your funds would soon be depleted.**

Our hormones mirror our age. Think inside out—like a reversed shirt, your deeply wrinkled face and/or gray and receding hairline are the other sides of an empty reservoir of hormones missing in action.

Primary hormones are anabolic. Physicians and researchers use this term to describe something that supports life and to describe the cell activity that helps your body build cells and proteins that give thickness and quality to your skin and organs. There are also, of course, catabolic hormones, which take part in the normal process of breaking down protein and cells.

During the first quarter of our lives, between the ages of 20 and 25, the balance of anabolic processes (build-up) reaches its peak. After the age of 20, there's a slight possibility that the body may grow a tad bit more, but after the age 25, growth is highly unlikely. By this I mean, when we're young, our entire being is growing, getting taller and larger, and our DNA developes to its fullest. At this stage we have a large net of positive anabolic hormones.

Between the ages of 30 and 35, the anabolic mechanism peaks and plateaus. Between 35 and 40, our anabolic hormones begin to stabilize. Thereafter, the balance of anabolic and catabolic starts to tilt slightly more toward catabolic. This means our bodies start to deteriorate in quality. The tissues and proteins in our organs dwindle away as our energy and vitality lessen more and more with time and hormone depletion.

From this point forward, we become slightly more catabolic than anabolic. From age 50 on, this shift happens at a much more accelerated rate. As you can expect to see in the coming chapters, our bodies are affected in so many ways when our hormones go into a drastic free fall. We lose most of the constructive building effects of "good" anabolic hormones every day. Take a look at yourself in the mirror and you'll see increased anabolic depletion through the lines and age spots on your face. You don't need fancy lab tests or a doctor to tell you that "baby, you ain't what you used to be."

Five Stages of Anabolic/Catabolic Process

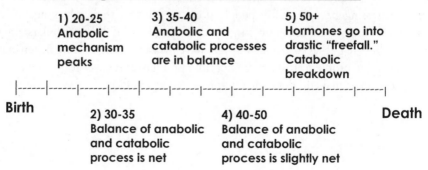

1) 20-25
Anabolic
mechanism
peaks

3) 35-40
Anabolic and
catabolic processes
are in balance

5) 50+
Hormones go into
drastic "freefall."
Catabolic
breakdown

|-----|-----|-----|-----|-----|-----|-----|-----|-----|-----|-----|-----|

Birth

2) 30-35
Balance of anabolic
and catabolic
process is net

4) 40-50
Balance of anabolic
and catabolic
process is slightly net

Death

Baby, you ain't what you used to be!

Q: "How can I reverse the aging process? If anabolic hormones can keep you younger longer, how can I make them stick around?"

Adrienne, 36

A: See a physician for a physical examination and laboratory tests to establish where you are in terms of hormones. You may have aged before your time. Hormones are biomarkers—you may be older than 36, or younger. Age partially depends on the level of your hormones. Get tested first, and then you can start panicking about which approach to take next.

Chronological age versus biological age

You're how old? No, I don't think so.

The essence of rejuvenation is evaluating lifestyle and it requires you to understand your bodily functions, primarily your hormones.

First, I want to establish that chronological age is the day and year of your birth date subtracted from today's date; it's used to determine exactly how many years you've existed. Chronological age cannot be controlled. If you were born in 1960 and it is 2006, you most definitely are 46. Biological age works differently. The inner you follows no rules. It doesn't say, "Well, if I was born in 1960, I must be 46." No, the inner you can be younger or older, depending on how you treat yourself. The first step to aligning how you feel with your "true" age is by balance. Thus, the balancers of the body must be kept steady and these balancers are hormones. You must be reasonable—you can't be 46 and look like you're 20, yet you can look like you're 35 and feel like you're 20. This is possible, and at the same time it is also distressing because many people don't use this to their advantage. We take antidepressants, seek cosmetic surgery and spend thousands of dollars on facial creams that are packaged attractively and have pleasing scents, yet we haven't tackled the real aging problem. Instead, we coat the problem and cover it up. We embellish the problem as makeup does an acne-prone teenager's face.

Samuel's Story

27-year-old Samuel is studying to join the seminary. People refer to him as the "friendly giant." He's 6-foot-5, which is taller than most guys. This also means there's a lot of focus on his abdominal and chest area, since most people are at eye level with these two areas of his body. Samuel's weight has increasingly become problematic, so he's embarrassed that people maintain eye contact with these areas instead of centering on his face.

Lacking muscle tone, Samuel looks effeminate. Not only does he speak in a soft voice, but he has wider hips and larger thighs than most guys do. A lot of people assume Samuel's sensitivity to be a part of his personality, but it's not. Over the years he's complained about appearing overly sensitive because of how he articulates himself. Samuel drags his words and takes longer than a few moments to complete a thought.

At 27, Samuel is at his prime. If anything, he should be bouncing off the walls with energy. How was he to be the future leader of a religious ministry without energy? That's like having a toothless dentist fix your teeth!

His lack of energy drove him to bed early and most of the time he would miss class in the morning because he'd sleep in. The guy was obviously depressed and definitely not in the best shape. As for his diet, I'd watch him finish up a whole chocolate bar in one office sit-in. He told me he did this often. Once, he said, he finished a box of 50 chocolates in one hour. I asked how and why he would do such a thing to himself. He responded that he's become so depressed he resorts to food, usually in the form of sweets.

A complete hormone panel was taken from Samuel, checking his progesterone, testosterone, estradiol and DHEA levels. His biomarkers revealed that he was closer to age 73 than 27.

Samuel is aging prematurely. What will happen to him? Which diseases is he likely to contract from his lack of immunity and from his current cardiovascular status? Are there ways to revive Samuel's hormones?

These are all disparities of chronological and biological aging. Samuel might as well have been born 50 years earlier! Chronologically he's 27, but biologically, he's closer to 80 than he is to 30. You may have experienced meeting someone like Samuel and have asked yourself, "What's wrong with this picture? These youngsters are moping around. They look so tired and stressed when they're supposed to be at their prime."

Seeing is believing

Image

Judging by the way he presents himself, if an employer were to interview Samuel, he or she would probably think he's a lazy bum. As part of the pre-hiring screening process, the human resources department usually schedules interviews so potential employers can see candidates instead of judging them by a sheet of paper packed with a timeline of achievements. A prospective employer wants to conduct an interview so he or she can look the person in the eyes and feel the grip of a handshake. Samuel drags his words, slouches while he sits and looks exhausted all the time. I said "ENOUGH!" to Samuel. I told him we need to get his inner and outer body working. Looking and acting the way he did, I was sure that no one was going to hire him and frankly, I couldn't imagine anyone having the desire to date him, either.

So, what can we do regarding the disparity between chronological and biological age? Do we have to live like Samuel? No! Can something be done; can someone help you prevent this? Absolutely!

STORYTIME with Dr. Tai: "GET OUT AND STAY OUT!"

The body has receptor sites for hormones that work very much like locks and keys. Natural hormones fit perfectly within these locks... synthetic hormones *don't*.

Though both keys resemble each other, they're dissimilar. Oftentimes both keys fool the lock-holder, but only one key is identified by the lock. In the very same way receptors are affected by certain hormones, synthetic hormones try to mimic natural hormones but often fail and go unrecognized by the receptor cell.

When a synthetic hormone (the "wrong key") enters a receptor site (the "lock"), the body signals an alarm, causing an extensive array of side effects. The body goes into a "lockdown" mode where it attempts to relieve the body of the uninvited trespasser by making other part(s) of the body suffer.

Avoiding the consequences

With age, we expect our hormone levels to drop and become less available. Consequently, we'll display the signs and symptoms of this by looking and acting like "old people." Regardless of economic status, appearance or intelligence, this process affects every man and woman. Remember folks, age doesn't discriminate! However, all too often, the ravages of lower hormone levels prematurely affect you and your loved ones. It's bad enough that as we age we lose the benefit of our hormones, but it's far worse to be a young man or woman with severe hormone depletion.

Nevertheless, with proper evaluation of your present hormone status by a professional, remarkable changes are guaranteed if you follow your physician's instructions. He or she will probably ask you to modify your lifestyle by modifying your diet and exercise plans and provide you with instructions for vitamin, mineral and bioidentical hormone supplementations.

Bioidentical hormones

By bioidentical hormones, I mean natural hormones, not synthetic. Please don't confuse the two, because they're a world apart in how they affect the body. Without stating the obvious, natural hormones are 100 percent compatible with your body. Synthetic hormones are often only six to eight percent compatible with your body. If over 90 percent of a synthetic hormone is incompatible, tremendous negative side effects that cause damage to your body and health may result.

> **Recap:**
> ◊ *Anabolic hormones* are hormones that help build cells and proteins.
> ◊ Your body's age (biological age) can differ radically from your calendar age (chronological age).
> ◊ Natural hormones are 100 percent recognizable by your body. Synthetic hormones are only partly recognized by cell receptors.

True and False
Natural and synthetic hormones

True: *Natural hormone supplements should replace depleted hormones.*

False: *Natural hormone supplements will cause your body to have negative side effects or to act unusually.*

A popular hormone fallacy that has been spread by physicians and laymen alike is that using natural hormone replacement can cause your own endocrine glands to become sluggish and eventually prompt them to break down. Nothing could be further from the truth! When your body's glands stop making a hormone, or decrease the production of a particular hormone because they are "too tired" to produce any more of the hormones they're accustomed to producing, natural supplement hormones assist them in making the hormones your body needs.

STORYTIME with Dr. Tai: *"Whoa...hormones."*

Imagine you had a small pony you grew up with. Over the years, as you've grown, the pony carried you wherever you needed to go. Think of your hormone producing glands in the same context. Like the pony, your glands have supported you through some of the toughest situations. With you, your pony grows into adulthood. Following you day and night, it turns into a faithful steed, and then something happens. Your faithful steed evolves into a feeble old horse that's too frail to carry even a bucket of water.

Once obedient, as your pony ages, it becomes more stubborn due to its inability to carry you. What do you do? You resort to discipline—you whip the poor animal!

This whip can be referred to as a (natural or chemical) secretagogue that's supposed to be getting your old horse to move again.

Endocrine gland exhaustion is a vicious cycle. The lower the level of hormones, the worse exhaustion can be for glands. The more your body demands hormones and doesn't get them, the more pressure is placed on those very same glands to produce when they're already exhausted and incapable of production. This increases stress, fatiguing glands and making them more likely to never produce hormones again.

You can't make a gland work any faster or any better than what your body's own mechanism of stimulation already has in effect. Every gland and every hormone has a chemical compound produced by the brain (called a natural stimulating hormone) which prompts a particular gland to produce the hormone your body requires. It's nature's already perfect balance.

If that stimulating hormone is not capable of making the target gland produce more of the hormone, it's because that gland is too tired and overworked to do so. When this occurs, no matter how many artificial stimulants you feed your gland, it's unable to produce any more hormones. In fact, forced continued stimulation has the tendency to only worsen matters.

The perfect solution to a terrible problem
Take away gland exhaustion!

A more reasonable solution to preventing gland exhaustion is to alleviate pressure before it has time to worsen. As with a diabetic that is unable to produce enough insulin, overstimulating insulin production would be both wrong and unfair. Instead, you give the body a little bit of insulin to relieve the fatigue of the pancreas. When you take the load off the gland, the gland has time to regenerate and repair itself.

Studies show that people who have stopped taking bioidentical hormones after many years have stronger working glands than people who've never taken them. Some endocrinologists believe that taking natural bioidentical hormones even before problems occur can prevent gland exhaustion. For example, if you started to take replacement bioidentical hormones at the age of 40, and you've used them for 10 years, by the age of 50 you spared your glands 10 years of stress. This results in producing identical hormones to your own at a much better rate than if you hadn't used bioidentical hormone replacement at all. However, give your own gland a few weeks to rev up its own production. After a short transition, it should be just fine.

⳥Dr. Tai's Anti-Aging Health Secret⳥

In order to spare glands from severe fatigue, start your anti-aging bioidentical hormone replacement as soon as you notice hormone depletion. Don't wait until you're totally depleted before starting replacement with natural bioidentical hormones. By then, it maybe too late for you to start bioidentical hormone treatment because your glands have almost withered away. I can't stress enough the importance of replenishing hormones beforehand.

In the future, don't be too surprised to see bioidentical hormone replacement being used by people as young as 30. The environment is growing increasingly polluted, and demands are ever-increasing as the economy seems to be skyrocketing with technological advancements. Life will only get more complicated. This can only mean that stress levels and blood pressures will go up with everything else.

This is why it would've been a smarter decision on our parts to have tested our hormone levels at the peak of our youth, instead of our clinging moments of desperation. However, we have not the time for regrets. Now is the time to do what you can! Intrinsic hormone abnormalities cause cravings for sugar and deficiencies in the metabolism such as hypothyroidism and DHEA scarcity. When hormone levels drop, you will begin to see an increase in weight gain (usually around the abdomen), which correlates with cardiovascular disease.

Find out how your body works and what it can and cannot handle. Natural hormones don't cause cancer, weight gain or heart disease. These side effects for hormone replacement are applied mostly to synthetic hormones only. There's been no researched evidence linking bioidentical hormones and diseases. However, an excess of anything can never be good, even in nature. Whether it be hormones, oxygen or water, too much of anything can eventually cause harm. Be careful and stick with the safest choices. You won't be sorry!

Chapter 2

Chronological Age vs. Biological Age

"We have a lot to do... People don't understand this. They think we're sitting around in rocking chairs, which isn't at all true. Why, we don't even own a rocking chair."

—Sadie Delany, 103, on her 101-year-old sister and herself

There are thousands of people in the world like the Delany sisters who are alive and well into their early hundreds. Journalists who have hiked to the mountainous districts of Ararat, Turkey and Damavand, Iran have reported to have visited 115-year-old men and women. When these men and women were asked how they've managed to stay alive for so long, despite tumultuous weather conditions and unpredictable harvests, they said they owed it all to how they felt and how often they've kept busy. The health and longevity of people throughout the world has been attributed to the blend of diet, climate, emotional well-being, stress and physical activity. Compared to how most Americans live, a mountaineer's living conditions would be considered well below the povertylevel. Born at the hands of midwives in huts made of decayed vegetable matter found in bogs, mountaineers' birthdates were remembered by seasons. Many "115 summers old" men and women have been said to have shown physical signs of attentiveness by responding when spoken to, laughing, talking and walking at a moderate pace. To people like the mountaineers of the Caucasus mountain range, age only matters if you're cheese.

But what about you? How old do you feel? Ask yourself and understand the difference between chronological age and biological age.

Chronological age

Again, chronological age is how old you generally say you are: this year subtracted from the year you were born.

Biological age
Steadiness of the body: Balance

As years progress, your health problems and appearance only worsen if your hormones continue to diminish and if you continue living a life chock-full of bad habits (e.g. sleep deprivation, high-carb diet, high cortisol levels, substance abuse in the form of cigarette smoking and alcohol consumption, etc.).

How youth is delivered

Hormones are the system's messengers. They control, make, regulate, send, take and give. Together, they work as the post office, FedEx, UPS and DHL in more than 150 different ways. This means that in order for the face and body to look vibrant and youthful, the delivery services must work together in synchronisity; they must have a plan and a schedule. They must have strong and dependable deliverers. Like a city, a body without organization will be chaotic.

Who are you going with?

In our present health care system, almost every instance involving our present health care system, synthetic hormones are chosen over bioidentical hormones, because of prescriptive or insurance reasons. Sadly, synthetic hormones are of primary choice because many people have been lured into thinking that synthetic hormones deliver rapid results to problems that have worsened with time. This may be true, but then so is the adage "what begins too soon, ends too soon." Bioidentical hormones can be used through liposome technology, which can be rubbed onto the skin, spritzed under the tongue (sublingually), or even inserted (by means of suppositories).

Lean on me

Since your hormones depend on each other to get various jobs done, if one collapses, the others must work more intensely to make up for its absence. If a hormone or a set of hormones work harder, the areas they were meant to serve will be neglected. One reaction triggers another—without one, you don't have the other, and eventually a person will suffer by becoming or appearing ill.

Hormone Deficiencies

Fact: *Statistically, more than 50 million women and up to 40 million men a year suffer from hormonal deficiencies.*

Translation: *Every year, more than 50 million women and up to 40 million men feel as old, or older than they are chronologically. Over 3500 women join the menopause group every single day in USA alone.*

Hormones grow scarce because of:

- Severe illness
- A history of major surgery, or surgeries
- Internal aging (over time self-neglect)
- Depression
- Stress
- A lack of exercise
- Inadequate amounts of sleep (decreased melatonin)
- Increased deadlines. The feeling of always being rushed, the feeling of being under pressure and under stress every day, all day (increased cortisol, decreased DHEA).
- Poor nutrition and major deficiencies of important minerals and essential fatty acids.

Only in America

The United States is among the few countries in the world where age isn't regarded as attractive. The "old" in America aren't graceful, nor are they beautiful. However, in countries like France and Italy, age is sexy. The difference between Americans and their Western counterparts are lifestyle and diet. An average day for an American consists of: working eight to ten hours; having a carbo-packed breakfast, lunch and dinner comprised of super-sized fast-food and refined sugars found in doughnuts, pastries, cake, smoothies, juices and sodas; and not exercising at all, or exercising too much.

Carbs that are consumed too often and too quickly will lead to higher cortisol levels, which can increase the pressures of stress even when stress isn't present. When the body triggers "high tension," the desire to eat is than increased by ten-fold; this leads to insomnia and obesity. Poor nutrition, fatigue, stress and a lack of sleep will destroy a person's hormones by exhausting the glands that produce vital hormones.

The last thing people want to do when they are tired is exercise. Speaking for myself, when I'm tired I feel like I'm strapped to a metal ball and chains. Muscles need to be put in use before they can build aerobic capacity, and how will that be possible for you to do if you're exerting all the energy you have by attempting to stay awake? This is neither possible nor expected.

Q: "I used to run. Over the years, I've stopped because I haven't had enough energy to run as much as I used to. I really have to push myself to get going, but as soon as I put on my running shoes I make my way back inside my house. I'm desperate. I'll refrain from eating only because I'm not exercising. I already have a belly, and I don't want to gain any more weight."

—Mark

A: Mark, you're not alone. Millions of people are like you. We need to learn to eat right,. Stick to foods low in glycemic levels, and make sure to get your hormones checked out. It seems to me your testosterone is aromatizing into estrogen. This means your testosterone is turning into estrogen (an abundant hormone in women). Because this has already been done, we need to keep the other hormones from turning into estrogen, keep testosterone where it's at and balance your estrogen with progesterone, so it doesn't create abnormal growths in your body.

Your body is tired because it's experiencing declines from every end. Eat a diet rich in greens, fish and red berries. Make sure you take the initiative to exercise. You don't necessarily have to run—instead, go for a brisk walk. Once you feel like you can, run. But for the time being, check yourself out and take it easy.

As I responded to the question from Mark, a market analyst from my hometown, I'm certain that his problem is a lack of hormones essential to a man's body. Besides a bit of general advice, I can't give him specific guidelines without a complete saliva hormone panel evaluation. Although it may seem as Mark's only problem is his inability to run, it's not! If he can't run, he can't muster the energy to work, run errands, or have sex with his wife. This is why a lack of energy is more serious than one may actually realize.

If you revisit Mark's question, you will notice only his name. I left his age out purposely. Reading his question may seem like a man in his sixties is asking the question, but Mark is 37, three years away from turning 40! I wanted you to see for yourself just how early hormones begin to diminish. If Mark feels like this at 37, what will he feel like at 60?

Dr. Tai asks:
What happens to such a "chronologically" young man like Mark?
Already he feels "biologically" old—so what happens when he becomes "chronologically" older? Will he be "biologically" older?

Aging is nature's way of preparing us for death. Many of us will begin to lose appetite, yet we'll gain weight. We'll experience trouble urinating, yet we feel urgency to go. Some of us will have to go more often than others, and some of us won't go as often as we should. The same applies for sleeping: Some of us will feel sleepy all the time, and others will feel sleepy and have trouble waking up. Hormones and chemicals will make our days such an enormous struggle that dying sooner may seem like a better idea than dying later.

"If I had the use of my body I would throw it out of the window."

—Samuel Beckett, *Malone Dies*

Biological signs of aging:

- Lack of energy
- Being overweight
- Lagging libido
- Nervousness/ shakiness
- Fatigue
- Skin lesions/ wrinkles, sun spots, sagging skin etc.
- Variable appetite
- Poor memory
- Digestive problems/ frequent diarrhea or irritable bowel syndrome/ constipation
- Sore joints
- Chronic pain
- Sleep problems
- Frequent allergies
- Low immunity

Being placed on a bioidentical hormone plan will help reverse the aging process within your body, so you look as young as you feel. Within this book, you will read about the different experiences people have had with replenishing their hormones. Here I'll give you a glimpse of what you should expect to read about in upcoming chapters.

Testosterone: The anabolic hormone responsible for high metabolism, muscle tone, muscle strength and sexual desire. Many people think that something is psychologically wrong with them when they lose testosterone levels. Contrary to popular belief, it's physiological before it's psychological.

What folks like you are saying about testosterone...

"My decreased sex drive began to take a toll on my marriage. My husband thought I was seeing another man because I didn't want to sleep with him. Worse yet, my husband started to doubt I loved him. Thankfully, I found out that my testosterone levels were lower than average. I was glad to know that I pinpointed the problem before it really started to upset my marriage.

"My poor husband thought of all sorts of things. I tried to tell him that it wasn't him, it was me. He found that to be too cliché to be true, but really it was me! When he found out what my problem was, he started taking an interest in his hormones, too. "

—Denise, 44

"My belly fat and chest size were both results of low testosterone."

—Mark, 37

"I lost a lot of the hair on my head, and I started losing the hair on my arms, underneath my arms, all over my body and even my eyebrow hair started to thin. It was a very sad time in my life, because beside the curves on a woman's body, I feel that a woman's hair defines her. Because I barely had any left, I couldn't do anything with my hair. I was relieved to find that I wasn't diseased—instead I had extremely low testosterone and thyroid."

—Nefrita, 56

Human growth hormone: The hormone we depend on to grow. Human growth hormone strengthens the immune system and provides energy to keep us going.

Sophia smiling with HGH...

"*You know, I've never been so depressed in my life! Everything was going pretty darn well for me, too—I couldn't pinpoint the problem! My daughter got married, my husband and I traveled frequently. I was a fire-cracker, but until recently, I'd developed anxiety issues. I'd make excuses not to go places. I'd call off parties with friends, and when I'd see my daughter I'd depress her with my demeanor. Not good, so I sought the help of my doctor and he told me exactly what was wrong. I was missing HGH, progesterone, and testosterone. I'd never think that hormones would play such a significant role in the way people feel. It's been a few weeks and I'm feeling better. Slowly but surely, I'm going to fight this feeling—I know I will!*"

—Sophia, 48

Estrogen: The hormone that tends to rise and fall the most throughout women's and men's lives. The body reacts greatly to the deficiencies and excessiveness of this hormone. Estrogen gives women eye moisture, vaginal lubrication, breast fullness and mental clarity. In men, estrogen influences the brain, protects against cardiovascular disease and has a major impact on bodily tissues.

It's known as the hormone essential to all the characteristics of female health. It gives glow and youth to women as it prevents wrinkles by promoting anabolic protein developed in the subcutaneous layer (the fourth layer of skin; see chapter on skin) important to collagen and elastin. The hormone works together with progesterone, as an excess can result in cystic or tumerous growths.

The girls on estrogen: mixed reviews...

"*Honest to goodness, I felt like my mirror was getting tired of me. I was tired of looking at myself. While I was going through menopause, I felt so shriveled-up and dry. You know those smokers that can finish a carton in one day? Well, I felt just like one of those chain-smokers. My skin was dry, my hair was dry, I felt dry.*
"*I lost the glow in my skin and pride in my body. I felt like sh_.*"

—Katarina, 53

"I found myself shopping for coffins. I thought I was going to die from breast cancer. Every time I visited my gynecologist, she found the same thing wrong with me—there were more cysts in my breasts. I remember crying. I hated my breasts. Men loved my breasts, but I hated them, because I'd developed too many problems because of them—until I discovered that it wasn't because of my breasts, it was because I was producing too much estrogen and not enough progesterone to level and neutralize the excess."

—*Ta'Rah, 34*

"Since the age of 19 I've been on birth control to regulate my periods. For some time the pill didn't pose any problems, but years later, when I got off of it, I saw my periods were becoming brown and stringy. This scared me, so I saw a doctor and I was told that the birth control pill produced too much estrogen for my body. The excess estrogen was also the reason for my re-occurring migraines."

—*Jen, 26*

DHEA: This anabolic hormone has actor-like characteristics. It's versatile and can take on a variety of roles at the same time by producing hormones while converting them into other hormones.

Researchers have linked cancer to a lack of DHEA. Animal studies have shown that DHEA supplementation helped prevent obesity and memory loss and stimulate longevity.

No DHEA in Dean...

"Losing my mind—literally, I was losing my mind! I began to forget things that were once so familiar to me. Birthdays used to be a cinch—I'd remember birthdays as I did faces. I realized something was wrong with me when I forgot my anniversary with my partner of four years. I thought maybe I was preoccupied, but I couldn't have been, because things really began to slow down at work. I run an online business and I'm always at home, so that wasn't the case. I've never been under insurmountable stress where it's affected my health or my state of mind. I've always been in control... until age hit me. Ironically, my doctor never made any mention that it could be my hormones until I saw a woman talk about her hormones on a daytime talk show. 'All right,' I said to myself, 'I gotta check this out.'"

—*Dean, 64*

Cortisol: Unlike the other hormones I've mentioned, cortisol is a catabolic hormone. An excess or a deficiency of it is the primary cause of neurovascular and endrocrine deterioration. Cortisol excess causes accelerated aging by continuously breaking down tissues, proteins and muscles as it exhausts the adrenal cortex and increases the level of sugar in the bloodstream. Cortisol demands for higher insulin level, very hard on the pancreas. Cortisol's consequences include osteoporosis and undesirable fat distribution. The indirect effect is on our immune system's NK cells as well as T cells, and increasing vascular hypertension, skin thinning and thyroid destruction.

Cortisol production factory: LaVon, single and stressed father of two

"One week I did 96 hours with no sleep. Boy Scout honor, no sleep. I thought it was insomnia, but I realized that it was a burnout. I'm a single father. I have two children; my wife left me three years ago. Frustration became me. I turned to drinking, smoking excessively, skipping meals—I totally lost myself. I had to do something else; I knew bad habits were going to catch up with me one day. I've dealt with all sorts of therapy for my mind; I needed to put my body in check and I did. I found out that I was blowing out my adrenals and thyroid by producing massive amounts of cortisol from stress.

"I've turned to supplementation and prayer. I go to church more often and I find praying a form of intense meditation. I feel so… ughhh, I don't know how to say this, but I feel like LaVon. I feel like it's really me."

—*LaVon, 33*

Adrenals: The adrenal gland produces powerful epinephrine, an emergency hormone that shows up in our actions when we're frightened. The adrenal gland also produces Cortisol, DHEA, HGH, melatonin and pregnenolone. When our nerves are sharp and the body is on high alert, it's because the adrenals are producing hormones that help us deal with anxiety and fear. Ultimately, false alarms from various hormones can elevate sugar levels, break tissues, and accelerate heart beats and aging.

Persian police officer lives dangerously...

"In my country there is much conflict, because the rich they are very rich, and the poor, they are very poor. I have to deal with very much stress because I am police. My aunt knows homeopathy and practices nutrition to help the people deal with problems naturally. She tell me all the time that people get sick too much from the medication they taking. I asking her one day, what my problem is, I get tired so fast. This threatens my life, because I have to be alert, you know? Awake! I say, 'Wake up, Abdallah!' My aunt, she tell me is because of fear. I fear too much and my body is always running."

—*Abdallah, 40*

Dr. Tai's looking back

Over the years, I've gathered snippets from what people have said to me about how their hormones have affected their lives. As you've read, that was some intense stuff. Hormones led Denise, a 44-year-old woman, to drive her husband to believe she was cheating on him because she had no desire to be intimate with him.

You read about 34-year-old Ta'Rah shopping for coffins because she was petrified of the cysts in her breasts. Abdallah the Persian police officer lives a stressful kind of life running around and following orders, where Ohio native LaVon experiences a different kind of stress from painful memories and daily challenges like paying the bills and feeding his children. All of these people are much older than they really are. If you were to go back and re-read the stories, add 10-20 years to them. Throughout the years, I've kept in touch with these people, and thankfully they've made 180-degree improvements. They all seem "hopeful" and excited for the future, but when I met them the word that seemed best to describe their situations was "hopeless."

Feel good with the right food

The most popular foods in American culture are pizza, white bread, sugary foods, cookies, sodas, cakes and all other foods high on the glycemic index. They're also foods that cause blood sugar levels to rise quickly, and subsequently fall quickly. Another food that I loathe to hear of is cereal. It's not even food! It's a dessert! A handful of sugary cereal is a dessert. It doesn't qualify as breakfast, yet sugary cereals have become so many people's breakfast, lunch, dinner and midnight snack. It's no wonder America's been looking so terrible—with wrinkled faces and a tag like "the world's fattest country." Our patriotism has been a defense mechanism used to guard against the slimmer, fitter bullies of the world.

More sugar results in more carb cravings. The more chocolate you eat, the more you'll want to eat. By avoiding sugary carbos (especially before bedtime), you can lower stress levels, lose weight and control the cortisol and insulin produced by your adrenals.

Slippery, sly, fried foods

Compelling you to doze off instead of accomplishing your goals for the day, oily foods can induce a tired, deadbeat feeling. People who've depended on fried and greasy foods for most of their lives can expect a heavier load of cleanup work than those who watched what they ate. By eating balanced meals packed with vitamins and minerals you'll feel like a cleaner, lighter person.

If you've been eating foods high in sugar, starch and grease you're risking a lifetime of good health for a few minutes of tastebud satisfaction. Sugar, carbo and transfats are all allergy, inflammation and diabetes inducers.

> **Dr. Tai's tip:**
> Next time you decide to take a bite out of a doughnut or a slice of oily pizza, ask yourself, "Would I feed my dog these foods everyday?"
>
> I'm only hoping your answer is "No!"

Dr. Tai's Anti-Aging Diet Plan:
(see weight loss chapter)

Decrease intake of high-glycemic foods like:

Cereal, sweet corn, pasta, crackers, rice cakes (whoever said these were healthy should be slapped), pancakes, toaster waffles, white rice, white bread, potato chips, all pastries, sweets and candy, most cereals, doughnuts, pizza, white bagels, chicken nuggets, fruit juices, bananas and carrots

Increase intake of foods with the following micronutrients:

Zinc, selenium and copper (Ionic charged minerals and 80 trace minerals)

Try adapting a high-protein diet mainly consisting of
vegetable, fish or lean meats

Don't be afraid to use grape seed oil and olive oil.
These are monosaturated oils that don't pose the same cardiovascular risks
of saturated fats. The best quality of olive oil is light virgin oil. It's been
shown to be effective against arthritis, cancer and heart disease.

If you must snack, eat light portions of snacks and a handful of unsalted,
unsweetened almonds, cashews, walnuts and macadamias.
(Manufacturers tend to overwhelm pistachios with salt.)

… and when eating, remember—

Portion control! Portion control! Portion control!

Inhale, Exhale. Inhale, Exhale. Inhale, Exhale. Inhale, Exhale.

How to do it right, ninja:

Breathe in through your nose. Watch your lower belly expand. (Hold for 10 seconds.)

Breathe out through your mouth. (Do at least 20 repetitions per day.)

Oxygen fuels your metabolic rate. Try to avoid the "Weekend Warrior Get-Well Program." Don't get all Zen on yourself for a Sunday afternoon and then go through living a rock star lifestyle for the rest of the week. Make breathing a habit. Breathing is a form of cranial and craniofacial therapy, which means breathing is exercise and food for the brain and spine. A specially low temperature fermented Cordyceps Sinensis is a terrific anti-aging herbal supplement, greatly improving the efficiency of respiration and oxygen transfer by over 40%. See Max-Performance Specialist.

Antioxidants

You can't have a complete anti-aging plan without antioxidants, the body's first line of defense against cell ravaging free radicals and excess Reactive Oxygen Species (R.O.S.) buildup. See AntiOxidant Specialist (take nighttime only).

How do they help?

Free radicals damage by fusing DNA and protein molecules. Because of this, other cells are unable to produce new strands of DNA. This process, called "cross-linking," results in the body's proteins acting destructively. By this I mean cross-linking causes aging, brittle bones, kidney/liver failure, wrinkles, cataracts and diabetes (since glucose fuels the process).

More critical to anti-aging than most people believe they are, antioxidants play a major role in aging. Without the help of antioxidants to protect against free radicals, white blood cells and digestive enzymes are ruthlessly attacked and destroyed.

The more cells are destroyed, the more molecular trash your body gathers and disposes of through fatal illnesses like cancer, vital organ failure, osteoporosis, a pathetically puny immune system, heart disease and senile dementia.

Without antioxidants, you can lose your mind and your pretty face. Key to understanding why you need protection against free radicals is, simply put, your health. Wrinkly faces aren't quite as scary as developing fatal illnesses like cancer, which results from what I'd like to call "cell betrayal."

Cell Bandits

Similar to something straight out a James Bond movie, cells that have been affected by a free radical invasion are held captive, so to speak, and forced to cooperate with their captors because they, unlike free radicals, are a much weaker kind of cell. It's been said that cells have "clocks" which determine their life spans. However, cancer cells incessantly reset their clocks, so that while other cells die (natural apoptosis), *they* continue to live.

Laboratories all across the world have conducted countless experiments on how to keep cells from resetting their clocks. Once cells reset their clocks, they'll continue to multiply, and like the car that'll eventually break down, the body will eventually do the same.

Dr. Tai gives an example: Cancer cells are like a vehicle without brakes; now only the accelerator is working. Can you imagine your car speeding along a highway or rushing down a hill with no brakes to stop? Well, that's a cell turned cancerous—once it had a natural brake to stop replicating and reproducing itself, but now all it can do and all it knows is to reproduce and grow without being able to stop.

"If I'd known I was gonna live this long, I'd have taken better care of myself."

—Eubie Blake

Wishing you longevity

It's up to you to live as long as you want to, and if you want to live a long, healthy and happy life, you must do everything in your power to protect your body. People are outliving each other, but they're also dying from more unexpected deaths. The average lifespan for men and women in the U.S. is somewhere in the upper seventies—it's safe to say an average of 78 years. However, I believe this number will change in due time.

In five years, 78 may seem far too young to die. It already seems too young to me, but they're only stats. (Please remember that with regard to health, almost everything you read is based accumulated statistics.) You are an individual with needs, and your needs will invariably differ from mine. You're just wasting time making assumptions about yourself based on statistics. The guidelines are generally the same for everyone: eat well, replenish your hormones, sleep well, exercise in moderation and drink as much water as you can possibly consume. What varies is how much of a supplement you'll need, if you need it at all.

Antioxidants protect us against pollution

As pollutants create a haze in the sky in even the most remote places of the world, it's outrageous to think a darkened atmosphere won't affect us in any way.

Antioxidants serve as protectors and neutralizers of all the smog you've inhaled so that what's been accumulated throughout time doesn't affect your lungs and weaken your tissues.

What do antioxidants do?

- Protect against cellular damage
- Guard against organ damage
- Prevent endocrine gland from exhaustion
- Promotes cellular repair, an especially important process in healthy cell turn-over. When dead skin cells slough off, you want healthy cells to move up. A diet rich in antioxidants shows itself off on gorgeous, soft, supple, fresh, young-looking skin.

> **Remember...**
>
> Another way to protect your cells is by replenishing hormones. Healthy cells can't be produced without functioning hormones.

Ow! I feel good!

In Michigan, our longest season is winter, and while everyone is sniffing and coughing away, it's a rare occasion that I become ill. Even while viruses have peaked in circulation and the weather becomes too cold for anyone or anything to survive, I'm whistling away in my office like one of Santa's elves. Since I began taking antioxidants, I've felt I've regained my strength. I've never felt this physically and mentally powerful before; not only because I continue to refill hormones, but because I take antioxidants.

I've logged the supplements I take on a daily basis. I suggest you adapt a similar plan for yourself. The antioxidants I take affect a broad range of problems that people experience. Through extensive research (much of it trial and error), I've sifted through supplements that are phenomenally effective. If you should choose a plan similar to mine, as a physician I advise you exercise caution with milligram intake. I suggest you consult your physician before following a supplementation plan that may not be suitable for your present state, especially if you have a medical condition.

Allicin (garlic): Allicin is the active ingredient in garlic. For centuries, the herb has been used to prevent and treat heart disease. It reduces hypertension and lowers blood pressure. Attention, all you varicose veined women: people with poor circulation should definitely consider taking a garlic supplement like pure allicin on a daily basis as it does an excellent job in making the blood flow. (Don't be fooled, dry garlic powder has no active allicin.) See MaxGarlicin Specialist.

Alpha-Lipoic Acid: One of the most powerful water and fat soluble antioxidants known to man, combine this stuff with a CoQ10 enzyme and you're on your way to glory. It boosts the power of other antioxidants. It prevents strokes, cataracts, cancer and it stimulates glucose disposal, so fat (when metabolized from sugar) is proportionately dispersed throughout a person's body. ALA recharges spent Vit A, E, and C. See AntiOxidant Specialist.

Ashwaganda: Also known as "winter cherry," ashwaganda improves the body's ability to maintain adaptation to various types of stress. An African antioxidant plant, it helps people who lack sleep and experience mental and physical strain on a daily basis.

Beta-Carotene (Vitamin A): Found in deep green salads and vegetables, beta-carotene is heavily involved in the aging process. According to clinical research, children who take beta-carotene have a quicker recovery period when taking the antioxidant. It does a multitude of things, primarily strengthening immunities and speeding up healing processes.

Boron: Used to enhance brain function, so you're not psycho-babbling about random topics which have absolutely no correlation with mattersofthemoment. Boron helps you focus and is important for people who are exhibiting signs of arthritis.

Cordyceps: A blade-shaped fungus that grows and thrives on the backs of underground caterpillars high in the Himalayas. With ample supply of cordyceps in my possession, I've created formulas which consist of the mushroom (fungus). If I could have placed cordyceps at the very top of my supplement list, I would have, but we're going in alphabetical order. I'm convinced that cordyceps can save and lengthen your life. For many years, doctors have used cordyceps to successfully treat people with immune, respiratory, circulatory and endocrine system disorders (which just about covers all of the systems). Cordyceps supports male potency and female vitality while increasing the levels of naturally produced antioxidants in the body. It enhances libido while promoting longevity (For more information on Cordyceps read my last book: Cordyceps Miracle.) You must use low temperature fermented Cordyceps and if possible, use the full complement of all the different Cordyceps species, ie. Ophioglosoides and Militaris. See MaxPerformance Specialist.

Green Tea: With antibacterial and antioxidant properties, green tea promotes youth and longevity. Asian women consume a lot of green tea. Just by looking at the clarity of their skin and the thickness of their hair it's safe to assume that green tea has done their bodies good (move out of the way, milk). Green tea protects blood vessels and strengthens the immune system by preventing free radicals from attacking innocent cells and preventing inflammation of all sorts.

Lycopene: Found in tomatoes, lycopene has been picking up momentum in the world. Increasingly, I'm seeing advertisements for this antioxidant and I like it. People need to know about lycopene. It should be promoted as it reduces the risks of myocardial infarctions or heart attacks and lowers high levels of cholesterol. Only cooked tomatoes have high lycopene content.

NAC (N-acetyl-l-cysteine): The anti-premature aging supplement, NAC, is great for preventing adult respiratory distress syndrome, liver damage (for all you once-booze-friendly bar-hoppers) gallstones, muscle fatigue, lung damage (smokers), brain injury and strokes. See AntiOxidant Specialist.

Vitamin C: Do you want look younger? Do you want to feel younger? Do you want to protect your heart? If you answered yes to all of my previous questions, then you need at least 1,000 milligrams of Vitamin C a day! Vitamin C has proven to work miracles on people who can't get enough of the sun and for people who've been exposed to harsh conditions. It's not uncommon to see hikers, travelers (especially those who frequent hostels) and students stock up on C. It's an essential antioxidant that works in a million different ways. Further studies are being conducted on this truly fascinating vitamin that continuously keeps amazing researchers, nutritionists, doctors, physicians, laboratory technicians and alternative medicine practitioners. For higher efficacy take Vit C bound to a peptide L-Glutamine. (See Max-Digestion Specialist)

So, back to my original question: How old are you?

Before you begin to roast marshmallows on the pile of calendars you burned from reading this chapter, make sure you transfer important dates onto a different spreadsheet, excluding your birthday. Find out how old you are by recognizing where most of your health ailments are rooted from.

Dr. Tai's tip: From time to time, try to test yourself. Try to recall names of places purposely. Try to retain information: Make a list of 10 common grocery items and see if you can remember what you bought from that list. Circle what you bought. Are you able to recall 60 percent? If you scored less than that, something in your routine needs to change before things get worse.

How does it happen? Main Supplements: Phosophytidylcholine, and phosphtiydylserine, two important brain hormones assist DHEA, prenenolone, and estrogen, which are hormones necessary for neuro-cell preservation. Anxiety and emotional upheavals occur when there is an imbalance of DHEA, estrogen, testosterone, prenenolone, and progesterone. If you're able to keep these hormones balanced, you'll be able to salvage your memory. See Sharp Memory and Brain Specialist.

Ask yourself...

- How's my vision?
- How's my depth perception?
- Have I become clumsier?
- How's my hearing?
- How many times do I have to ask someone to repeat?
- Can I remember things easily?
- Can I recall names of people, places, memories, etc.?
- How often do I write notes to myself?

And be honest about this....I mostly complain about...

- joint pain
- muscle pain
- headaches

- trouble breathing
- chest pains
- uneasy stomach
- constipation
- lax bowel movements
- hair loss
- feeling lethargic (weary)
- negative change in attitude
- violent skin reactions

Assessing your current physical condition will give you a good idea of how old you are. However, make sure to pay specific attention to your vision, memory and strength.

Vision: It starts with the eyes. If you're constantly adjusting your prescription, this is a problem. The tiny muscles behind the eyes control movement and adjust precision and accuracy. Vision is a specific sign that you're aging; with age, the muscles behind the eyes become weaker.

Memory: Brain cells shrink approximately 6-8 percent after the age of 40. With age, special neurons that used to interact with each other cut communication. It's like the cells in your brain have all been good friends for years, and then, one day, they get fed up with talking to each other. When neurons refrain from communicating this can be considered as a form of catabolic destruction that'll eventually require you to perform different acts of "mental gymnastics."

Strength: Typically, after the age of 30, you'll begin to lose 1 percent of muscle mass. Muscles deteriorate, sapping away strength. If you're begin to experience shortness of breath and have trouble lifting groceries into your car, your hormones are long overdo for a reboot, especially testosterone levels.

Skin: With regard to visible signs of aging, the skin confers and suggests how old you are. Innately, we've programmed the eyes to play a guessing game with a multitude of things, making assumptions about everything we meet. People are usually the subjects of our analyses. Scientists have divided aging into two categories: internal and external. They have said that you can only control external aging by monitoring your surroundings, staying away from the sun, and negative habits like smoking, poor eating and a lack of exercise. The very same scientists have said that internal aging cannot be controlled. I beg to differ. You can do numerous things to control what's happening inside of your body by strengthening aging cells and balancing hormones. The only internal factors that are beyond your scope of powers are genetic factors. If you've inherited a characteristic from family members, altering DNA is something only your creator can help you with. Aging skin shows wrinkles, bags, tiny blood vessels, dullness, deep facial grooves and permanently etched expressions. See Dr. NanoDerma Skin Care.

Chapter 3

Counting your hormones: Easy as 1, 2, 3
Saliva Testing

Your trusted mirror has confirmed the fact that you're aging. This can only mean you're missing hormones, but which hormones? The next and most important step of bioidentical hormone treatment is testing for a hormone count.

As if you don't have enough decisions to make, deciding which test to take to measure your hormones can be tough. I've tried alleviating extra stressors by offering you the best way to check your hormones, which is through your saliva.

Through extensive research and laboratory trials, I've come to realize that saliva hormone testing is by far the simplest and most accurate way to determine metabolic factors and biological age. With the help of a trained physician or expert health worker, you'll learn how to achieve and maintain a biohormone balance. Needless to say, no one should be careless and use supplements without understanding how to balance them. Your physician will customize a life-long natural supplement plan tailored to you and only you.

Step 1: Acknowledging you have a problem not sure where this fits in?
Step 2: Knowing how hormones work
Step 3: Seeking expert advice to evaluate your available hormone count

Hormonal Testing and Monitoring
"If you can spit, we can test"

Vocabulary you should know:

Free hormones: Unbound by protein; ready to be used. These hormones are functioning, alive and active.

Bound hormones: Inactive and unusable hormones

The saliva panel is my favorite screening tool for determining an accurate hormone count. Like a saliva panel, the urine and blood tests can also determine your hormone count. However, unlike hormones found in blood and urine, hormones found in saliva are free and unbound by protein. This means saliva analyses would reflect the exact markers of your own working hormonal activity. Saliva hormone testing is the only easy test through which you can directly and accurately meausre Free Unbound Active hormones.

37

Hormones, by nature, are the very life force of our existence. They circulate within our bloodstream in the form of bound and unbound hormones. The bound hormone fraction is a biologically inactive hormone that is connected to cortisol-bound globulins (CBG) and sex hormone binding globulins (SHBG). Both are glycoproteins that bind to sex hormones DHEA, testosterone and estradiol. These bound hormones make up more than 95 percent of the total hormones that circulate throughout our bloodstream. Therefore, any measurement of essential hormones in our blood is a reflection of an immensely large number of inactive hormones, meaning that in order to achieve an accurate hormone report, multiple blood drawing attempts are required.

Unbound by any other protein or globulin, free hormones make up a rather small fraction of hormones that circulate throughout a person's body. Free hormones are completely available for immediate use by organ and tissue receptors for the maintenance of the body's activity.

These small yet essential portions of free hormones represent only 1 to 5 percent of the total concentration of hormones in our blood, whereas in the saliva hormones exhibit quite a presence. Free and unbound hormones show through saliva testing, making it the most accurate and painless way to obtain a correct hormonal status report. Affordable and convenient, saliva samples are collected by one's spitting into capsule sized tubes. They're then sent to laboratories for evaluation. Within days, the patient's physician is contacted with the results on the free hormone (active and useable) count.

Saliva is produced by three sets of major glands:

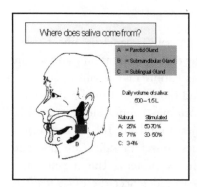

As it travels towards the salivary glands, saliva is produced when components of the blood and lymphatics pass through three membrane barriers.

The *parotid* gland located in front of our ears on the outside portion of the mandible produces 30-40 percent of saliva; when stimulated it produces 70 percent.

The *sublingual* gland is located within the oral cavity underneath the tongue. It produces 25 percent of our saliva; when stimulated it produces 50-70 percent.

The *submandibular* gland located under the jaw produces 15-25 percent of saliva.

The daily range of the amount of saliva produced is approximately 1.0 liter (1 quart) per day. As we age (especially under abnormal circumstances, e.g. internal and external stress) saliva output decreases to about 500 ml. (1 pint) per day.

> **Recap:** Saliva is produced when components of the blood pass through a membrane barrier as they travel towards the salivary glands.
>
> Think of the coffee filter you use to make your morning cup o' joe. Your "blood" would be Columbian roasted coffee grinds. The "membrane" would be the paper filter you insert into the coffee maker. The product would be your daily dose of energy: coffee (without the grinds), or, in this case, "saliva" (without bound hormones).
>
> Free hormones are only 300 mw, which means they're small enough to cross the membrane barrier from the entire body to the mouth.
>
> Free hormones appear in saliva. When blood is tested free hormones are mixed with bound hormones.
>
> Sex hormone binding globulin (SHBG) is a glycoprotein that binds to sex hormones, specifically DHEA, testosterone and estradiol. Other steroid hormones like cortisol are bound by transcortin. When determining levels of circulating estradiol or testosterone, a measurement of these hormones would include a fraction of "free" and inactive hormones. Saliva hormone testing would only measure free hormones.

The blood filters through salivary glands as it passes through a tight junction of acinar cells. Any hormone less than 1,900 molecular weight (mw) is able to cross the filtration membrane. Free hormones typically weigh only 300 mw, and because free hormones are so lightweight, they can easily pass from blood to saliva. Average albumin (a.k.a. bound hormone) weigh 66,000 mw, cortisol-binding globulin weigh approximately 50,000 mw, and SHGB sex hormone weighs 115,000 mw. Therefore, only free/unbound hormones can actually cross the junction from the body to the mouth, leaving behind all globulin and albumen bound hormones in the blood and the free and unbound hormones in the saliva.

Slimy and sure: It's in your saliva

There's a balanced agreement between blood and saliva. By this, I mean the ratio between saliva and hormones is always constant. For example, in a blood test, testosterone shows up as 100 to 1 (100:1). This means blood shows 100 times more testosterone than saliva would ever show. Sensitivity and accuracy issues arise when such a large number appears in testing; "100" represents the total number of hormone, both unbound and bound in saliva hormone testing.

Complicated when contaminated

Ubiquitous complications such as blood and food contaminations in saliva can cause an inaccurate determination of hormone count. In a clinical study conducted to show the effects of food and drink consumption while testing progesterone levels, test results were altered measurably before and after a patient consumed milk. These results proved just how much eating and drinking can obscure the presence of hormones.

No eating and drinking before testing

Inaccuracy can be controlled by **not** drinking or eating two hours before testing. You may not be aware of saliva contamination, since it could be a blood-related problem. This too can be a problem that's difficult to distinguish, given that blood exceeds the saliva by 50-100 times in hormone levels. Particular attention should be given to avoid blood contamination in the saliva testing sample, especially for those whose gums bleed often.

Research has determined that blood contamination is visible to the naked eye when it approaches 0.156 percent. Its equivalent laboratory testing of the containment of blood at 0.156 percent contributes to approximately 3 to 7 percent of the total hormones being evaluated. Generally, this is the acceptable cut off rate for blood contamination in blood sampling, making it a laboratory technician's duty to reject any saliva samples contaminated by the slightest amount of blood.

Blood contamination can also be prevented by avoiding brushing and flossing your teeth two hours before samples are collected. Saliva hormone testing is non-evasive, painless and convenient because it can be done any time of the day or night.

Old-school & new-school

By comparison, saliva hormone testing is relatively newer than serum and urine testing, yet it's been gaining momentum and acceptance because of powerful appeal, practical usage and simplicity. Only 25 years old, its presence in mainstream medicine has had a considerably lesser amount of published information on its clinical usage than that of blood and urine hormone testing. Crucial in hormone testing, saliva sampling allows for multiple sampling collections to be taken throughout the day, thereby making it possible to get accurate reliable assessments of hormone concentration. Because hormones are produced in spurts, collecting saliva at various times of the day can determine the highs and lows of your hormones. For example, the hormone melatonin is higher in the evening than it is in the morning. Conversely, cortisol is higher in the morning than it is in the evening. You see, it's important that you not rely on a single random sample to evaluate your hormonal status. By taking five saliva samples (a sample every three hours throughout the day), your statistical chances of obtaining accurate hormone results are high.

Urine Testing:

A urine test is conducted by urinating into a special urine container. *Urine tests measure clarity, odor, color, pH levels, protein, glucose and ketones to reveal clues to various conditions.*

Pros:

- Urine can easily measure estrone(E1), estradiol (E2),estriol (E3), DHEA and metabolites, testosterone, pregnenonlone, progesterone metabolites.
- Relative cost: $250
- 24-hour collection makes timing re: hormone dose less critical

Cons:

- Urine samples must be collected throughout the day. Urine sampling calls for 24-hour collection, making it inconvenient and disastrous.
- 3-4 weeks to get results
- Fewer labs available to run tests

Serum testing:

Blood is drawn from the veins using a needle and syringe. *Blood tests are done to obtain cells and extra-cellular fluid from the body to check its health.*

Pros:

- Readily available, shortturn-around time on results
- In use for a long time
- Relatively standardized results.

Cons:

- Provides information on hormone level only during the moments blood is drawn.
- Can be expensive
- Bound vs. free are calculated, not directly measured. May be inaccurate depending on SHBG levels.
- Drawing blood is painful causing false (higher) levels of cortisol (stress hormone) due to the pain patient endures.
- Does not take into account the hourly fluctuations of hormones.
- Blood must be drawn at the laboratory by a professional technician, nurse or doctor

Cotton Salivates:

Requires patients to salivate on a cotton roll that is wrapped around a plastic retainer.

Pros:

- Especially convenient for children (below age 5), older patients (80+) and patients with specific abnormalities, as string on cotton rod serves as a choking preventative.

Cons:
According to the investigative report of Dr. Garrence Trier (2004, June) "The use of cotton salivates resulted in erroneous cortisol values."

- Garrence found that cotton substances are able to interact with cortisol by creating an affinity binding. In conclusion, it's best to avoid usage of these cotton devices in saliva hormone sample collection.

Saliva hormone testing pros and cons

Studies on saliva testing are finally becoming more abundant as it becomes a more widely accepted practice. From the pharmacokinetic perspective, there is a lack of published information involving the medical phenomena involving various types and ranges of salivary delivery systems (i.e., transdermal hormone delivery shows an enhanced salivary presence).

The saliva sample collection poses minimal disturbance to the patient's lifestyle. These collections can be taken under any circumstance and are suggested to be taken during various concurrent symptoms, e.g. during stress attack episodes, weakness, dizzy spells, and before and after intense physical activities like playing sports. Saliva testing is simpler, convenient, non-evasive and much more appealing. It doesn't require a professional to draw blood because if you can spit, we can test.

What's normal and what isn't?

These exacting and specific timing correlations of hormone release give the patient and the physician a unique perspective on the pathodynamics of disorders, diseases, or perhaps normal, physiological functions that were unable to have been detected in previous examinations. This innovative approach to testing will open a brand-new horizon in our current knowledge of hormones. It will be evidence of the incredible variations of hormone waves and the dynamics of human disease and activity.

Saliva hormone testing allows for multiple sampling collections to be taken throughout the day, thereby making it possible to get extremely accurate reliability assessments of hormone concentration, in spite of diurnal fluctuations.

In human physiology, diurnal fluctuations are due to 120-minute (timed intervals) hormone spurts throughout a person's day (depending on the hormones). In addition, saliva hormone testing is a diurnal profile of the daily dynamics and structure of various hormones peaks and troughs.

Hormone fluctuations

Some hormones go through long-term fluctuations, such as monthly profile fluctuations of estrogen and progesterone (i.e., the menstrual cycle). For seasonal variations, in the summer, because of longer daylight hours, the body's testosterone reaches its peak, as opposed to the winter when the days are shorter. The difference in light affects certain hormones, i.e. melatonin, hence creating different levels of mood swings and sleeping patterns.

Practical experience has proven that single collection samples of hormones taken at random will give false and erroneous results. This is why it's highly imperative for a collection to include more than five saliva samples taken during different times of the same day. To avoid erroneous results, saliva should be taken one hour after waking in the morning and every three hours thereafter.

Saliva hormone testing allows for specific hormones to be tested. It isn't a calculated sample, but rather a direct quantitative measurement of active free fraction hormones without the interference of bound hormones.

Saliva collection

The sample collection process is non-invasive, painless and convenient. The procedure allows doctors to evaluate a mixed saliva sample from multiple collections to get an actual value of hormones with distinct diurnal fluctuations.

Whether you're testing one hormone, or a panel of different kinds of hormones, such as DHEA, progesterone, estradiol, estriol, and testosterone, five collection samples must be taken throughout the day for accurate quantification of the results.

Exception: For Cortisol, there are two choices of tests:

First hour and last hour test: This two cortisol test gives you the minimum vital information you need to evaluate the cortisol level. First collection is taken at one hour after you awaken for the day. Second collection is taken at sleeping hour.

Five collection test: This five cortisol test give you comprehensive information of your cortisol level throughout the day. The first collection is taken at one hour after you awaken for the day, and one collection every three hour thereafter for the remaining of the four collections.

Almost all laboratories follow the same procedure, and most laboratories require people to follow the same instructions. When testing saliva, you will be provided with plastic vials or, as they are sometimes called by laboratory technicians, "Sali-cap collection tubes."

Each vial will come with a plastic straw to spit into and a pack of labels to record your name, date and time when each saliva test was taken. Because hormones fluctuate, it is of extreme importance to document each saliva sample with *exact time. Timing must be precise; no approximations or guesstimates are allowed.

Special Attention

Saliva specimens contaminated with food or blood will cause abnormal and inaccurate test results. Laboratories are not responsible for this error. You must make sure that the specimens are clean and non-contaminated.

On label write:

- Date of collection: month, day and year
- Time of collection: hour and minute(s)
- The most obvious, your name. You'd be surprised how many people forget to write their names.

Precautions:

If you're experiencing oral bleeding your saliva test will be rejected once it's reached the laboratory. Therefore, avoid taking the test if you're aware of the slightest possibility that saliva may be contaminated with blood.

Discontinue hormone supplementation for 24 hours prior to collecting saliva samples.

Don't eat, drink, or smoke an hour before each saliva sample collection. Water is fine; however, anything else poses a problem with regard to testing accuracy.

Also, many people send in there saliva samples with ice packs. No ice packs are necessary. Altering temperature can pose the threat of inaccurate results.

Directions:

Precisely one hour after you've woken, take your first saliva test. Reach for your first vial-- spit, label and set aside. *There's no need to refrigerate; it's advised to keep vials at room temperature (70- F).

The second saliva sample should be taken three hours after your first collection was taken. Do the same: spit, label and set aside. When spitting, use the straw as a suction device. Place the tiny straw against tongue, draw saliva from tongue and eject into straw. You can't reuse a straw; as soon as one is used, throw it away.

Saliva must fill at least half the vial. Cap the tube tightly after filling to avoid leakage.

You will need to do this three more times throughout the day, totaling five collections. Each collection must beexactly three hours apart . Saliva samples should be sent for testing as soon as possible within 2-3 days.

How saliva is tested:
New technology—Luminescent Immuno Assays (LIA)

In the past, saliva hormone testing was done by using Radio Immuno Assays (RIA) and Elisa Immuno Assays (Elisa); originally designed specifically for serum (blood) testing, Elisa and RIA immuno assays were later changed for saliva testing by using specific laboratory after-market adjustments.

The Luminescent Immuno Assay was the first form of saliva hormone testing designed and created specifically for measuring and testing hormones through saliva.

Direct measurements

To obtain measurements of hormone levels, a specific photo spectrometer allows ultra-sensitive light to be achieved by way of illuminescent amino assays.

The hormones in saliva react with LIA reagents and emit a light, which directly measures the precise level of hormones. One hundred times more sensitive than the current routine method of testing known as RIA, with LIA's glowing light, lab technicians can count and examine each specific hormone that a person possesses. Luminescent technology inhibits cross sensitivity between target hormones and other hormones that aren't meant to test. Well below the picogram range, LIA has the capacity to measure the smallest particles.

Approved

The Federal Drug Administration (FDA) has cleared saliva hormone testing kits used for assessing cortisol, progesterone, estradiol, and testosterone, and is currently in the process of clearing DHEA. The FDA cleared reagents and has passed the FDA 510(k) process by validating the testing procedure.

Sticking around

Saliva hormones are, by nature, small non-polar molecules which have physical charges. Often, they have a tendency to stick to plastic materials opposite from their physical electric charge.

Glass is completely absorption-free and carries minimal static electric charge. However, the common plastic container is made of polyethylene plastic (PET), which is highly absorptive and carries an electrostatic charge. It's highly absorptive of certain hormones, specifically progesterone, which is electrically charged. Likewise, the stopper (also made of polyethylene) plays a highly absorptive role by binding together a large amount of an already small pool of hormones present in the saliva specimen. The saliva collected in a PET container may arrive at the laboratory already changed resulting in a false measurement of hormone levels, making your results inaccurate long before it's tested.

> **The Saliva Collection Container**
>
> Saliva Hormones - Small non-polar molecules that stick to plastic material
>
> The best plastic material has been observed to be Ultra-Pure Polypropylene, not recycled plastic. Polypropylene is highly absorptive and is used especially for Progesterone, a highly non-polar hormone.
>
> Stoppers made of polypropylene are high absorptive.
>
> Glass seems to be completely absorption free.

To minimize the interference of saliva's interaction with materials, recent procedures use polypropylene (PPL) tubes to avoid the tendencies of certain hormone's attachment to container materials.

Advantages

The saliva sample collection poses minimal disturbance to a patient's lifestyle. Again, these collections are advised to be taken under a variety of conditions and circumstances (e.g., working, playing, relaxing and stressing). These exacting and specific timing correlations of hormones give the researcher and physician a unique perspective into the pathodynamics of disorders, diseases, or perhaps normal physiological functions that were unable to have been detected in previous examinations.

∾DR. TAI'S ANTI-AGING HEALTH SECRET∾

I'm certain that saliva hormone testing will open a brand-new horizon in our current knowledge of hormones. Because of multiple sampling collections, saliva testing will not be solely used for hormones, but to also test for abnormalities and disease.

Saliva hormone testing can give incredible evidence of many human waves and dynamics because of the multiple sampling collections, which are taken throughout the day, thereby making it possible to get extremely accurate reliability assessments of a variety of concentrations, despite diurnal and nocturnal fluctuations.

SECRET II

"Be wiser than other people, if you can;
but do not tell them so."
—Lord Chesterfield

Chapter 4

Synthetic vs. Bioidentical Hormones

I've been fooled many times by the similarity of cubic zirconia and diamonds. I can't tell the difference, but unfortunately, my wife can. She has a keen eye. To the untrained eye (such as mine), a cubic zirconium (CZ) appears to be identical to a diamond. But it doesn't take neither a gemologist nor a jeweler to mark the chief dissimilarity between high-priced diamonds and CZs. One is real, and the other... isn't.

Diamonds, the world's strongest rocks are pure and can take thousands of years to form. CZs take merely hours. People like CZ. They prefer diamonds, but they buy CZs because they're affordable. But reasonable prices have never guaranteed quality or any customer's satisfaction; exercise prudence when shopping for an item of lesser value and go for quality, not quantity, especially when it concerns your personal life. Just as CZs have a higher likelihood of breaking before a diamond will, synthetic hormones will let you down before natural hormones will. Do as you wish, but I'm trying to save you one sad face and another doctor's office visitation.

Fake vs. Real: Which would you prefer?

- Monopoly money or *real, cold cash*
- Plastic flowers or *real flowers*
- Silicon breasts or *real breasts*
- Acrylic sweaters or *cashmere sweaters*
- Synthetic or *bioidentical hormones*

My point...

Just as geological deposits like caves make diamonds, your body makes hormones. Bioidentical hormones are made from the exact same compounds that produce hormones in your body (bioidentical literally means "identical to your biology"). Do not confuse bioidentical hormones with phytohormones. Phytohormone supplements are, at times, combined formulations of herbal extractions and natural chemical substances. At other times, labels that read "phytohormones" are oral supplements that possess the ability to support the bioidentical hormone that you may be lacking. Bioidentical hormones work differently—they give you what you need, when you need it, with hardly any side effects.

51

Key and Lock

To further elaborate, bioidentical hormones are like keys to locks. Specific hormone molecules are like specific keys— only a hormone (as in one kind) matches the lock (hormone receptor site).Just as a particular key is needed to open a door, a particular hormone is needed for your body to function properly. When a hormone and a receptor correspond with each other, they set off a chain of events that allows you to go on with your life, normally and healthfully.

> **Change the grooves on your keys and see what happens...**
>
> Will your car start?
> Can you open that door?
> Does anything start, open, or unlock?
>
> You have to find an identical key that fits before you can do anything or go anywhere.

Phytohormones

Phytohormones comparable to red clover and black cohosh aren't identical to your body's hormones. The hormones found in these plants have to be converted inside your body by way of mixing with stomach acids and going through a process of chemical digestion before they can mimic hormones. It would take years of consuming plants like red clover and black cohosh to have the same beneficial effects of taking a bioidentical hormone supplement.

Most plant extracts (phytohormones) work on keeping cell receptor sites busy so that the body's tissues require less hormone production. Bioidentical hormones replenish lost hormones while fortifying already-existing hormones. Bioidentical hormone supplements support specific hormones that you may lack or have an excess of. (For example, for an estrogen excess, take bioidentical progesterone. For a testosterone deficiency, take bioidentical testosterone.)

Synthetic hormones

Synthetic hormones, or pharmaceutically produced hormones are FDA-approved because of financial reasons that allow exclusive marketing for a certain drug. There's money in pharmaceutical drugs--it is a multi-billion dollar market. People like chemicals because they think that chemicals deliver rapid results, so companies invest in chemicals and marketing their products via emotionally appealing television commercials that plead with the hearts and minds of Americans.

I couldn't agree more with consumers—synthetic hormones do bring about rapid results—rapid results with dangerous long-term effects. With synthetic hormones, you should know that you may be damaging some parts of the body in order to remedy another part. Is this really what you want?

Pharmaceutical companies have an absolute corner on the market. They produce a hormone that is 90 percent (or more) like a bioidentical hormone, but only in chemical structure and *not* in function, receptor compatibility or normal metabolism. By creating a 10 percent difference, pharmaceutical companies can claim exclusivity in the marketplace—creating a new patent for an innovative chemical creation. They make it look similar to a hormone but the body reacts very differently with negative side effects and potentially dangerous end metabolites, as shown in countless indepth published research.

Basically, pharmaceutical industries can't patent drugs made from the same molecular structures as the kind found in your body. From a business perspective, it's important that these pharmaceutical companies continue producing patents for synthetic hormones. Why? Because chemical formulas generate enormous revenue and colossal profits.

Evidence

In the last several years, millions of people taking synthetic hormones have said that their bodies were starting to act strange. Going nothing short of haywire, within a matter of months, their regular internal functions became irregular. This doesn't surprise me—as with my key and lock example, synthetic hormones are very different from the hormones our bodies produce. However, the part that isn't similar is completely rejected, creating metabolic aberrations and severe long-lasting side effects.

The body exerts a great deal of energy trying to metabolize substances it can't recognize, resulting in irreversible long term damage to tissues and DNA.

Powerful Reasons to consider Natural Hormones

1. Relief of symptoms
2. Prevention of memory loss
3. Improvement to heart health
4. Prevention of osteoporosis
5. Increase cell repair and growth

Dr. Erica T. Schwartz, author of *Hormone Solution*, and I share a similar philosophy when it comes to synthetic hormone—synthetic and bioidentical hormones possess greater differences than they do similarities.

"Synthetic hormones are simply no replacement for natural hormones. After many years of getting poor or no results with conventional capital HRT in my practice, natural hormones proved to be more effective and safer than any other treatment I have seen or used."

—*Dr. Schwartz*

Clinical Studies

In 2002, a study was conducted on healthy (free of life-threatening illnesses) post-menopausal women which examined the risks and benefits of synthetic estrogen and progesterone. During the trial, 26 percent of the study's participants who used synthetic estrogen and progesterone were at risk of developing breast cancer. (Women's Health Initiative research team. "Risks and benefits of estrogen and progesterone in healthy post-menopausal women." Journal of the American Medical Association, 2002; 288:321-333.)

The Journal of Clinical Endocrinology and Metabolism published a study conducted by researcher L. Hofseth (et al.) on "The effects of synthetic hormones on women." Hofseth and his team of fellow researchers found that hormone replacement therapy using estrogen and madroxy progesterone acetate (synthetic progesterone) increased the chances of epithelial proliferation (growth underneath the first layer of skin) in a group of post-menopausal women. If it wasn't for the progesterone used to control the growths developed from an estrogen excess, the study's participants were again at risk of developing breast cancer. (Hofseth, L., "Hormone replacement therapy regimen and breast cancer risk." *Journal of Clinical Endocrinology and Metabolism*, 1999; 84: 4559-65.)

Dr. Neal Rouser, author of *Natural Hormone Replacement for Men and Women: How to Achieve Healthy Aging*, commented on the Women's Health Initiative (WHI), one of the largest and longest-running studies America has experienced thus far. Dr. Rouser said synthetic estrogens pose dangers women should pay heed to.

"In my practice of prescribing natural hormones to women for five years, I have never seen the problems and side effects as we have seen with synthetic hormones. Why not replace the body with natural biologically identical hormones? Anything besides natural hormones, as we have seen with the recent discontinuation of the WHI trial, is dangerous to a woman's health."

—*Dr. Rouser*

Fill in the blank:

1) **Synthetic hormones are made from…**
   A) **Coal tar**
   B) **Horse urine**
   C) **Chemicals that will potentially cause cancer**
   D) **All of the above**

Correct answer: D, all of the above

Powerful Negative Side Effects of Synthetic Estrogen

1. Premarin made from horse's estrogens, equilin and equilenin.Side effects: burning on urination, allergies, joint aches, and pains. Ahlgrimm, M., *The HRT Solution*. 1999; New York: Avery Pub.

2. Synthetic Estrogen is not compatible with your body's estrogen receptors. Sinatra, S., "Heart Sense for Women." Washington DC; *Lifeline Press*, 2000.

3. Estrogens derived from horses urine may stay inyour body up to 13 weeks, in contrast to your natural estradiol, which is eliminated from your body within a few hours. Ahlgrimm, M., *The HRT Solution*. 1999; New York: Avery Pub.

4. Horses estrogen is 200 times stronger than natural estrogens.Collins, J., "What's Your Menopause Type?" Roseville, CA: Prima Health 2000.

Dr. Tai's Something to Think About

Would you feed yourself a substance similar to that you'd "feed" your car? Petroleum-based chemicals?

A dash of this, and a pinch of that
Ingredients in synthetic hormones

The so-called "estrogen equivalents" sold annually to millions of women across the world are made from the urine of pregnant horses. Synthetic hormones are produced in laboratories and are mostly made from hydrocarbons, more commonly referred to as coal and tar derivatives. Among the hundreds of kinds of synthetic forms of hormones readily available, the attempted reproduction of testosterone, methyltestosterone, is made of ammonium ions. Truth be told, when in an alcohol form, methyl can be used as an industrial solvent, sort of like antifreeze. Chemically manufactured, methyltestosterone is nowhere near a reproduction of natural testosterone. Synthetic hormones like methyltestosterone and estrogen are multifaceted—they're complex formulas that can do a number on your body. As a filter, our bodies sometimes have difficulty processing complex forms of drugs. Conjugated estrogens like pregnant horse urine mixtures have approximately 30 different forms of estrogens, which only animal bodies can make the most of. Our human bodies are much more complex organisms and can experience difficulty adjusting to derivatives Mother Nature intended only creatures with hide to possess.

Hormones derived from animals are 200 percent more potent than necessary, which can cause the body to act in very aggressive way, e.g. developing certain forms of cancers, strokes and thrombophlebitis (blood clots). I'm convinced that synthetic hormones aren't safe, yet somehow they've been approved by the FDA. Throughout the book you'll begin to see why I emphasize taking bioidentical hormones over any other kind of hormone.

Potential side effects of synthetic hormones

- Weight gain
- Depression
- Various forms of cancer
- Hormonal imbalances
- Memory loss
- Disease
- Loss of mobility
- Loss of libido

Bioidentical hormones

Active extractions from natural sources like soy beans and yams are good sources of bioidentical hormone. These extractions are identical in molecular structure to that of human hormones. The potential is becoming clearer in natural hormone replacement therapy in that research has defined the lines between synthetic and natural hormone replacement. This is also the reason why so many doctors are making the switch from synthetic hormone therapy to natural hormone therapy.

Regardless of what medical trends appear to be, ultimately you have a choice. It's your body and your decision, but before you decide, allow me to ask a rhetorical question—would you choose a cubic zirconium over a diamond?

Potential side effects of bioidentical hormones

If monitored, side effects of any kind are rare and uncommon.

FACT: 90% of Post-Menopausal women with breast cancer have never taken any kind of hormone therapy at all. Ahlgrimm, M., *The HRT Solution.* 1999; New York: Avery Pub.

Chapter 5

Hormone Delivery

When I was in school, I was taught that hormones could be delivered only through injection; fortunately, that's not the case today. Bioidentical hormones can be administered in a variety of ways and there are enough choices to make anyone go a little cross-eyed.

Currently, these methods include injections, dermal patches, gels, lotion, pills, tablets, rings and sprays. This chapter focuses strictly on how hormones are delivered and dispersed throughout a person's body. I'm hopeful that this chapter will also help you understand which method of taking bioidentical hormones is right for you.

Would you rather be...

fed ?
rubbed?
sprayed?
injected?
- or -
slapped?

As I'm certain you'll notice, I prefer more painless methods like sublingual sprays and transdermal liposome creams. However, I would like to educate you on your choices. You do have choices, after all, and my job is to give them to you. I just hope you choose a gentle method that'll deliver rapid results.

Hormone departure time: As soon as possible
Hormone arrival time: Arrive when departed

My philosophy has always been that taking care of yourself should be a pleasure, not a pain. Hormone delivery is just as important as the hormone itself, because it's all about how it gets where it needs to be and when the hormone actually arrives at its intended destination. It's like going on a trip--the important thing is that you're going. Great! But how? How will you go? Will you travel by train, plane or car? Will you walk? Will you ride your bike? Can you afford a plane ticket, or is it more cost-efficient if you drive? If you drive, will you get there on time? All of these things matter. Just as important as it is for you to get where you need to be, it's just as important for your hormones to do the same. Unless your hormones get where they need to be when they need to be there, the only place you'll be is in bed, and we don't want that, do we?

Negative Side Effects of Oral Estrogen

   Vliet, E., "New insights on hormones and mood," Menopause Mgt. 1993; 6/7:140-146)

1. Increases blood pressure
2. Increases fatty triglycerides
3. Increases estrone (E1)
4. Increases incidence of gallstones
5. Elevates liver enzymes
6. Decreases available Growth Hormone
7. Binds tryptophan and interferes with serotonin necessary for calmness and happiness. *Hays, B., "Estrogen amd depression," Institute for Functional Medicine, Inc., 2002; p. 269-270*
8. Increases sex hormone binding globulin (SHBG) and decreases available testosterone
9. Increases carbohydrate cravings. *Pansini, F., Ann NY Acad Sci 1990; 592:460-462.*
10. Increases weight gain. *Pansini, F., Ann NY Acad Sci 1990; 592:460-462.*

Dr. Tai's rating legend	Side effects rating
Excellent: ***** Good: **** Average: *** Below average: ** Terrible: *	Excellent: * Good: ** Average: *** Below average: **** Terrible: *****

Dr. Tai's Ratings
Convenience: *
Cost: *
Effectiveness: *****
Side Effects: ****

Injections

Most supplements used for hormonal replacement have started as injections. These treatments are delivered to a person by using a sharp syringe that squirts out various kinds of bioidentical hormones. Doctors usually aim for the arms or the butt. Ouch!

Pros	Cons
• Rapid delivery • Direct administration into blood • A cool plastic bandage	• Are painful • Require doctor's visits • Are expensive (requiring weekly or monthly visits plus the cost of the injection itself) • Are time-consuming • Dosages prescribed may be too high for a given individual's physiologic makeup

If your hormone levels are particularly low, you may have to visit your doctor more often and it will cost more money. The procedure is often painful, and as adults, we can hardly expect to receive lollipops for being good boys and girls. Sorry.

Injections: More than necessary

Besides being inconvenient, costly, and time-consuming, injections can give you more of a dosage than you actually need. Before your bioidentical hormone injection, your levels would obviously be very low. With an injection, a specific hormone level can be higher than your body can tolerate. Moments after an injection, hormone levels can rise up to several hundred percent of your natural optimum level, which means that receiving an injection would be like eating three meals in one hour when you're supposed to eat three meals over the course of 12 hours. Typically, you would get sick. (I would either vomit or fall asleep from over-stuffing myself.) The same example can be applied to bioidentical hormonal injection. From a subnormal state, you quickly reach levels that exceed normal, and this abrupt change can upset your body. It will take days before excessive hormonal quantities are neutralized by a gradual depletion.

Testimonial

"For three years I've been going to anti-aging medical clinics to receive weekly injections of human growth hormone (HGH). Had I known there was a way to avoid injections, I would have. They were painful and left bruises on the body I was trying to perfect. It was expensive, and although helpful, a series of awful experiences. I'm now taking a supplemental form of HGH (called HGM by Health Secrets USA), and I use DHEA and testosterone cream. People frequently mistake me for my early 30s, when in my early 30s, they thought I was in my late 40s."

—*Robert, 47*

"In September 1996, my husband was diagnosed with adult onset diabetes. Besides that, he experiences severe food allergies and is required to receive his EpiPen auto-injection whenever he comes in contact with anything from the nut family or the sea. It's been difficult seeing him the way he is and I'm sick of syringes. I cringe at the sight of needles of any kind; his allergies and diabetes have swayed me to abandon knitting and sewing.

"I see the face he makes when I inject the needles into his thigh and it troubles me to see him in pain. Whenever I am given the choice to stay away from injections, I do. Publicly, I want to profess my hate for injections and when I started replacing my hormones, I totally ruled out injections as an option. My phobia of needles has caused problems at hospitals.

"Fortunately, with the way I've been feeling from bioidentical hormonal therapy, I don't see myself in any clinic's or hospital's waiting room."

—*Kayla Dee, 51*

Dermal patches

Transdermal patches are like stickers. The skin is waterproof; however, it's not oil-proof. Dermal patches use skin-compatible oily material that can pass through the skin's top-layer, the epidermis, making its way through the skin's sub-layer, the dermis.

Dr. Tai's Ratings
Convenience: ***
Cost: *
Effectiveness: ****
Side Effects: ***

Pros	Cons
• Fast delivery • Direct administration into blood	• Frequently fall off • Can cause itching & irritation • Can be painful • Limited selection of patches • Expensive

As you can see in the table above, the cons of dermal patches are much less numerous than those of injections. However so, I find dermal patches to be just as inconvenient. By and large, dermal patches are used for patients who are lacking testosterone and estrogen (two hormones that stimulate the development of masculine and feminine characteristics). They aren't commonly used for other forms of hormone therapy. They're rare, and you have to keep track of changing patches on a regular basis. Hormone patches are very similar to nicotine patches—for those of you who have tried to quit smoking, hormone patches are similar--requiring daily attention.

Dr. Tai's Ratings
Convenience: ***** **Cost:** ***** **Effectiveness:** ***** **Side Effects:** *

Gels and Lotions

As a form of hormone delivery, topical solutions have become increasingly popular. They're painless and have effective results. All you have to do is pump, rub vigorously and spread widely, hold off for a few moments before getting dressed, and out the door you go. I prefer gels and lotions over patches and injections.

Pros	Cons
• Convenient • Inexpensive • Painless • Overuse unlikely • Hormone levels replenished at a pace the body determines	• Can be messy • May elicit an allergic reaction in those with exceptionally sensitive skin • Must be used daily

As I've stated in the section devoted to dermal patches, the skin is waterproof, which means that gels and lotions wash off. Not only do topical solutions wash off, they rub off on clothing. You'll be getting less for your money if gels, lotions, creams or any other topical solution aren't made with *liposome technology*, the only one that accomplishes skin penetration within minutes.

Gels and Lotions: Liposomes

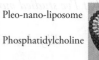 Liposomes cross the skin's barrier because they are carried in gels or lotions that contain micro-encapsulation the skin can recognize. Liposomes are micro-encapsulated phosphatidylcholine. Skin and skin cells are also coated with phosphatidylcholine, which means your skin assumes that those liposomes are a part of its own.

Unlike gels and lotions that don't have liposomes, bioidentical hormone gels and lotions are carried through the top layer of skin and transported into your blood, making creams with liposomes almost 1000 percent more effective than any other 24-hour time-released formula. Additional studies have concluded that 95 percent of liposomes reach target cells by diffusing through the skin and entering through the blood stream.

In a 2002 study conducted at the University of Ljubljana, Slovenia, dermal therapy researchers concluded that liposomes "considerably improved the effectiveness of drugs," by "influencing the rate of transfer and efficacy of the drug's actions."

Benefits of "above the skin" bioidentical hormone delivery
Patches and topical solutions: Gels, creams, lotions, etc.

1. Lower the possibility of SHGB formation in the liver
2. Bypass the liver in the initial introduction of naturally supplemented hormones
3. Are 10 times stronger than oral forms of delivery
4. Can be customized specifically for your needs via dosage adjustment

Testimonial

"My wife of 19 years regularly slathers her face in all manners of creams, balsams, unguents, balms, conditioners and lotions. She said it helps reverse the aging process— utter decay. She's still lovely without these creams—a bit wrinkly, perhaps—but all these cold creams in fancy jars are a marketing man's invention. None has done what they've promised except for the creams that are made from liposomes. The effects are remarkable and I've monitored her usage, only because I find the effects fascinating. I ask her if she's been using the liposome cream. She's taken aback by the idea that I've studied our bathroom cabinets so well."

—Eliyahu, 43

Pills, tablets and capsules

Despite a bad aftertaste, pills, tablets and capsules are effective. Oral consumption of any sort of bioidentical hormone supplement only requires a tall glass of water, making it a painless and a far quicker form of hormonal replacement delivery than injections or topical solutions.

Dr. Tai's Ratings

Convenience: *****
Cost: *****
Effectiveness: *****

Side Effects: *****

Pros	Cons
• Convenient • Inexpensive • Painless • You can reduce or increase dosages depending on how you feel (i.e., if two pills a day aren't helping, you may want to try four; if four pills a day feels like too much, you can reduce it to three and so on	• Overdosing is a possibility • Oral consumption leads to minor SHGB formation (binding globulins resulting in fewer free anabolic hormones)

Dr. Thierry Hertoghe commented on oral forms of hormones in his book *The Hormone Solution: Stay younger longer with natural hormones and nutrition therapies* (Three Rivers Press, 2002). He said, "Taking any estrogen orally even natural estrogen puts you at risk of accumulating too much estrogen in the liver. That stimulates the production of too many binding proteins (SHGB) which don't get just the estrogen, but, also, many other hormones making them inactive and creating other deficiencies."

Dr. Hertoghe is right—the production of too many sex hormone-binding globulines (SHBG) can eventually cause problems for your liver and result in lower levels of free and unbound hormones. SHBG is a glycoprotein that binds to sex hormones, specifically DHEA, testosterone and estrogen. Other steroid hormones such as progesterone, cortisol, and other corticosteroids are bound by *transcortin*. When determining levels of circulating estradiol or testosterone, either a total measurement can be done that includes the "free" and the bound fractions, or if using saliva testing, only the "free" hormone can be measured. Too many SHBGs makes most other hormones bound or useless. If the result of the test is that the net active free hormone is at a lower level than you started out with (because your body produced more SHGB as a result of taking oral hormones), then you're losing ground. The net free hormones are less even if the total hormone level is higher than in the beginning.

Sublingual sprays

Last, but certainly not least, the sublingual spray is my favorite method of hormone delivery for a variety of reasons—a few pumps under the tongue will give you your dosage for the day, and with the least amount of cons, sublingual sprays score five stars in almost every category.

Dr. Tai's Ratings

Convenience: *****
Cost: *****
Effectiveness: *****

Side Effects: **

Pros	Cons
• Bypasses the liver • Is transmitted directly into the blood • Convenient • Inexpensive • Painless • You can reduce or increase dosages depending on how you feel (i.e., if two sprays a day aren't helping, you may want to try four, etc.) • Sprayed directly under tongue: good for people who have trouble swallowing capsules • Suitable for traveling. You can take it with you everywhere, leave it in the office, keep it at home or stash in your purse	• Overdosing is a possibility • Because the liver filters all oral supplements, you may exhaust it by taking pills, tablets or capsules for an extended peiod of time. • Oral consumption leads to the creation of SHGB

Like most cultural, personal and professional circles, medical crowds have their own jargon. Doctors refer to sublingual sprays and transdermal liposome creams as instruments of *First Pass Technology*. This means that sublingual sprays go directly through the blood while bypassing the liver! That's right—no SHBGs with sublingual sprays! The natural bioidentical hormones go into the bloodstream through the vessels underneath your tongue. This particular technology is shown to create less SHBG binding because the skin continuously absorbs much smaller amounts more closely to the physiological production of our own body.

Similar to some topical solutions, sublingual sprays use phosphatidylcholine micro-encapsulation, which means that bioidentical hormones are transported directly through the sublingual blood vessels found under the tongue. From there, the active components of the spray are carried throughout the entire body before they reach the areas where they're needed most.

ᲜᲝDR. TAI'S ANTI-AGING HEALTH SECRETᲜᲝ

Each and every one of your symptoms will require a different dosage from a different hormone. Emotional, physical and mental stressors can effect hormone consumption and absorption. This is why you may require different dosages of a certain hormone if you've undergone a traumatic experience like a death in the family or job lay-off. Contrary to this, if you've been in rather high spirits, you may require less of a dose. For example, if you've noticed the sex in your relationship has been getting better, you may be happier because you've become more active. In this case you may have to lower the dosage of hormonal supplementation only because your body has reached stabilization. Please monitor your symptoms so you can adjust the dosage for your needs and your doctor can better understand what you need more or less of.

SECRET III

"The fact was I didn't want to look my age.
But I didn't want to act the age I wanted
to look either. I also wanted to grow old
enough to understand that sentence."
—Erma Bombeck

Chapter 6

Dehydroepiandrosterone (DHEA): *A weakly androgenic steroid secreted largely by the adrenal cortex, but also by the testes; a precursor of testosterone.*

What to Expect

What is DHEA?

How is DHEA produced?

Who should use DHEA?

Functions of DHEA

DHEA deficiency

DHEA and cancer

DHEA and sugar

Testing DHEA

DHEA Self-assessment

Taking DHEA

Anti-aging Health Secret

"My favorite DHEA studies"

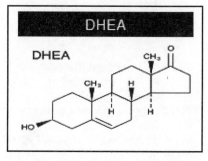

—Stedman's Medical Dictionary

Finally, DHEA has been getting the acknowledgement it deserves! Picking up momentum through marketing, advertising and a surge of various vitamins and supplements, DHEA is becoming more broadly used in the battle against age resistance. Unlike HGH, DHEA is safe to use in larger doses because the body has it in abundance. It's also possibly one of the most versatile hormones as it converts into other hormones like testosterone and estrogen.

Where does it come from?

Like cortisol, DHEA is a hormone manufactured by the adrenal cortex, a small triangular gland that sits on top of both kidneys. At age 50, the adrenals produce half the DHEA they once did. After 25, your body begins to lose 2 percent every year, more or less.

DHEA: the "big kid on the block"

DHEA is considered the "father" among hormones just as the Pituitary gland is among glands. Together with pregnenolone (considered the mother of all hormones) affecting nearly every organ in our body including our brain, DHEA is an anabolic hormone that possesses the ability to repair and construct tissues.

Conversion

DHEA is converted into testosterone, and oftentimes through aromatization it's converted into estradiol. DHEA and DHEA-S are mutually interchangeable through the process of sulfating; however, the concentration of DHEA is 500-1000 times lower than that of DHEA-S.

> **DHEA: Gas tank ½ empty**
>
> —Full at 25
> You lose 2 percent thereafter
>
> —By 50, half is gone
> You continue to lose 2 percent
>
> —By 75, you're out of luck if you don't replenish.

Secretion

DHEA is secreted through the adrenal cortex (in both men and women) and approximately 10 percent of DHEA's plasma is secreted from the ovaries (only in women). ACTH from the hypothalamus-pituitary axis (HPA) affects the production of DHEA, which has a pulsatile/ circadian-like variation just as the cortisol hormone does.

Functions of DHEA. Ahlgrimm, M., *The HRT Solution* 1999; New York: Avery Pub.

1. Decreases blood cholesterol
2. Decreases fatty deposit in blood vessel
3. Lower incidence of blood clots
4. Improves bone growth
5. Weight loss
6. Improves brain function
7. Improves sense of well being
8. Better stress management
9. Supports your immune system
10. Improves cell repair
11. Decreases allergic reactions

Effects of DHEA

DHEA works on central nervous system excitability. Because of this, the hormone has a tremendous effect on the libido and the general well-being of individuals. When DHEA acts on the central nervous system, its effect is 5 to 10 times greater than in plasma. Increasing DHEA improves the quality of sleep as it boosts a person's energy levels and increases stress-handling abilities.

Doc's lingo explained

*Lymphocytes: A white blood cell formed in lymphatic tissue throughout the body.

*Monocytes: A large mononuclear leukocyte that normally constitutes 3 to 7 percent of the leukocytes of the circulating blood and is normally found in lymph nodes, spleen, bone marrow and loose connective tissue.

Having a positive impact on depression, memory, thinking and cognition, DHEA has a powerful effect on the immune system through the lymphocytes*. As an antioxidant, DHEA decreases the production of free radicals by its effect on monocytes.*

Effects of bioidentical DHEA supplementation

Bioidentical DHEA supplementation shows increased production of testosterone and androstenedione, IGF-1, IGF-BP and a decrease of IGF-BP3. Upon undergoing proper and correct supplementation of DHEA, most patients with low levels ofDHEA improve in their perception of physical and psychological well being and increase lean body mass, decreasing fat.

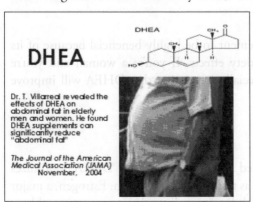

DHEA

Dr. T. Villareal revealed the effects of DHEA on abdominal fat in elderly men and women. He found DHEA supplements can significantly reduce "abdominal fat"

The Journal of the American Medical Association (JAMA) November, 2004

DHEA and DHEA-S

DHEA and its twin brother DHEA-S (as you can see, I like "family" analogies), which is a metabolized sulfate molecule from the liver, constantly work together in creating a balance for the body. From that special vantage point, DHEA is able to produce testosterone and estrogen. Because of DHEA's social role, by way of producing other hormones, supplemental DHEA takes on an especially important role in not just anti-aging medicine but in anti-obesity, anti-anxiety, anti-diabetes and a new one—anti-heart attacks.

Let's Get Ready to Rumble!

To my right—we have men...

During andropause, DHEA serves as a powerful androgen formation, supportive of producing natural testosterone in the body. It has a positive effect on aging men suffering from:

- declining muscle mass
- increased body fat around the waist and the middle of the body
- libido reduction
- fatigue
- dry skin
- energy loss
- strength loss

The prospect of improvement by using DHEA replacement and its positive effect on testosterone production bears the potential of bringing happiness to every aging male. With bioidentical supplementation of DHEA, men will turn into lovers instead of fighters.

To my left—we have women...

Women will find DHEA replacement to be highly beneficial because of its powerful anti-depressant and anti-anxiety effects. If you're a woman and you're reading this, I know you'll find it especially interesting that DHEA will improve libido and boost your skin's thickness.

For backup, here's research...

In 2000, Dr. Baulieu reported that supplemental DHEA optimizes improvement in serum estrogen as well as testosterone in women. Estrogen, a major female sex hormone, has a lot to do with how sexually active a woman is and how firm her skin is.

Benefits of DHEA

Lieberman, S., *The Real Vitamin and Mineral Book*. NY: Avery Pub. 1997

1. Muscle strength and lean body mass
2. Improves immune function
3. Improves quality of life
4. Improves sleep
5. Boosts feelings of wellness
6. Decreases joint pain
7. Improves sensitivity to insulin
8. Lowers fatty triglycerides
9. Stops damaging effects of stress

STUDYING DHEA

- Researchers have reported that DHEA shows promise for potential improvement in cardiovascular disease and arterioscleroses. These vascular complications of fatty deposits and plaques the arterial wall's inner lining causes diminished blood flow, nutrients and oxygen throughout the heart and the entire body.
- Studies conducted on rabbits at John Hopkins University in 1988 have shown that supplemental DHEA improved the severity of arteriosclerosis. Results showed nearly 50 percent of plaque shrinkage in the inner lining of blood vessels. These very same clinical studies have shown that higher levels of DHEA confer improvement in cardiovascular protection for men as they did in rabbits.
- Research conducted at the University of California, San Diego with 1029 showed a significant reduction (up to 25 percent) in the risk of cardiovascular disease in men.

What's up, Doc?

*Five out of five stars: Experts give DHEA two thumbs up, way up!

Dr. Baulieu and his research team in Paris conducted a study using DHEA. After testing DHEA's effects on a group of women, he found that they reported having a greater desire to have sex more often, which was probably due to developing more energy, therefore greater self-esteem (energy and self-esteem go hand-in-hand).

Dr. Baulieu checked up on his "Golden Girls" and found that after long-term use of DHEA they made fewer complaints about their osteoporotic conditions.

(Baulieu, E.E., et al. "DHEA Sulfate and aging contribution of the DHEA age study to socio-biomedical." *Proceedings from the National Academy of Sciences USA, 2000;97(8)4279-4284.)*

In 1995, at the New York Academy of Science, Dr. John E. Neffler, a physician at the Medical College of Virginia, said he considers DHEA to "represent the biomarkers of healthy aging."

Dr. Bulbrook from England reported that women developing breast cancer have very low levels of DHEA. These low levels of DHEA can appear as much as nine years prior to the diagnosis of breast cancer. Dr. Bulbrook found in a study of 5000 women that 27 women developed breast cancer because they had low levels of DHEA.

DHEA and Cancer
The Real Deal: Studies That Can Save Lives

1) Temple University, Dr. Arthur Schwartz, professor/researcher

A number of reports suggest that DHEA has an extraordinarily positive effect on cancer. The extensive laboratory research conducted by Dr. Arthur Schwartz of Temple University validates this. By gathering cell cultures, Dr. Schwartz saw the amazing results DHEA had on cancer patients. He saw that when cancer patients were given DHEA via their diets, the cells which were unaffected by cancer became stronger.

Inspired by this, Dr. Schwartz subsequently conducted more extraordinary research using live animals--mice that were predisposed to breast cancer. He noted in his experiment that the mice without DHEA suffered and most of them died, while the mice that had been supplemented with DHEA were free of tumors.

Dr. Schwartz did two additional studies in 1981 and 1984 where he reported on two separate and different strains of mice where he found a 75 percent and 100 percent reduction in cancer after 8 months. In one of his more prolonged studies, he found a 50-75 percent reduction in the cancer rate in these mice after 15 months.

Dr. Schwartz reported that DHEA supplementation protected mice from forming cancer in tissues, skin, lungs, breasts, intestines and the liver. (Schwartz, Arthur. "Cancer prevention with DHEA." *Journal of Cellular Biochemistry,* 1995;

59(S22):210-217.)

Studies on people and animals can and will differ greatly, but I think it's safe to conclude that if DHEA has such a positive effect on mice with cancer, it can only strengthen human patients with cancer. If you have a history of cancer, please check with your doctor before using bioidentical DHEA.

2) Dr. McCormich and Dr. Rao, doctors/ authors

In 1999, Dr. McCormich and Dr. Rao found that rats supplemented with DHEA and exposed to cancer seemed to be resistant to further developing other forms of cancer (e.g. prostate cancer).

The doctors stated in their study that "DHEA inhibits prostate cancer induction both when chronic administration is begun prior to carcinogen exposure, and when administration is delayed until pre-neoplastic prostate lesions are present."

> Three doctors (Dr. Schwartz, Dr. McCormich and Dr. Rao) concluded that DHEA protected cells in mice from turning cancerous.

The two authors were able to find that DHEA worked as an effective contributor to prostate cancer prevention. (McCormick, D. L. and Rao, K.V.N., et al. "Chemoprevention of hormone dependent prostate cancer in wistar unilever rats." *The Journal of European Urology*, 1999; 35: 464-467.)

DHEA and Sugar

I've seen and read about the phenomenal ability of DHEA to deal with diabetes and glucose metabolism. Evidence proves that DHEA may, in fact, be able to help or even reverse the abnormal metabolic problems of diabetes. Because DHEA is able to increase insulin sensitivity of receptors, it can improve the transport of glucose across cell membranes, specifically for improvement of energy and stamina and lowering the fatigue factor that ultimately helps to delay and improve the abnormal sugar metabolism of diabetes.

Research has shown that one of the many extraordinary abilities of DHEA is that it restrains the negative effects of G6PDH, an enzyme known for its yielding factor. G6PDH turns glucose into fat cells; DHEA redirects the enzyme, turning it into energy instead of fat

G6PDH + SUGAR= FAT
+SUGAR
  \
  + DHEA
   \
  = ENERGY (instead of fat)

DHEA and Sugar
Studies

In July 2003, *The Journal of Clinical Endocrinology and Metabolism* reported the findings of two Japanese research projects. DHEA was given to 24 men with elevated cholesterol levels for 12 weeks. Each of the 24 men was given 25 mg of DHEA; a separate group received a placebo.

The study showed that DHEA improved two physiologic functions that declined with age:

1) Endothelial function
2) Insulin sensitivity

These changes may follow the development of insulin resistance, and the researchers reported that the levels of age-related decline in DHEA are associated with a decrease of insulin sensitivity, which also occurs with age.Shortly thereafter, the participants were assessed for endothelial function.

Blood samples were drawn to assess insulin sensitivity. The subjects who received the DHEA supplementation showed vasodilatation of the brachial arteries that increased significantly over the course of the course of 12 weeks, whereas the placebo group remained at base line levels.

The Japanese researchers noted the subjects taking DHEA supplementation had a fasting plasma glucose level that was much lower, demonstrating increased insulin sensitivity. Blood vessel dysfunction (endothelium) causes vessels to dilate; therefore, DHEA deficiency inhibits the potential to cause cardiovascular disease.

> **Conclusion:** *DHEA can significantly minimize progression of cardiovascular disease on an older aging population. This is why I use DHEA as a heart disease preventative. If I were you, I'd consider it, too.*

DHEA in blood: "Where the river runs wild"

DHEA is commonly available throughout pharmacies, grocery stores and local health food stores. It's not expensive to purchase DHEA tablets; however, it's my belief that oral consumption of DHEA may lead to complications.

My thoughts based on research:

1) DHEA taken orally travels through the stomach, into mesenteric arteries, and finally to the liver where it's metabolized.Between 90 and 95 percent of DHEA will be filtered and discarded by the liver, leaving you with no more that 5 to 10 percent of usable DHEA. What's worse, DHEA causes the liver a great deal of stress because it isn't digested easily.

2) It may be that the well-established principle of sex hormone binding globulins becomes a greater threat and complication during oral consumption of DHEA. When taken orally in large doses, DHEA causes an alarm to go off in the liver, whereupon the sex hormone binding globulin* (SHBG) may go into hyper production, tripling the level in order for the liver to neutralize excess DHEA.

Naturally, the liver doesn't know any better. All it knows is that it is being bombarded and overwhelmed by DHEA so it will do what it does best, which is neutralizing excessive hormonal amounts. The problem with SHBG outpour is that SHBG doesn't really know or care what hormone is being binded, so it may end up binding not just DHEA but also testosterone and other essential hormones. As a result, you will have lower levels of available free hormones across the board.

When utilizing DHEA, the best approach to take is First Pass Technology, transdermal liposomes. Through this mechanism, DHEA is protected by micro encapsulation of liposome and instantaneously absorbed and delivered through the sub-dermal vasculature.Instead of waiting several hours to be metabolized by the liver, with liposomes, DHEA is transported directly into the bloodstream where it can be disposed of within minutes.

DHEA testing

Salivary testing is a very convenient and inexpensive way of checking DHEA levels. As a precautionary step, saliva tests should be taken before you begin to take bioidentical DHEA to ascertain the exact level of bioidentical supplementation needed.

Salivary testing measures only free DHEA (in preference to the serum test which may be measuring the total DHEA of the free and bound DHEA, as serum testing is basically useless, especially when testing for DHEA). Only saliva testing reveals accurate assessments of DHEA levels for transdermal bioidentical DHEA supplementation.

Male DHEA pg/ml Test Result Reference				Female DHEA pg/ml Test Result Reference			
AGE	ASSESSED BIOMARKERS	ASSESSED OPTIMUM RANGE WITH SUPPLEMENT	ASSESSED OPTIMUM RANGE WITH TRANSDERMAL	AGE	ASSESSED BIOMARKERS	ASSESSED OPTIMUM RANGE WITH SUPPLEMENT	ASSESSED OPTIMUM RANGE WITH TRANSDERMAL
20-29	300-330	300-350	350-3500	20-29	270-300	250-300	300-3000
30-39	270-300	300-250	350-3500	30-39	240-270	250-300	300-3000
40-49	240-270	300-250	350-3500	40-49	210-240	250-300	300-3000
50-59	210-240	300-250	350-3500	50-59	180-210	250-300	300-3000
60-69	180-210	300-250	350-3500	60-69	150-180	250-300	300-3000
70-79	150-180	300-250	350-3500	70-79	120-150	250-300	300-3000
Over 80	100-150	300-250	350-3500	Over 80	80-120	250-300	300-3000

DHEA Saliva references

Note: The above are DHEA saliva testing reference tables for men and women. The far left column represents the age a person is according to their level of DHEA hormone found in saliva. Persons using transdermal DHEA (i.e., liposome or patch) will have a higher Assessed Optimum Range with Transdermal (found on far right column) than if supplemented taken through injection or orally (see Assessed Optimum range with Supplement).

Persons on any kind of hormonal therapy must cease hormone supplementation prior to testing. If supplementation is continued, results will appear several hundred percent higher than assessed optimum range. High results for people using transdermal liposome are completely normal. If this applicable to the reader, one can calculate biomarker age by dividing result number by eight. Again, calculation is applicable only for persons using transdermal liposome hormone therapy.

DHEA Self-Assessment	
Symptoms of DHEA Deficiency Note: *If supplementation has already been taken *increase* dosage if following symptoms are experienced:	**Symptoms of DHEA Excess** Note: *If supplementation has already been taken *decrease* dosage if following symptoms are experienced:
• Depression • Poor Stress Management • Lack of Stamina • Moodiness • Dry Eyes • Osteoporosis • Memory Loss • Bone, Joint, Muscle Pain	• Facial Hair • Oily Skin • Acne Pimples • Bossiness • Impatience/Anger • Irritability/Mood Changes • Deepening Voice

Taking DHEA

DHEA should be used in a transdermal liposome.

Here's one more reason why:

Dr. C. Labrie (et al.) performed an experiment administering DHEA transdermally. Dr. Labrie concluded that the transdermal route of delivery was ten times more effective than the oral route. Dr. Labrie and her researchers concluded that her data shows high bioavailability of percutaneous DHEA as measured by its androgenic biological activities. (Labrie, C. and Belanger, A., et al. "High bioavailability of DHEA administered percutaneously in the rat." *Journal of Endocrinology, 1996; 150: S107-118.*)

Besides Dr. Labrie's research, a variety of other studies show that transdermal administration of DHEA on postmenopausal women for six months resulted in significantly increased density and mineralization of the hip bone. This has a positive effect on osteoblastic activity of bone and has clinical uses such as increasing supplementation of DHEA for osteoporosis. Some authors have reported that an increase in DHEA levels will lower the rate of accidents caused by osteoporosis.

Testimonial

"Twenty years ago, if you had asked me how I'd feel today, I probably would have responded with a sarcastic 'I probably won't be around to tell you.' At 40, I was headed downhill. I was the butt of every old-person joke one could think of. In the engineering plant where I worked, my colleagues started every gag with, 'You know you're old when you start to look like Gary.'

"Ten years ago, my wife started to become progressively more concerned with her appearance. She tried everything. She bought books, spent all of 'my' money on visits to the dermatologist, bought facial creams, cleansers and moisturizers sold by every Tom, Dick and Harry who promised to erase the marks off her face. Well, nothing worked like the hormones she started taking. Let me tell you, her doctor ran a few tests on her and determined what kind of hormones she needed. The fourth or fifth time she visited her doctor, I decided to tag along, and somehow, the lady convinced me to 'replenish my hormones.' I'm 63 and for the past thirteen years I, along with my wife, have been firm believers that hormones can offer you a heaping of help.

"My wife uses bioidentical estrogen and progesterone. Recently, she decided to take testosterone and pregnenlone.I've been taking an estrogen defense, testosterone and DHEA. It is to my understanding that DHEA replacement covers a lot of hormones since it aromatizes. I started with DHEA and just kept on adding. Now I'm taking an estrogen defense to guard against testosterone aromatizing in estrogen.

My brothers (all younger than me) complain about their bones and joints hurting. I'm the only one who has nothing to say at the poker table. When the guys are complaining, I'm explaining that because of DHEA, life just gets better."

—Gary, 62

Directions

DHEA is produced by the adrenal gland and is at its highest level early in the morning. Adrenals produce DHEA in two-hour spurts, meaning that levels fluctuate throughout the day. I believe that most physiological approach for supplementation of DHEA is to apply transdermal DHEA early in the morning upon rising.

Daily supplementation of DHEA is a vital and powerful program for anti-aging hormonal balance. It stimulates the androgenic repair function of DHEA hormone. You can start with 25 to 50 mg of transdermal DHEA daily, skipping Saturday and Sunday if you wish. Women typically use less DHEA—you must customize the dosage for your own body.

Your goal should be to maintain a physiologic DHEA level equivalent to that of a person who is 30 years old. Customize the dosage to how much you require, but most importantly, how much you can tolerate. (See Deficiencies and Excess symptoms.)

Again, I'd like to remind you that an excess of DHEA (or any other hormone) can be potentially dangerous. Every few months, your family physician or health care worker will help you monitor DHEA levels via testing making sure that you're taking appropriate levels of bioidentical supplementation.

✍DR. TAI'S ANTI-AGING HEALTH SECRET✍

DHEA supplementation is one of the most important anti-aging hormones. DHEA serves as a protector for your immune system and keeps energy levels high. Because DHEA plays a significant role in the way we feel, bioidentical supplementation of the hormone does a nice job in making us happy. DHEA protects mostly all nerves, thus it shields the cardiovascular system and brain.

Bioidentical supplementation will give you more energy, improve your well-being and give you a greater ability to cope with chronic stress that could potentially accelerate aging. DHEA has been researched and clearly shown to work well with cortisol (stress hormone preventing adrenal fatigue). Because of DHEA's protective and reparative hormone ability, it balances the powerful effects of cortisol on our organs, muscles and bones. DHEA is certainly one of the most powerful protective anti-aging hormones we have at our disposal. Make sure your DHEA levels are equivalent to a biologically aged 35-year-old's. If they are, a lack of energy, libido loss and stress will all be feelings of the past.

"My favorite DHEA studies"

* For additional studies see references

1) *American Journal of Physiology, November, 1997; 273(5 pt 2): R1704-8.*
   * DHEA has a protective effect against accumulation of visceral fat and development of muscle. DHEA also shows insulin resistance in rats fed a high-fat diet.

2) *Annals of New York Academy of Sciences, December, 1995; 774:271-80.*
   * High levels of DHEA may retard the development of coronary atherosclerosis and coronary vasculopathy.

3) *Journal of Clinical Endocrinology and Metabolism, June 1994; 78(6): 1360.*
   * In DHEA studies, serum levels were restored to those found in young adults (25+) within two weeks of DHEA replacement.
   * DHEA-increased serum levels of androgens (androstenedione, testosterone and dehydrotestosterone) were observed in women.
   * There was a small rise of androstenedione in men.
   * DHEA raised serum levels of IGF-1 (HGH more on this in Chapter 8)
   * Perceived physical and psychological well-being rose by 67 percent in men and 84 percent in women.

4) *Journal of Clinical Investigations, August, 1998; 82(2): 712-20.*
   * DHEA is a steroid that blocks carcinogenensis, retards aging, and exerts antiproliferative aging properties.
   * Low levels of DHEA are linked to an increase of developing cancer or cardiovascular disease.
   * High levels of DHEA inhibit the development of atherosclerosis.

Chapter 7

Pregnenolone: *A steroid that serves as an intermediate in the biosynthesis of numerous hormones.*

—Stedman's Medical Dictionary

In the hormonal revolution, pregnenolone is a dinosaur. It's one the oldest hormones and has had the longest lifespan within a person's body. Directly derived from cholesterol, pregnenolone helps the conversion of over 150 steroid hormones. For this reason, I've developed an increasing concern for people that have a desire to lower their cholesterol levels, because without adequate cholesterol, there would be virtually no hormone production.

People with low cholesterol generally have a pregnenolone deficiency, and they experience symptoms that affect the preservation of memories. Alzheimer's, dementia and senility are illnesses of the brain which result from an absence of pregnenolone within a person's body.

Making the acquaintance of people who have lost much of their memory is something I can't tolerate well. It's very unfortunate for those taking care of elders. I feel for those people and it concerns me for people to further develop illnesses of the brain. Alzheimer's is a favorite plot for many scriptwriters because it's compelling and emotionally draining to watch people forget the names of those who devote their lives to caring for them. When I see shows with this plot, I have a tendency to switch channels. I can't stomach them, and this is why I've devoted much of my time to advocating (if you will) methods to further retain memory and mental energy. Without a functioning mind, we are, in a sense, useless.

What to expect
Pregnenolone
What is pregnenolone?
Functions of Prenenolone
How is pregnenolone produced?
Stress and the brain
Prenenolone research
Self-assessment
Taking pregnenolone

I've always asked myself, what good am I if I can no longer make contributions to the world? What good am I if I can no longer teach or learn or give? Who am I if I can't remember my family, my past, and my experiences?

With every day, we age; nobody gets any younger. And despite the fact that at times I wish I could freeze time for myself, I wouldn't wish to immobilize the hands of time for anyone else. I want my grandchild to grow; I want to see her become a high school graduate, a college graduate, a mother, a beautiful woman. I want to see my students become successful doctors; I want to hear about the lives they've saved. I want to live long enough to see everyone's successes and experience these narratives as they're told. I want to experience all of these things so badly that I've realized that getting old just isn't so bad, just as long as I can remember everything, and I want to do this for as long as I can.

> **The optimum level of Pregnenolone is at 35 years of age. By the age of 75, you will have lost 65% of your Pregnenolone.** Roberts, E., Pregnenolone from Selye to Alzheimer's. *Bio Chem Phama 1995. Vol..49, No.1.Pg. 1-16.*

Before I begin...

I find it amusing that researchers (who are some of the world's most technical, as well as logical people) pick up where others have left off. One would assume that in science, everyone starts at the base. Science is supposed to be a grassroots system, where practitioners in the field of medicine find the source of a problem and work their way through. Astonishingly, this isn't the case. Many researchers, medical practitioners and doctors take the simplest route out—they treat the problem and attempt to make a quick escape from the patient's life, just until their funds are secure. When their bank accounts appear to be lower than usual, this is when the follow-up call is made. I refuse to be one of those doctors. To act in such a way would be an insult to my upbringing, concentrated work ethic and, most importantly, my concern for people's well-being. If hormones had a family hierarchy, cholesterol would be Grandmother (Source) and pregnenolone would be Mother, the one that all the other hormone family members come from.

How pregnenolone is made

When cholesterol is synthesized from the liver and changed in the adrenal cortex (the two glands that sit above the kidneys), it creates pregnenolone. As with all of your other hormones, pregnenolone production slows with age. When pregnenolone drops, the outlook is grim, because pregnenolone provides the materials for other hormones to grow and multiply in number.

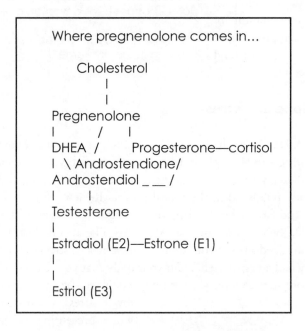

Where pregnenolone comes in...

Cholesterol
    |
    |
Pregnenolone
| / |
DHEA /   Progesterone—cortisol
| \ Androstendione/
Androstendiol _ _ /
| |
Testesterone
|
Estradiol (E2)—Estrone (E1)
|
|
Estriol (E3)

Functions of Pregnenolone

1. Improves excitation and inhibition of the nervous system
2. Increases resistance to stress
3. Improves physical and mental energy
4. Increases nerve transmission and memory
5. Reduces pain and inflammation

Pregnenolone making sense

Pregnenolone, like cortisol (also produced in the adrenal glands), works diligently to improve our body's ability to deal with stress, which one of the most damaging and devastating problems, with the potential to cause a compilation of diseases and symptoms that can shorten our lives and destroy our health.

> ### Dr. Tai's "Think Outside the Box"
>
> The word "pregnenolone" has the prefix of "preg-" like pregnant. It births other hormones as a woman does a child.
>
> Hmmm...could that be the reason behind its wacky name?!

Pregnenolone and stress

In 1943, Dr. Hans Selye became increasingly curious about how pregnenolone produces calming effects. A pioneer in research, the lab veteran conducted studies on mice and then on humans testing the sedative effects of pregnenolone. Dr. Selye wrote in a study published in the Pineal Journal Review, "Pregnenolone hormone reduces stress and fatigue by repairing the damages of stress and fatigue."

What Dr. Selye meant by that was stress, like a torn shirt, tears easily once someone has initiated a rip. If you've already experienced stress to the greatest extent, it's most likely had a negative effect on your body that you've been unable to mend. By adding more stress, you're worsening the damage. By using a supplement that lowers stress, you're repairing damage while preventing potentially volatile future reactions.

> ***Stress includes:**
>
> traumatic health problems
> chemical oxidation
> emotional stress
> environmental (noise pollution, temperature intolerance, etc.)

Dr. Selye explained that pregnenolone was able to control the damaging effects of stress through neutralizing excess cortisol. He said that the overproduction of cortisol is the result of relentless stress and abnormalities in metabolizing sugar. Thus, replenishing depleted pregnenolone can help you avoid severe depression and all of the other symptoms associated with too much cortisol like water retention, insomnia, over-eating, weakened immunities and destabilized liver functions. (Selye, H., et al. "Potentiation of a pituitary extract with pregnenolone and additional observations concerning the influence of various organs on steroids, metabolism." *Pineal Journal Review, 1943; 10(2):319-28.)*

Pregnenolone and memory

Besides helping people cope with stress, pregnenolone affects the brain more than anything. Decades ago, in the 1940s, researchers obsessed over pregnenolone (they had every right to). Their curiosity regarding the parent hormone led them to discover something miraculous in a laboratory filled with white little mice.

One group of mice was left alone, while the others were injected with pregnenolone. The group injected with pregnenolone made their way through a maze faster than the group that wasn't injected. Do you want to know why the injected mice got to the finish line before the mice that were left alone? Sure you do. After conducting a few of the same studies, the researchers concluded that pregnenolone helped the mice remember their way around the maze! This led the researchers believe that pregnenolone has a lot to do with the brain's most sophisticated roles—memory.

Recently, because of data that's been collected over decades of research, pregnenolone has been proven to contribute to increased intelligence, learning, memory and alertness. Since our vision is directly associated with our brains, if this leads you to ask whether the amount pregnenolone has anything to do with our ability to see and perceive, I must say that you are undoubtedly correct!

Remember this

In Dr. William Regelson's *The Super-Hormone Promise: Nature's Antidote to Aging* (Pocket Books, 1996), Regelson included a study by a St. Louis University School of Medicine researcher, Dr. Rahmawhati Sih, who conducted several studies on men and women to test the effects of pregnenolone.

Dr. Sih administered a pregnenolone capsule to small groups of men and women. Hours later, the groups that took the capsule were asked to take two examinations testing their ability to recall and reiterate. The men performed better in multiple-dimensional thinking, while the women demonstrated enhanced verbal recall.

Unquestionably, pregnenolone's main contribution to the body is improving the neurological function of our brain, our memory and our thought concentration, which in turn, can affect our mood. Ask yourself just how frustrated you get when you can't remember someone's name.

"The old forget. The young don't know."
—German proverb

A diet of too much saturated fat and trans-fatty acids interferes and blocks the natural pathway of Pregnenolone. *Yanick, P., Prohormone Nutrition, Montclair, NJ: Longevity Institute International, 1998.*

Record recall

In 1992, researcher J.F. Flood (et al.) tested the memory-enhancing effects in male mice using pregnenolone and steroids metabolically derived from it. He found pregnenolone helps the neurotransmission of the nerves. When reviewed, his study read that neurons communicate with each other through electrochemicals. Therefore, by having higher levels of pregnenolone, you're able to think clearer by recalling information with less delay (Flood, J. F., et al. "Memory-enhancing effects in male mice of pregnenolone and steroids metabolically derived from it." *Proceedings from the National Academy of Science of the United State of America, 1992; 89:1567-71.*)

Changing moods

Before Flood came McGavack, a researcher in the early '50s who, through extensive research, found that pregnenolone was lower in individuals who were diagnosed with mental and emotional disorders.

McGavack helped patients undergoing internal kismet by placing them on a bioidentical pregnenolone supplementation plan. Weeks after supplementation, McGavack found that his patients weren't as depressed. (McGavack, T., et al. "The use of pregnenolone in various clinical disorders." *Journal of Clinical Endocrinology and Metabolism, 1951; 11: 559-77.*) Awww, doesn't that make you want to smile?

Mr. Popularity

I make sure to tap into the medical world as much as possible. I'm a member of more than a dozen medical societies, and I've subscribed to at least 70 different science and medical publications, newsletters, journals, etc. While people ask

Dr. Tai's "In addition..."

Studying pregnenolone while driving the message home

In addition to controlling stress, pregnenolone has been revealed to have positive effects directly correlated to arthritis. Pregnenolone has been found to help with swelling, inflammation, joint and muscle pain—most, if not all, of the symptoms related to arthritis. (Freeman, H., et al. "Therapeutic efficacy of pregnenolone in rheumatoid arthritis." *The Journal of the American Medical Association, 1950; 143: 338-44.)*

In addition to helping patients control arthritis, researcher R. Davison (et al.) found that pregnenolone supplementation has had helpful effects on immune diseases lupus and psoriasis. (Davison, R., et al. "Effects of pregnenolone on rheumatoid arthritis." *Archives of Internal Medicine, 1950; 85: 365-88.)*

Jeeves, *I* ask PubMed for the most recent clinical studies. Through observation and consistent monitoring, I've found that pregnenolone has become a progressively popular hormone in laboratories. As time progresses, we're learning more and more about the body's major hormones. However, two things are certain: Pregnenolone will help you think and control stress.

Pregnenolone Self-Assessment	
Symptoms of Pregnenolone Deficiency Note: *If supplementation has already been taken *increase* dosage if following symptoms are experienced:	**Symptoms of: Pregnenolone excess** Note: *If supplementation has already been taken *decrease* dosage if following symptoms are experienced:
<ul><li>Loss of short term memory</li><li>Forgetfulness</li><li>Fuzzy thinking</li><li>Depression</li><li>Reduction in perceived brightness of color</li><li>Pessimism</li></ul>	<ul><li>Edginess</li><li>Feeling uptight</li><li>Frequent worry</li></ul>

How to use it, when you use it

I've observed that using DHEA and pregnenolone together is a lot more effective than just using pregnenolone alone. Together, I've found that DHEA and pregnenolone are profoundly well received by the adrenal cortex as well as the rest of the body. Pregnenolone and DHEA should be used in the form of a liposome cream. This way, the application is absorbed transdermally, so it avoids your liver causing no rebound effects and a reduced likelihood of over-consuming, so you don't experience the side effects I've previously mentioned (tension, edginess, and anxiousness).

Positive Effects of Pregnenolone: Arthritis, Depression, Memory Loss, Fatigue & Moodiness. *Smith, W. Pamela, HRT The Answers. Healthy Living Book, Inc. Traverse City, MI*

༝Dr. Tai's Anti-Aging Health Secret༝

As you've read in my previous chapters, and as you'll continue to read, I am my own guinea pig. I've tried everything before I've suggested that you try it. Yes, I am a man, and I realize that you (the reader) may be a woman, but I want you to remember that every body is made up of both male and female hormones. Pregnenolone is the base of all of these hormones—therefore, I think it to be extremely crucial (regardless of your sex) that everyone replenishes lost pregnenolone levels. Because of age, some people may require more than others, but nevertheless, pregnenolone is the first hormone that you should be concerned with, and it's the first hormone that you should seek to replenish. For a sharp memory, decreased mental fatigue, better stress adaptation, and enhanced concentration, I suggest you try adding pregnenolone to your bioidentical hormone replacement program to sharpen your memory and improve your vitality.

SECRET IV

**"It takes a long time to grow young."
—Pablo Picasso**

Chapter 8

Human Growth Hormone (HGH): *A protein hormone of the anterior lobe of the pituitary, produced by acidrophil cells, that promotes body growth, fat mobilization and inhibition of glucose utilization*

—Stedman's Medical Dictionary

"I've used human growth hormone for a year and six months. Since I've used HGH, I've lost weight and am convinced it's helped my skin. It's done something to me and my nieces tell me every day. I've had the energy to do what I want; I don't make any more excuses and have seen that I've been more outgoing."

"Although I love kids, I was unhappy working at the same high school as a secretary. Eight years ago, after my partner died, my love for dogs grew exceedingly. My two retrievers have given me all the company and love I need. A little after notifying the school of my leave, I decided to take up dog training courses."

"I'm two months away from being a certified dog trainer. Obtaining my certification from a dog training school, I will be certified to train dogs to search for narcotics, protect their families, and lead the blind."

"I'm very excited, and have, in a way, started over again. I feel like a new woman and that's a good feeling. If it wasn't for the HGH and various other bioidentical

What to expect
Testimony
What is HGH?
What is IGF-1?
Functions of HGH
Who should use HGH?
HGH deficiency
Testing HGH
Self-assessment
Side effects of excessive HGH use
Results
Anti-aging Health Secret
"My favorite HGH studies"

hormones, at 64, I don't think I would have developed the courage or confidence to do what I did. Instead of retiring, I went to school and started a career I know I'll excel in."

—Chante, 64

HGH

When Ponce de Leon set off to sail the seven seas in search of the awe-inspiring Fountain of Youth, he inevitably failed, instead discovering one of our 50 states (not so bad for failure). Hundreds of years have passed since his quest, and for just as long, we, as people, have mimicked the Spanish explorer by conducting our own personal quests of striving to find ways to Feel Stronger, Look Younger and Live Longer.

The Fountain of Youth does exist. It may not be a body of water in a wild rainforest or a magical potion, but it does indeed exist, or rather, it did and always has. This legendary youth-restoring antidote is nothing more than a hormone replacement system with its most powerful hormone being HGH, the human growth hormone.

Ladies and gentlemen, HGH has left the building

After childhood, HGH levels peak and throughout the rest of your life, your body will maintain a low level of HGH. Without this hormone, age begins to look like it sponges every ounce of resilience from us. Like blood in a glass of water, it curls and works its way throughout the interior of the glass turning the water pink. Age does something similar, and it affects every part and portion of our bodies. Contrary to cliché, age discriminates as it seems to concentrate on our face. Nevertheless, it also takes a toll on our body by shrinking muscles, bones and blood vessels, causing us to make conscious effort to do the simplest of things like standing up straight. Anti-aging involves more than just your exterior—it requires reshaping your interior.

What people are willing to pay?

Known as the battery hormone, growth hormones can cost more than the batteries of your car. Twenty thousand dollars per year will buy you growth factors that will improve skin elasticity, energy, fatigue and increase mental clarity, thus promoting creativity. Children advancing to adolescence have the highest levels of human growth factors. Adults who take human growth factors have revealed that they feel younger, more sociable and have a greater desire to be active. Literally, HGH impacts every cell in our body as a "master hormone"; it's what makes us grow. This is probably why people go "gaga" for HGH.

VROOM! HGH driving force in growth

> **Albeit, as a small compound HGH has extraordinarily powerful effects on the body.**

Human growth hormone is made in the pituitary gland, deep inside the brain just behind the eyes. It's a microscopic protein substance that is secreted in short pulses during the first hours of sleep and after exercise. Made throughout a person's lifetime, HGH is plentiful during youth. It stimulates growth in children and plays an important role in adult metabolism.

It's a simple protein made of 191 chain amino acids that are in a polypeptide formation. HGH is responsible for controlling most of the major functions in our bodies. It's especially important to know that as a peptide, its delicate nature is overly sensitive and can be destroyed by gastric acid found in saliva and stomach acids.

Manufactured in the anterior frontal lobe of the pituitary gland (a small pea-sized gland located at the base of the brain), HGH is secreted in large waves and spurts around the time you fall asleep. HGH's most intense activity occurs between 10 p.m. and 4 a.m. Its production is closely related and affected by the Human Growth Release Hormone (HGRH).

The "working" growth protein: IGF-1

HGH is released into the bloodstream and taken to tissues, where specific receptor sites in organs throughout the body are identified and then locked in. There's a specific key-and-lock relationship where growth hormones are attracted to certain receptor sites. Most of human growth hormones are delivered into the liver where the liver cells (through its metabolic process) convert them into insulin growth factor-1 (IGF-1) and insulin growth factor-2 (IGF-2), epidermal growth factor (EGF), vascular growth factor (VGF), nerve growth factor (NGF), and transfer growth factor (TGF).

> **Recap:**
>
> HGH is produced in the anterior frontal lobe of the pituitary gland, located at the base of the brain. HGH is a simple protein made of 191 amino acids. HGH's most productive activity occurs during the night, while you sleep.

After age 30, both the amplitude and the amount of HGH decreases with age. So do the frequency of spurts. IGF-1 blood levels in adults range from 200 to 500 ng/ml (nanograms per milliliter).

Yet, one-third of individuals over 50 years of age show abnormal levels (less than 200 ng/ml). During a person's growth spurt, HGH levels are at their maximum and somatomedin-C (another name for HGH) will be measured well over 600- 800 ng/ml. Yet for men and women under 40, less than 5 percent have levels below 250 ng/ml!

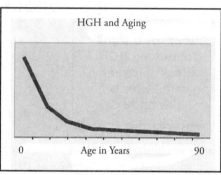

HGH and Aging

0   Age in Years   90

When IGF-1 levels fall below the adult normal range, muscle and bone strength and energy levels most likely will decrease. Tissue repair, cell re-growth, healing capacity, upkeep of vital organs, brain and memory function, enzyme production, and revitalization of hair, nails and skin will also diminish. When we age, decreasing growth hormone levels go hand-in-hand with the loss of pituitary production of HGH due to surgery, infection or accident. We instantly suffer many profoundly ill effects.

Lifespan

HGH is extremely difficult as well as inaccurate to be measured in the laboratory due to its very short lifespan. IGF-1, however is a different story,produced in the liver, actually has an 18 to 20-hour half-life and can therefore be measured by laboratory tests. The levels of IGF-1 are much more constant and reliable for practical clinical use. IGF-I also appears to be the key player in muscle growth. It stimulates both the differentiation and proliferation of myoblasts as well as amino acid uptake and protein synthesis in muscle and other tissues. Growth hormone has important effects on protein, lipid and carbohydrate metabolism. In some cases, a direct effect of growth hormone has been clearly demonstrated. In other cases, IGF-I is a critical mediator, and in still others it appears that both direct and indirect effects are at play. By age 50, half of the growth factors levels are depleted; by 80, almost all are gone.

Recap
- The liver converts HGH into an insulin factor also known as somatomedin-C into six additional growth factors: IGF-1, IGF-2, EGF, NGF, TGF and VGF.
- Children have approximately more or less of 600 ml, while adults have less than 200 ml of HGH.
- If IGF-1 falls, muscle and bone mass fall.

Dr. Tai's "Do-it-yourself" Testing levels of HGH

Step 1: Pinch your skin.
Step 2: Pull it up.
Step 3: Let it go and see how fast it returns to its original position.
Step 4: Try these same steps on a child or teenager. (Whoever you choose, try not to hurt the poor kid. We all get a little carried away with the pinching).
Step 5: Compare the time it took for your skin to return to its original position vs. the kids.

As you age, your skin will take longer to return to place.

Chondrocytes

IGF-I stimulates proliferation of chondrocytes (cartilage cells), resulting in bone growth. Growth hormone does seem to have a direct effect on bone growth in stimulating differentiation of chondrocytes into bone cells. A powerful tool in the treatment and prevention of osteoporosis!

Es para tu? Es para mi?

With less than a year of treatment, studies have shown that medically supervised HGH therapies can turn back the clock on the effects of aging by as much as 10 to 20 years. HGH is an important tool to adding years to your life along with rejuvenating your body physically and mentally.

Lacking HGH

Growth hormone production drops at least 15 percent every ten years. We see a reduction of the amplitude of the growth hormone with nightly pulses of growth hormone secretions.

As you lose HGH, you have an equivalent loss of IGF-1. Once you lose HGH and IGF-1, concentrating will be difficult and you'll most definitely lose the desire for more physical activities like having sex and exercising. You'll begin to see a different you, a lazier, fatter, more depressed version of yourself.

Because of decreased cardiac output, heart X-rays show that an HGH-deficient patient has reduced left ventricle mass and a decreased shortening of the heart muscle. The exercise capacity in a person lacking HGH (which probably includes all of us) is 25 percent less than those with the essential hormone in abundance, hence muscle mass and muscle strength loss is also predominant.

Losing your mind? No, you're just losing HGH

The biomarker IGF-1 decreases significantly in the cortex of the brain as we age, which in turn decreases learning ability and spatial memory and delays responses, causing impaired psychological well-being and potential neuropsychiatric manifestations. Memory impairment can also lead to depression, loss of vitality, fatigue, and social isolation.

Because people are losing essential hormones like HGH, some researchers believe that this causes lower self-esteem, which may lead to depression and

> **Study: HGH turning fat into muscle**
> In a study conducted with 24 HGH-deficient adults over a six-month period, there was marked improvement in lean body mass when a minimal amount of HGH was administered. Researchers concluded that HGH increased positive protein synthesis, thus improving muscle mass and muscle function as well as muscle strength. In these patients, there was a significant decline in fat mass around soft internal organs (visceral) as well as around the waist, compared to the arms, neck and legs. Without exercise, patients lost over 3 kilos (6 pounds) of fat within that period and gained 3 kilos of muscle!

social isolation. Pessimistic perceptions regarding the self can negatively impact relationships both in the home and office. One may quit a job or break up with partners, friends and spouses.

Duh! Dendrites

IGF-1 affects dendrite growth and repair. There is significant loss of dendrites in the aging brain; neurons die, and so do glial cells. Less active and whole nerve cells affect the neuro-electrical signals that make logical thinking and memorizing possible.

"Ahhh! I'm shrinking! I'm shrinking!"

Growth hormone deficiency results in lower bone mineral density, lower bone mineral content and therefore increased risk of osteopenia, osteoporosis and osteomalacia. The primary mechanism is that growth hormone IGF-1 stimulates osteoblastic activity, the activity of bone cells depositing calcium in the bone, making it stronger, denser and harder, fabulous in the prevention and treatment of osteoporosis. See Human Growth Matrix and Bone Specialist.

Testing HGH

Before you start to use HGH/IGF-1, I advise you see a physician to run an IGF-1 laboratory test in the morning, an hour before you eat breakfast. Consider measuring IGF's bound protein version—IGFBP-3, a protein that neutralizes into active IGF-1, and at the same time decreases the level of free IGF-1. Again, only the free hormones that are not bound to a binding globulin or albumin can be used. More than 95 percent of our hormones that run through our blood are bound and useless. Oral doses of any hormones pass through the GI tract and the liver, causing a very high elevation of hormone binding globulins, leaving very little net free hormones by depressing triggering hormones. Oftentimes, blinding globulins are indiscriminate about which hormones they bind.

Study: Got HGH?

In clinical studies, human growth hormone replacement shows a significant increase in bone GLA-protein, a very sensitive indicator of osteoblast function and improvement of the vertebral (spinal) bone density. The study concluded that corticobone increased up to 5 percent over a 12-month period of growth hormone therapy among patients.

HGH a pill?

I don't care how clever an advertisement is—don't fall for HGH in a pill, because it doesn't come in a pill! Most often, HGH is injected. The actual usage of human growth hormone can only be made available through injections that must be dispensed by your physician. After you've consulted your physician, he or she will give you a prescription for an HGH injectable divided into dosages per week. Amounts should be small as they're considered to be safer. You may inject HGH using hypodermic diabetic syringes along the sides of your stomach (sides nearest to your bellybutton).

While pinching your skin, you can give yourself an injection every night when you go to bed or early in the morning when you wake up. Some doctors will recommend two or three shots throughout the day. This is entirely up to you.

Your doctor can give you guidelines, but only you can evaluate the side effects. Most importantly, give your doctor feedback. With this information, both you and your doctor will be able to decide if you should increase or decrease the units injected. After letting ample time pass after injections, make sure you have your physician monitor your IGH-1 and IGF binding globulin 3 (IGFBP-3).

Syringe side effects

Due to the normal physiology of the human body which produces hourly spurts of human growth hormone and converts it into IGF-1, once-daily injections do not emulate nature and therefore tend to produce serious side effects such as carpal tunnel syndrome, arthritis, joint pain, water retention and hypertension.

Many doctors are trying to lower the dosages of human growth hormone per day to get the maximum amount of benefit with the fewest number of side effects. Reports of therapeutic benefits are mixed. Some people are absolutely elated with the results, while others, looking for weight loss, do not get as much result as they expect given the perceived trouble and cost.

Secretagogues

Some have tried taking the route of secretagogues. These are supplements taken from amino acids and other natural compounds to stimulate the secretion of HGH. In recent years, secretagogues seemed to have done a nice job in stirring controversy. I was curious about these wishy-washy reports of whether they worked, so I tried an HGH secretagogue. Regrettably, it gave me a blister outbreak on my upper and bottom lip. This was a minor form of herpes, and I hadn't had a blister outbreak in the last 20 years! The reason behind the outbreak is because most secretagogue formulations are made up of arginine, and blisters are typical side effects of the combinations as it may stimulate viral replications.

IGF-1 to the rescue!

Mmm hmmm. Though it isn't HGH in the purest form, it's pretty darn close. Human Growth Matrix (by Health Secrets USA) is a sublingual spray with all the growth factors you'll need. You can take this supplement in the morning and at night. You may spritz twice in the a.m. and twice in the p.m. People report they get a wonderful response by increasing the dosage in the first or second week.

Technology Breakthrough: New Deer Antler Extract

The formulation is made up of natural water-extracted deer antler--a natural source of IGF-1 that is known to keep people young. Not just anybody—people like emperors and members of the nobility have been using deer antler for ages. In the last 25 years, a great deal of effort has been put forth by a number of scholarly institutions to research and extract IGF-1 from deer antlers extract. Through special water extraction, IGF-1 has been extracted from deer antlers successfully.

Growth Factors

Laboratory technicians collect very small fractions of essential growth factors: epidermal growth factor (EGF), neural growth factor (NGF), transfer growth factor

(TGF) and vascular growth factor(VGF). These factors were difficult to isolate and extract because the molecules are very small and easily lost in the process; the molecular weight of most growth factors is between 300 to 2000 mw. Human Growth Matrix (see sources) is a microencapsulation of natural IGF-1 from a water extraction of deer antler in a liposome carrier that is sprayed sublingually. When we spray IGF-1under the tongue, our blood absorbs it in the upper GI tract where it doesn't get digested and broken by the digestive acids and juices. Human Growth Matrix is a new and improved delivery system of liposomes. Using nanotechnology, the delivery of HGH to the body has never been so affordable. You get the benefits of human growth factor without the expense or the inconvenience of HGH injections.

For specific conditions like severe arthritis, traumatic injury or inflammation, you may want to increase the human growth matrix dosage to three or four spray pumps, used once in the morning and again in the evening to help with inflammation and pain control.

Six Human Growth Factors
1. IGF-1 (Insulin Growth Factor I)
2. IGF-2 (Insulin Growth Factor II)
3. EGF (Epidermal Growth Factor)
4. VGF (Vascular Growth Factor)
5. NGF (Neural Growth Factor)
6. TGF (Transfer Growth Factor)

> **Dr.Tai's Injury**: Due to an accident (which was bound to happen if you've read my introduction), I tore my left shoulder, popping it out of the socket. After a year of taking Human Growth Matrix with Max Pain Specialist, an anti-inflammatory supplement, I was back to my regular self with total return of 99% of my shoulder function. (You may also add MaxArthro Specialist if you wish.)

Side effects of HGH injections
Growth hormone is a very powerful hormone which can have bad side effects if taken incorrectly. It is not, however, a dangerous hormone. If you take it correctly and monitor the results, only side effects like water retention, prostate pain or carpal tunnel syndrome should result.

Edema
Retention of water or edema isn't as serious a side effect as one would expect. Edema disappears if dosage is lowered or once the body adjusts to the increase in growth hormone.

Carpal tunnel syndrome

Carpal tunnel syndrome is a pain in the wrist caused by small bones in the wrist rubbing against each other. It occurs after a few months of taking too much growth hormone. I imagine this is because the small bones are crowded with increased edema or high amount of growth hormone. The symptom is preventable by monitoring the result of taking growth hormone, and is normally reversible by discontinuing or lowering the dose being taken.

Gigantism

The worst possible proven disease is acromegaly, or gigantism, which is an unnatural growth of bone mass and thickening of the skin which caused by a great excess in growth hormone. Acromegaly occurs naturally in persons that have pituitary tumors that cause them to release growth hormone without control.

Not only is it necessary to take blood tests to monitor results, it is also foolish to take a dose much above what is the normal physiological standard. At the start of a program, taking 1 i.u. per day of HGH is the most you should take unless your doctor advises more, and you should not increase this dose unless you take a saliva test that shows you can safely increase it.

Low dose growth hormone treatment with diet restriction accelerates body fat loss, exerts anabolic effect and improves growth hormone secretory dysfunction in obese adults. *Kim KR, et al. Horm Res 1999;511(2):78-84.*

Benefits

One of the greatest benefits of HGH is increased energy. Because most of us experience reduced energy as we get older, we often encounter physical activities that we can no longer participate in. With HGH/ IGF-1 supplementation, that's not necessarily true anymore.

Other benefits of HGH are: greater cardiac output, amplified muscle mass, enhanced memory, enhanced libido, better sleep, increased burning of fat, improved profile of cholesterol, stronger bones and muscles, sharper vision, an enhanced immune system, re-growth of hair, more agile and thicker skin, better disease resistance, increased positive mood, rapid wound healing, lowered blood pressure, improved social skills, and restoration of the essential organs of the body like kidney, heart and liver.

HGH Self-Assessment	
Symptoms of HGH Deficiency Note: *If supplementation has already been taken *increase* dosage if following symptoms are experienced:	**Symptoms of: HGH excess** Note: *If supplementation has already been taken *decrease* dosage if following symptoms are experienced:
• Waist and hip fat • Loss of muscle • Loss of strength • Increased fatigue • Bone and joint pain • No sexual interest • Anti-social behavior • Skin thinning/sagging/ wrinkling • Lack of libido	• Carpal tunnel syndrome • Sudden arthritis pain • Water retention • High blood pressure • Prostate pain/enlargement • Aggressive behavior

---

∽DR. TAI'S ANTI-AGING HEALTH SECRET∽

It's well known that as we age there is a decrease of HGH affecting all the hormonal functions of the body, organs, and metabolism. These have generally magnified effects on the body. As we age, we lose tissue hydration and water from our body, actually seeing visible signs of wrinkles and dry skin. If you compare a young person's body water content with that of an elderly person's, you will notice 10 to 14 percent more water content in the tissues. This is a huge difference with extraordinary consequences. HGH replacement can give you skin so plump and moist you won't be able to keep yourself from reminiscing about "the good old days."

If you overdose on HGH, though, you can develop hypertension, joint pain, water retention and swelling, and these are just some of the less serious side effects. HGH is not a hormone you want to mess around with. Use a minimum amount for optimum hydration. And if you suffer from cancer,or are in remission, HGH and IGF-1 are not for you!

We don't have clinical evidence of conflict between HGH/IGF-1 and cancer therapies and multiple studies show no cancerous effects from IGF-1. Nevertheless, as a precaution, I don't recommend HGH or IGF-1 if you have a history of cancer.

"My favorite HGH studies"
*For additional studies see references

1) *Geriatrics, November, 1999; 54(11): 62.*
   - HGH increases visceral fat tissue, which has a direct effect on age associated insulin resistance and cardiovascular disease. The increase of visceral fat in older persons is associated with decreased levels of estrogen, testosterone and growth hormone.

2) *New England Journal of Medicine, October 1999; 341:1206-1216.*
   - HGH restores normal body composition, improves muscle tone and normalizes serum lipid concentrations.
   - HGH improves quality of life, including energy level and mood.
   - After six months of treatment metabolism increased by 6 to 11 percent.

3) *The Journal of the American Medical Association, August, 2000; 284(7): 861-866.*
   - HGH decreases by 75 percent from adulthood to midlife. HGH loss is complete by age 40.

Chapter 9

Testosterone: *The most potent naturally occurring androgen, formed in greatest quantities by the interstitial cells of the testes, and possibly secreted also by the ovary and adrenal cortex.*

—Stedman's Medical Dictionary

Testosterone

What to expect

What is testosterone?

How is it produced?

Functions of Testosterone

Andropause and menopause

Testimonial

Testosterone in women

Misconceptions about testosterone

Testing for testosterone

Taking testosterone

Self-assessment

Anti-aging Health Secret

Contrary to popular belief, testosterone isn't just found in guys. In fact, everyone has testosterone, and we're healthier and stronger with more of it. In 1889, Charles Edouard Brown-Sequard, a French physiologist, injected an extract made from guinea pig and dog testicles into himself. Sequard wasn't aware of what he was injecting until he felt the combination's after-effects. Days later, he felt sharper and stronger. In his memoirs, he noted that he had increased mental energy by recalling things he thought he'd forgotten. Soon enough, Sequard realized that he felt the way he did because of the chemicals within the animals' gonads. Since then, testosterone has become a hormone that almost everyone has heard of, but unfortunately it's a hormone that's blamed all too often for black eyes, bruises and oversized muscles. So, does testosterone control a man's behavior? It's a debate that's been waged in scientific and social circles for decades. Testosterone is, after all, the hormone of desire.

Testosterone 101

Indeed, testosterone isn't the only male hormone (androgen); however, it is the one that is predominant within men's bodies. This is why men have a larger build, larger bone structures, broader shoulders, and facial hair (some have more than others). When estrogen levels begin to drop during the first stages of menopause, testosterone also suffers. As a result, when women have their ovaries removed for medical or personal reasons, testosterone is lowered along with estrogen.

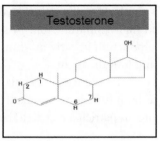

Testosterone is produced by the Leydig cells in the testes. Generally, testes produce about 3 to 10 mg of testosterone a day; however, during puberty, testosterone is at its peak. After the age of 25, these levels decline. Every ten years after age 25, you lose more than 10 percent of your testosterone levels, and by 80, you have less than 10 percent of what you once had. The precipitous change in the level of testosterone begins at the age of 40. Like a roller-coaster, you ride all way up to the top—testosterone production during adolescence. Then while still securely fastened into your seat, you feel the descent. After 40, you start to pick up momentum, riding with falling velocity, and by 80, you've made it back to where you started—you have the same amount you had when you were a child.

In women, testosterone is secreted by the ovaries and adrenals.

Our bodies essentially depend on the production of adequate levels of testosterone to create all the positive traits we need as men and women. Testosterone production is the end result of a long chain of events that starts way up in the center of our brains.

Step 1: The hypothalamus begins the process by producing gonadotropin releasing hormone (GnRH) and then, in small pulsating spikes, releasing it into the bloodstream. GnRH is deeply influenced by a number of neural transmitters produced by our bodies in the form of endorphins and epinephrine.

Step 2: Within the pituitary gland, luteonizing hormone (LH) and follicular stimulating hormone (FSH) are what give more of a given hormone to one sex than the other. Luteonization and follicular stimulation is especially important in the production of testosterone because it stimulates the proper glands to produce it.

Step 3: After the introduction of luteonizing hormones and follicular stimulation, testosterone is bifurcated, and functions differently in men and women. For pituitary hormones in men, it works more as a leuteonizing hormone than as a follicle stimulator. Leuteonization is what affects men's testes, where the specific specialized cells called leydigs (as previously mentioned) produce testosterone in high amplitude and in spurts throughout the day, with much higher levels of production in early morning and a slightly lower production later in the afternoon and into the night.

In women, leuteonizing and follicular stimulation works in different ways, as both functions stimulate different receptor sites in organs like the ovaries. Other organs participate as well, but to a much lesser extent.

Step 4: The newly processed and produced testosterone respectively produced from organs and glands travels far and wide throughout the entire body.

"X" Marks the Spot

The egg and sperm each donate a single sex chromosome to the embryo: an X chromosome from women and a Y chromosome from men.

- If the combination of these sex chromosomes is XX, then the embryo will be female.
- If it's XY, the embryo will be male.

It's not until the sixth week of development that XX or XY embryos are defined; before this, the human fetus is sexless. One interpretation of this is that all embryos begin as female. The introduction of testosterone makes the difference, influencing the growth of male genitalia, while the female component of the "indifferent" genitalia degenerates and atrophies.

In the bloodstream, testosterone comes in three specific varieties:

- Approximately 40 percent is bound to albumin, a very large molecule.
- 55 percent is bound to a protein called sex hormone binding globulin (SHGB).
- Finally, 3-5 percent is called "free testosterone," a rather small molecule of pure active and useable testosterone hormone that is ready to go to work and create the marvelous effects it has on the youthful physiological qualities of both men and women.

Functions of Testosterone

1. Increases sexual desire and libido

2. Stimulates feelings of emotional well being, self confidence, and motivation. *Persky, H., Arch Sex Behav 1978; 7(3):157-173*

3. Increases muscle mass and strength

4. Improves memory. *Vliet, E. Women Weight and Hormones, NY; M. Evans & Company 2001.*

5. Growth of pubic and underarm hair

6. Improves muscle tone and skin sagging. *Brincat, M., Br. Med. J. 1983; 287(6402):1337-1338*

7. Decreases body fat

8. Prevents osteoporosis. *Davis, S., Curr Opin Obstet Gynecol 1997; 9(3); 177-180*

9. Anti-Depressant; Elevates brain's norepinephrine. *Vliet, E. Women Weight and Hormones, NY; M. Evans & Company 2001.*

Testimonial

"I got the impression that it was OK to be overweight if no one was going to see you in the nude. It's six years since I've seen the beach and my wife and I haven't been intimate in months.

"Before we decided to stay together, my wife Ava and I slept in separate bedrooms. I used to think we stayed together for the same reasons most people stay together—the kids and out of convenience. We know each other; we really don't understand each other, but we respect each other. I'm loyal, because I have no desire to be intimate with anyone. I think if I was physically capable to show someone I love them, I'd try to make love to my wife.

"My friends have all experimented with erection formulas and I was too embarrassed to give them a try, especially since I've heard claims about heart failure in men. I went through a strict diet excluding sugars from snacks and meals, and I finally saw my doctor. My doctor informed me that my testosterone level was down. All it took was a glance at my chest size and my large, wide waist and hips. I asked him if there was a way he could help me. He said that he could offer me synthetic testosterone or natural testosterone. Curious to know which was best, I asked for a list of pros and cons, and I from what I perceived, it seemed like he was leaning towards natural testosterone.

"I got the hints he dropped and I decided to use the natural testosterone. I've lost inches all over my body and I'm continuing to lose. I'm 6-foot-2-inches tall and used to weigh 237—today I weigh 198. I've slowly lost my breasts and I feel more energetic.

"I see the way my wife looks at me, and gosh, she's so beautiful when she smiles. Really, I feel like I'm in my 20s all over again. I can't wait to see how I evolve months from now and I can't wait to find out what the new me does to our relationship."

—*Ryan, 47*

Andropause: Fact or Fiction?

Dr. Robert S. Tan, author of *The Andropause Mystery: Unraveling the Truths about Male Menopause* (Amred Consulting, 2001) describes andropause as being "a cruel reality."

According to Dr. Tan, in the U.S., five million men suffer from andropause and 60 percent of them are over the age of 65. (Personally I think those statistical numbers are way too conservative.) As men age, they lose hormones just as women do. When this happens to women it's referred to as menopause, and the male equivalent to this is andropause. For women, menopause marks the end of the menstruation cycle. Although men have no visible marker for andropause, they just know because they feel differently, and because they feel differently, they act differently. Physical, mental and emotional changes are associated with andropause and each change tends to emerge gradually. During menopause, women complain about hot flashes, depression, night sweats, mood swings and a loss in sexual desire. Men go through similar pains once they've reached the andropause stage.

Frightful Forty:

Most men will have lost 15 pounds of muscle by 40.

Between 40 and 60, the average man will lose more than 15 percent of bone.

50 percent of the American male population will experience erectile dysfunction in their life.

This could also be one of the reasons why America's divorce rate among aging couples is higher than ever before. Sex oftentimes can rule a relationship or cause its demise. Because andropause causes excessive weight gain and loss of libido, men generally lose self-esteem. In other words, andropause can have emotional, mental, physical and psychological effects.

Testosterone: Girl's Club V.I.P.

Testosterone is well known for its role in male puberty: It promotes the growth of the reproductive tract, increases the length and diameter of the penis, stimulates development of the prostate and scrotum, and causes the sprouting of pubic and facial hair. However, I feel that all too often we tend to give even things like hormones general connections. I want to try to eliminate this common misconception as much as possible. When you think estrogen, try not to think of it as a "she." Do the same for testosterone; when you think of the hormone, try not to think of it as a "he." It turns out men and women produce exactly the same hormones in different amounts. Men's bodies generate more than 10 milligrams of testosterone per day, 20 times more than women (an average of 1 milligram per day).

A young woman at her prime (about 25) may have more testosterone than a man in his 60s. What defines her as a woman is the overwhelming amount of estrogen she possesses at the same time. This is what balances the testosterone in her body and gives her stamina and endurance, which is more than likely to develop into a spirited and upbeat personality.

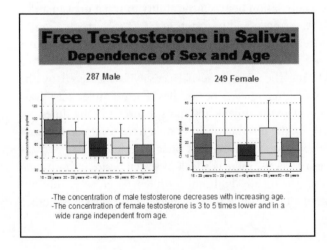

-The concentration of male testosterone decreases with increasing age.
-The concentration of female testosterone is 3 to 5 times lower and in a wide range independent from age.

As women age, their levels of circulating testosterone gradually decline. The effect can be especially felt in women around menopause, when they also experience a precipitous drop in estrogen. The symptoms of a "deficiency" or loss of testosterone can include a loss of vital energy and feeling of well-being, a loss of familiar levels of sexual libido, sensitivity of nipples and genitals, a thinning of pubic hair, and a lack of confidence and depression. Other impacts may include a "flatness" of mood, dry skin, brittle scalp hair, and loss of muscle tone and strength. It's understood that testosterone also contributes to the health of a woman's vulva, regrows the vital tissue of the clitoris, and can play a role in curbing osteoporosis by helping maintain the density of our bones. And if that isn't enough, it can influence our cognitive function (memory, logic, etc.) as well. The opposite happens to men—as the level of testosterone drops, what little testosterone is left changes into estrogen. Aromatization (changing from one hormone to another) leaves men and women with higher levels of some hormones than others.

Feeling sexy

In both men and women, testosterone increases the desire for sexual activity. Although estrogen can also have a libido-enhancing effect in women, testosterone's effect is far greater. Over the years, researchers have found that testosterone levels influence a person's cognition, sexuality and sex roles, occupation, personality, emotions, competitiveness, childhood behavior, facial expressions, relationships and more. Sexuality and libido are affected by much more than our biology. Let's not forget stress, boredom, anxiety, disinterest and exhaustion. But researchers have agreed that the wipe-out of sexual desire can result from a critical reduction in testosterone. In both men and women, clinical studies show a greater correlation than was previously thought on the level of free and active testosterone and sexual activity. There appears to be a correlation between the ability to reach orgasm and a combination of higher DHEA, estrogen and testosterone.

Likewise, for men, sexual activity as well as erectile dysfunction becomes apparent as the level of testosterone declines past the age of 30 (when our testosterone levels are at their peak). During those years, sexual activity is measured by the number of encounters of sexual intercourse a person has. For example, a 25-year-old who is in a relationship or is married generally has sex three to four times per week. As testosterone levels drop, the number of times men have sex drops to about half, which means at 50, you're lucky if you have sex once a week.

With a loss in testosterone levels, there is a lack of sexual desire in both men and women. Men develop the "roving eye syndrome," while women enter the "no-man" zone. They don't want anyone to touch them, especially not their husbands.

Dr. Tai asks "Did you know?"

If you have sex three times a week, you have it 156 times a year. Having sex once a week equals to 52 times a year.

Protect Your Testosterone Level:
Major causes of Low Testosterone

1. Menopause
2. Childbirth
3. Chemotherapy
4. Surgical menopause
5. Adrenal Fatigue
6. Endometriosis
7. Depression
8. Severe Stress
9. Birth Control Pills
10. Anti-Cholesterol medication
11. Anti-Androgen medication

Testimonial

"I am a woman that thought I was asexual! Seriously, I thought something was wrong with me. I've been married for twelve years and I started to get sick of my husband. I was scared by the whole comfort issue. I started to look at him like family instead of my lover/friend/partner. True that a person ages with every year, but I'm entirely convinced that nothing could be farther from the truth—I feel younger than I did fifteen years ago. I know it's the testosterone supplement I started taking months ago, because since then, I've been bursting with energy. I feel so bright! I'm happier, livelier, and at 55 I tutor math and science while running a cabinet-making business. Besides all of that, I run, walk, cook and clean. I feel like an excellent wife and mother and an accomplished professional. Everything is just going great for me and I'm convinced it's the testosterone that has brought the energetic woman back to life. The desires to please and to be pleased have always been there, yet I know now that they've just been hiding. My arousal time has reached an all-time record. My husband has to look at me a certain way and moments after I'm eager to just jump into his arms. I realize he doesn't look like David Hasselhoff, but I accept him for who he is, and who he is turns me on!"

—Nicky, 55

Let's take a break...

If you're a guy, you know your testosterone levels are depleting if...
- You can cry whenever and wherever for anything – even a commercial
- Your chest is a 32A+ cup size
- You don't care where your wife is going, just as long as you don't have to go along
- You wear your pants so high, tightening your belt becomes uncomfortable under the armpits.
- You've lost a lot of muscle and your idea of weight-lifting is standing up.
- Your memory is shorter and you're complaining longer.

If you're a gal, you know your testosterone levels are depleting if...
- It takes twice as long to look half as good
- You finally get your head together but your body is falling apart
- You realize caution is the only thing you care to exercise

OK, now let's get serious...

Due to a lack of testosterone, both men and women complain of losing depth perception. Many of my friends and collegues have grumbled about becoming clumsier. It's not that they're clumsier, it's that they're losing their balance because of hazy depth perception. They trip, fall off stairs, trample over their feet and are constantly bumping into objects. On one occasion, a friend of mine whom I've known since med school told me he apologized to a store mannequin after he had bumped into her (it). He was convinced it was a person even after he had turned around. I couldn't contain myself, I had to laugh, but I knew it wasn't very nice.

As in my friend's case, this is what happens when you lose testosterone. You don't know where you're going, and it's not that anything is wrong with your eyes. It may be, but generally it's not. Your sense of perception has become fuddled; this is primarily because nerve electrical charges to muscle reaction time are much slower. As muscle reaction time becomes slower and slower, you continue to lose testosterone.

Take for example my patients who are top executives. I mean, these guys are sharper than steak knives and quicker than red foxes, and they've obtained the recognition they deserve from years of hard work of designing and drafting clever business plans and strategies. Their memories are photographic; they'll never forget a face. At least, I used to think so. Just recently, I had a few of the guys over for some dinner and wine and to my surprise, two out of the three complained about making serious mistakes in memos, at meetings and during presentations. One of the two said something that really affected me. He said, "I have a reputation to maintain; I can't continue making these mistakes. My employees, who are all younger than I am, are beginning to think my position was a hand-me-down and I'm a cackling idiot."

"Wow," I said to myself. This is serious, and this poor guy needs help. From corporate genius, business legend/mogul/tycoon, my old buddy had turned into a confused, insecure and frightened old man. What's happening here? Well, it's testosterone. Mental and emotional capacities change, which could create a permanent change in personality.

Testosterone has a total and general effect on all the organs and systems in your body, which includes your cardiovascular health, the elasticity of your blood vessels, and the production of nitric oxide, a powerful compound that regulates blood vessel dilation and health as well as kidney and liver immunity.

More or less

Different body types require different amounts of testosterone supplementation. A larger, more muscular person will require more testosterone than a person with a smaller build. Similarly, the same applies for hair growth. Men with a darker beard and body hair growth (e.g. on the chest, back, shoulders, legs, arms—typically anywhere where hair grows) will have a greater need for testosterone than men who have less hair or thinner hair. This also applies to women who have larger distribution of muscle and greater hair distribution. Most experienced clinicians get a pretty good idea of how much or how little testosterone a person needs judging by their characteristics. However, this doesn't mean you should (or they should) bypass a physical examination, i.e., a prostate check and cardiovascular and blood pressure tests.

Testing for testosterone

From symptoms, signs and age, if suspicion arises of a possible loss of testosterone levels, then a blood, urine or, more practically, a saliva testosterone test can be performed to evaluate the present levels. After receiving test results that have validated and verified your levels of testosterone, your physician or health worker may consider putting you on a supplemental testosterone program.

The beginning stage of taking bioidentical testosterone involves taking smaller doses at first and then gradually increasing the amount that is needed to create a balance between testosterone and your other hormones. The other route your physician may take is to place you on an herbal extraction program, which consists of, again, herbal extractions that act as secretagogues that convert into testosterone via a natural biochemical process. At any age, bioidentical replacement therapy programs are extremely important for both men and women suffering from a loss of testosterone levels, especially if you or anyone you know is showing signs of hormone loss. Whatever you do, make sure you check it out and start early—don't wait until you're totally depleted.

Testosterone Saliva Reference

Male Testosterone pg/ml Test Result Reference				Female Testosterone pg/ml Test Result Reference			
AGE	ASSESSED BIOMARKERS	ASSESSED OPTIMUM RANGE WITH SUPPLEMENT	ASSESSED OPTIMUM RANGE WITH TRANSDERMAL	AGE	ASSESSED BIOMARKERS	ASSESSED OPTIMUM RANGE WITH SUPPLEMENT	ASSESSED OPTIMUM RANGE WITH TRANSDERMAL
20-29	145-155	140-165	250-2000	20-29	45-49	40-60	100-300
30-39	140-145	140-165	250-2000	30-39	40-45	40-60	100-300
40-49	135-140	140-165	250-2000	40-49	35-40	40-60	100-300
50-59	130-135	140-165	250-2000	50-59	30-35	40-60	100-300
60-69	125-130	140-165	250-2000	60-69	25-30	40-60	100-300

*Note: The above are Testosterone saliva testing reference tables for men and women. The far left column represents the age a person is according to the level of Testosterone found in saliva. Persons using transdermal Testosterone (i.e., liposome or patch) will have a higher Assessed Optimum Range with Transdermal (found on far right column) than if supplemented taken through injection or orally (see Assessed Optimum range with Supplement).

Persons on any kind of hormonal therapy must cease hormone supplementation prior to testing. If supplementation is continued, results will appear several hundred percent higher than assessed optimum range. High results for people using transdermal liposome are completely normal. If this applicable to the reader, one can calculate biomarker age by dividing result number by eight. Again, calculation is applicable only for persons using transdermal liposome hormone therapy.

Taking testosterone

Attention should be given specifically to anyone who is taking testosterone hormone supplements orally. As I explained in previous chapters, with oral administration, hormones are absorbed through the GI tract and through mesenteric arteries. It's taken into the liver where it is processed and metabolized. The liver, being the main filter, will automatically create sex hormone binding globulin (SHBG) to neutralize incoming excessive testosterone; therefore the increased level of SHBG will bind and neutralize testosterone the individual has taken. If you're running a blood test, and you show an increase of total testosterone, it's because SHBG has partially neutralized the small amount of free hormones you actually have; your tested levels will show a misleading 10 percent increase. Therefore, your net gain is nil, nada, zilch, zero.

Injections

An alternative for bioidentical testosterone supplementation is through injections. Many people are given one shot weekly or one shot every two weeks, and some a single shot a month by their physicians. The latter is fairly common. When you receive an injection, it'll last you approximately two weeks to a month. Oftentimes, the body receives "bolus," a medical term meaning a "large quantity" of testosterone levels. Because your body wasn't accustomed to these extra levels of testosterone, this may cause side effects. Remember my roller-coaster analogy— think of it as your body constantly experiencing highs and lows of testosterone. Once your levels are down again, you need to go back and keep on filling.

Creams

Applying natural bioidentical testosterone transdermally is a better way to go. I prefer it over taking it orally or via injection (ever since I was a kid, I've hated injections). Through liposome technology, testosterone is microencapsulated and can be rubbed vigorously on all areas of the body like on your arms, behind your knees, or on the thighs. Spread the cream across the largest amount of skin and rub vigorously until the cream is gone.

Important Information: When using Testosterone transdermal cream, be sure to rotate the application area of the skin, utilizing arms, torso, thighs, and legs on both sides of the body to avoid increased hair growth in an area.

Dosages

Testosterone is at its highest level in the morning and oftentimes we see a slight peak later in the afternoon or early evening. Like all hormones, testosterone is produced in spurts throughout the day, approximately every two hours. So, daily dosages of small amounts of transdermal testosterone are much closer to the pattern in which our bodies normally produce testosterone and will be absorbed into your body slowly throughout the day.

Transdermal dosages are very small and are used on a daily basis, or as needed. There are fewer side effects with creams, lotions and gels than there are with other alternatives (i.e., injections or taking tablets). Oftentimes, men apply creams on their chest; older men (60+) should do this especially if they see the size of their breasts is increasing.

Natural ingredients

In addition to using testosterone, men whose breasts are growing should use defensive estrogen neutralization by supplementing with aromatise inhibitors, I3C or DIM, and resveratrol from fermented grapes. (All three of these ingredients are found in Health Secrets USA's Estrogen Defense.) Women should apply the testosterone gel or cream, around estrogen, to the pelvis, surrounding the vaginal area and between the legs close to the vaginal opening. I've heard many doctors say that application in this area helps strengthen their patients' vaginal muscles, increasing clitoral sensitivity (results in amplifyinging libido sensitivity) and improving bladder control while strengthening pelvic muscles. Women using Testosterone Transdermal Liposome cream must apply the cream, rubbing vigorously in different areas of the body in a clockwise rotation, every day of the week—moving to a new body area on consecutive days. This prevents the accumulation of testosterone on the skin in any given point of application.

Natural supplements to lower testosterone levels are Saw Palmetto, flower pollen, isofalvone, and Glucophage.

TESTOSTERONE Self-Assessment	
Symptoms of Testosterone Deficiency Note: *If supplementation has already been taken *increase* dosage if following symptoms are experienced:	Symptoms of: Testosterone excess Note: *If supplementation has already been taken *decrease* dosage if following symptoms are experienced:
<ul><li>Flabby weak muscles</li><li>Low Self-Esteem</li><li>Loss of Muscle Mass</li><li>Lack of Energy and Stamina</li><li>Loss of Coordination & Balance</li><li>Loss of Confidence</li><li>Mental Fatigue</li><li>Decreased Libido</li><li>Lack of Orgasm or Sex Drive</li><li>Weight Gain</li><li>Depression</li><li>Thinning Hair</li><li>Fatigue</li><li>Dry-Skin–Thin and Lacking Elasticity</li></ul>	<ul><li>Too Aggressive and Pushy</li><li>Bossiness/Anxiety/Agitation</li><li>Oil Facial Skin</li><li>Over-confidence</li><li>Acne Eruptions</li><li>Increased Facial Hair</li><li>Constant Anger</li><li>Decreased HDL</li><li>Irregular Menstrual Periods</li></ul>

☙Dr. Tai's Anti-Aging Health Secret☙

If you choose to take oral testosterone, your physician may give you 30 to 100 mg daily of testosterone deaconate. Injections are 100 to 200 mg testosterone inathate or cytionate every two weeks. Dosage for women is approximately 10 percent of the men's dosages. My advice for women who wish to avoid testosterone's side effects is to use concurrently with natural transdermal estrogen as a balancer; by using estrogen at the same time, you can neutralize testosterone's potential side effects. Excess testosterone side effects can include over-aggressiveness (bossiness), a bad temper, insensitivity, acne formation, the feeling of being over-sexed, and facial hair growth on both men and women. Additional and more severe side-affects include insomnia, heat intolerance and the possibility of tachycardia and arrhythmia (irregular heartbeat rhythm). Decrease dosages to half and wait two weeks if symptoms don't improve. Reduce to half of that half again, and keep reducing until all unwanted symptoms disappear.

SECRET V

"The man who is too old to learn was probably *always* too old to learn."
—Henry S. Haskins

Chapter 10

Estrogen: *Generic term for any substance, natural or synthetic, that exerts biological effects characteristics of estrogenic hormones such as estradiol. Formed by the ovary, placenta, testes, and possibly the adrenal cortex, as well as by certain plants.*

—Stedman's Medical Dictionary

What to expect

What is estrogen?

How is it produced?

FSH and LH

Functions of Estrogen

PMS

Different kinds of estrogen

Postpartum

Perimenopause

Menopause

Estrogen in men

Natural vs. synthetic

Testing for Estrogen

Self-assessment

If there was ever a woman's "Top 10 Hormone List," estrogen would be ranked number one. Estrogen is a superstar; it's held the spotlight for decades. But in recent years it's done more than that—it's been the audience of its own show. Women, the physical embodiments of massive reservoirs of estrogen, are worrying because they have more or less estrogen than they need. In the late '90s, instead of lanky models cascading front covers, estrogen became the topic of discussion. This was because people began to see and understand the importance of the hormone more than ever. Balancing estrogen is necessary in bioidentical hormonal replacement and should actually be a woman's first step to any hormone replacement program. It's the hormone which makes the eyes glossy, the breasts full, and, most importantly, the hormone that brings clarity to mind. It uplifts and stabilizes the mood and makes a woman feel "herself." With an estrogen equilibrium, women have described being in their "element" by feeling sexier, more sensual and, most importantly, comfortable.

There really isn't a hormone more quintessential to woman than estrogen. It's the sex hormone that delineates the curvaceous forms of a woman's body while shaping and forming breasts and maintaining skin's softness and firmness.

How is estrogen produced?

When the ovaries mature, the two pea-sized glands produce estrogen. A special signal is sent to the brain via the hypothalamus and pituitary gland that causes ovaries to release eggs and also to produce progesterone.

As a young woman reaches puberty, estrogen production increases, which later causes her breasts to develop and her menstrual cycle to begin.

Menstrual cycle

During menstrual cycles, estrogen generates the proper womb environment for early embryo nourishment. Estrogen levels remain relatively the same for the first 25 years of a woman's physiological adult life, after which they will decrease consistently. Since the number of ovules available to mature decreases as women age, the formation of estrogen also decreases.

Menstrual cycles prepare the body to accept an ovum and if and when the ovum is fertilized to implant itself into the uterus. This, my friends, is when pregnancy occurs. During pregnancy, no symptoms are the same—all women feel, respond and relate in different ways during this stage all the way from conception through postpartum.

If an ovum isn't fertilized, the inner lining of the uterus sloughs off, causing bleeding, which cleanses the system and starts a new cycle. Bleeding is uncomfortable, and excess bleeding can in fact cause problems within a woman's body, i.e. endometriosis (see progesterone deficiency).

Estrogen's Function

1. Endometrial tissue development
2. Follicle development
3. Breast growth
4. Vaginal tissue support
5. Sexual characteristics
6. Heart Protection
7. Prevention of atherosclerosis
8. Increased blood viscosity

FSH and LH

The body produces estrogen as a result of signals by the hypothalamus: the follicle-stimulating hormone (FSH) and the luteonizing hormone (LH).

In men, FSH and LH are necessary for the formation of sperm and the synthesis of testosterone. It's not surprising, then, that men sometimes show the same symptoms as women.

Growing up with estrogen

Estrogen determines skeletal formation (wider hips), fat distribution and weight gain. Mothers can speak for their daughters, if they can't remember for themselves. Before high school (around the time when puberty hits its prime), girls are twig thin; their legs are the size of pencils, and their arms are the size of children's wrists. After the age of 13, a physiological evolution usually takes place right before a person's eyes. Growth takes place, and little girls turn into young ladies. This is all because of estrogen. However, many girls grow in some areas more than others; they can gain 20 to 30 pounds during puberty, which is also accredited to estrogen. Not only are their complaints about weight gain, but menstrual cycles begin, which are usually accompanied by mood swings and food cravings. Every hormone has its good and its bad sides. Women need estrogen for sensuality and lubrication, yet because they need it so much there are times they'll probably suffer from having too much.

Playing a part in menstrual cycles and pregnancies

I have no words to describe how much I respect women for what they go through, especially during menstrual cycles. Throughout my life, I've been fascinated by the whole cycle and just how well most women can tolerate the condition. Typically, women's periods cycle about every 28 days to signal the ability to conceive. During those 28 days, a myriad of

Dr. Tai's "Did you know?"

Estrogen plays an IMPORTANT role in pregnancies. Estrogen prepares the uterine lining for the embryo to grow into a fetus and then into what becomes a healthy newborn baby.

How?

Estrogen pads the uterus with tissues and blood, so that the future "bebe" has the space it needs to grow properly, healthfully and safely.

problems may occur. In due course, premenstrual behaviors like mood swings, and crying spells may worsen and increase in severity. Unfortunately, due to increasing levels of estrogen, 35 percent of women in America suffer from PMS symptoms. This means millions of American women complain about their menstrual cycles.

Periods have become the roots of arguments, misunderstanding and behavior that can create emotional scars and cause irreversible damage to women's bodies and personal relationships. But it's a fact of life, ladies: Without periods, there would be no babies, no you and no me.

Testimonial: PMS

"In a nutshell, I'd have to say I'm empathetic, disciplined, understanding, civilized and a person of good humor. However, at a point in my life, it seemed like all those characteristics had deteriorated and I had become nothing but an irritating tyrant, especially to my fellow staff.

"I advised my coworkers to ignore me when I displayed episodes of dramatic outburst. I said, 'It's my health talking, not me.' We'd joke about my request, but really to me it was a very sensitive and serious topic. Unfortunately, my sudden outbursts and villainous attitude worsened with time.

"So, I saw my physician and his advice only drove me crazier. He recommended analgesics for pain, sedatives for stress, antidepressant, and even birth control pills to help moderate my very obvious PMS symptoms."

"I started getting impatient with my doctor. I wanted to know what my problem was. I cried. A day later, I went to a clinic for saliva hormone testing. They wanted to measure the daily levels of my hormones. From the tests, it became conclusive that my estrogen levels were extremely high relative to my progesterone level.

"My doctor prescribed 14-28 day progesterone and I was able to finally get off birth control. Since then, my symptoms have become more livable, and as for my coworkers, they still like me."

—*Maya, 27*

Interesting Facts of Low Estrogen

1. Women who smoke have lower estrogen than those who do not smoke. They also have more menopause symptoms. *Michnovicz J. Int'l Clin Nutr Rev 1987; 7(4):169-173.*

2. Severe stress suppresses estrogen production. *Vliet, E. Women Weight and Hormones, NY:M. Evans & Company, 2001.*

3. The true cause of hot flashes is fluctuating estrogen rather than a constant decrease in estrogen. *Hays, B., "Solving the hormone replacement dilemma in perimenopause." Gig Harbor, Washington 2001.*

4. Diets of high fat increase level of estrogen and the incidence of breast cancer. *Ahlgrimm, M., The HRT Solution,. 1999; NY: Avery Pub.*

5. Estrogen can decrease heart disease by almost 50%. *Nabulsi, A., et al., NEJM 1993; 328:1069-1075.*

Estrogen: The Three Musketeers

Bioidentical hormone replacement is trickier than most people think, especially when it comes to estrogens. Estrogen comes in three forms—this is what makes it plural (although it's more commonly known as estrogen). For this reason, when replenishing lost estrogen levels, you must also concern yourself with Estrone, Estradiol and Estriol; when doctors refer to estrogen, the three estrogens are involved. Estrogen is a name used to refer to three different bodies with similar molecular structures and names which vary in age (in essence of enduring lifespan) and tasks (internal obligatory undertakings).

Remember:

Estrogen is divided into a number of different forms, but there are three specific kinds you should try to remember: Estrone (E1), Estradiol (E2) and Estriol (E3). All three hormones perform at the same level as estrogen, but in slightly different ways. Estriol makes up approximately 10-20 percent of the total estrogen pool while estrone and estradiol share approximately 80 percent.

Three Estrogens:

- **Estrone (E1):** Mainly produced and released during menopause. Follows the decline of estradiol. Estrone is produced by the ovaries and by conversion of body fat. The more fat you have, the more estrone you make; it's also made in the liver, which converts estradiol to estrone. Since estrone can be converted back into estradiol, estrone serves as a reservoir the body can use for its primary form of estrogen. After menopause, body fat continues as a source of estrone, so it wins the estrogen race by default.

- **Estradiol (E2):** The main hormone produced during menstruation produced by ovaries, it's the biologically active form of estrogen from puberty to menopause, Estradiol is 12 times stronger than Estrone, and 80 times stronger than Estriol. Produced in the ovaries, it's the biologically active form of estrogen that acts at the cell receptor sites throughout your body. It influences over 400 of your body's functions. This is the form of estrogen that starts declining after 35 and finally reaches low levels after menopause. It affects the heart, blood, bones, brain, skin, hair, vagina, bladder and organs. It causes women to gain weight in certain areas like hips and thighs; it deals with fat distribution. High levels of E2 Estradiol increases risks of breast and uterine cancer.

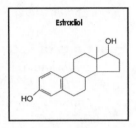

Important Functions of Estradiol
   Vliet, E. Women Weight and Hormones, NY:M.Evans & Company, 2001.

1. Maintains potassium, calcium, magnesium, and zinc levels
2. Improves blood HDL
3. Lowers bad LDL
4. Lowers total cholesterol
5. Lowers triglycerides (When using transdermal Estradiol supplement)
6. Decreases platelet aggregation
7. Improves growth hormone production. *Fonseea, E., Menopause J. North Amer Men Soc 1999; 6-1:56-60.*
8. Improves serotonin levels
9. Improves bone metabolism
10. Improves sleep
11. Decreases fatigue
12. Maintains memory

- **Estriol (E3):** Generated during pregnancy. After pregnancy, estriol is produced in very small amounts. Estriol shows evidence of breast cancer protection. When replenishing estrogens, getting an adequate amount of estriol can relieve mood, memory and fragmented sleep, without causing the user to worry about overconsumption or overproduction. Estriol is the most benign of all estrogens, causing the least amount of problems with regard to breast and ovarian cysts.

Asians and vegetarians have higher levels of Estriol and statistically lower occurrence of breast cancer. *Laux. M., Natural Woman, Natural Menopasue. NY: HarperCollins, 1997, p.20*

Functions of Estriol

Estriol found effective in menopause, lowering hot flashes, insomia, and vaginal dryness. *Heaad, K., "Estriol safety and efficacy," Altern med Rev 1998;3(2):101-13.*

Improves growth of G.I. good bacteria lactobacillus. *Stamm, W., NEJM 1993; 329(11):753-56.*

Increases good HDL and decreases bad LDL. *Lauritzen C., Horm Metabol Res 1987; 19:579-584.*

Maintains vaginal pH, prevents urinary tract infection. *Collins, J., What's Your Menopause Type. Roseville, CA:Prima health, 2000.*

Protects and treats breast cancer. *Lauritzen C., Horm Metabol Res 1987; 19:579-584.*

Estriol occupies Estrogen receptor sites in the breast.

Important Fact: Unlike Estradiol E2, Estriol E3 does not protect bone, heart, or brain. *Vliet, E. Women Weight and Hormones, NY:M.Evans & Company, 2001.*

Impress your doctor by asking about your E1, E2 and E3 levels, instead of estrone, estradiol and estriol. It's quicker and simpler.

Estrogen evolution

With time, and under certain conditions, each hormone has the capability of evolving into another version of itself: Estradiol can become estrone. Estrone can become estradiol, and eventually, both estrogens find an equilibrium amongst themselves, without affecting estriol.

Estrone, estradiol & estriol explained

Estriol, a predominant form of estrogen during a woman's pregnancy, is a benign form of estrogen, regardless of how abundant it can be in a woman's body. It goes through spurts, dominant during pregnancy and subsequently loosening its grip afterwards.

Two forms of estrogen that support each other, estrone and estradiol, have higher effects in the ovaries, uterus and breasts than they do anywhere else in a woman's body. When estrogen cells grow into a cyst or fibrous tumor, they assemble, and can take shape of a fist, forming a benign tumor. (See estrogen and cancer.) Research shows that estrone and estradiol increase and accelerate cells to reproduce more rapidly which may result in big problems; conversely, with estriol, women rarely experience abnormal growths of any kind.

Lifespan

The lifespan of these estrogens is approximately one month. Some estradiol is converted into estrone, a weaker estrogen. When both estradiol and estrone are secreted into the bloodstream and travel, they are in turn grabbed by the estrogen receptor sites. Cells that are sensitive to all estrogens stimulate new and different estrogen cell growth. In the ovaries (a major conversion site for hormones), all three forms of estrogen reach their peak levels prior to ovulation. The levels diminish during the second phase of the menstrual cycle and plummet just before menstruation. The body goes through a constant process of renewal and conversion: cells turn into tissues, bone, fat, marrow, etc. and hormones turn into other hormones.

2 and 16 Metabolites

Estrogen is broken down into two types of metabolites by enzymatic conversion. These two metabolites are: 2-hydroxyoestrone (protective estrogen) which has been reported as anti-cancerous, (*Bradlow, H., J. Endocrinol 1996; 150 (suppl): S259-S265.*) and 16-hydroxyoestrone, (destructive estrogen). 16-hydroxyoestrone is mostly found in breast tissues and is notorious for increasing breast and ovarian tumors (more on this later, see "Bioidentical estrogen in food").

Bioidentical Estrogen in Food: Mmm, metabolites

When estrogen is metabolized, it releases two metabolites: 2 (OH) and 16 (OH). In Dr. Bradlow HL (et al.) experiment "2-Hydroxyestrone: The 'good' Estrogen" published in a 1996 issue of the Journal of Endocrinology, Bradlow found that estrone metabolizes more 16 (OH) than estradiol and estriol.

What does that mean? Well, for one, 16 (OH) is the bad kind of metabolite, the kind that, when metabolized, can change and corrupt DNA synthesis. Dr. Bradlo concluded that 16 alpha (OH) can cause breast cancer. (Dr. Bradlow H.L.

---

et al. "2-Hydroxyestrone: The 'good' estrogen." *The Journal of Endocrinology, 1996; 150: s259-s265.*)

To better avoid your chances of estrogen metabolizing into 16 (OH), consume foods that metabolize into 2 (OH) instead of 16 (OH). Cabbage and broccoli, for example, have been shown to increase the necessary kind of estrogen for a woman's body. Both vegetables contain "indole-3-carbinol" (one of many metabolites). Whoa, long word—I don't expect you to remember that, don't worry. However, I do expect you remember that indole-3-carbinol functions as a major estrogen protector.

In Dr. Kabat's (et al.) "Urinary Estrogen Metabolites and Breast Cancer: A Case Controlled Study" for the Preview of Cancer Epidemiology Biomarkers, he highlighted that 73 percent of his study's breast cancer participants showed higher levels of 16 (OH) than 2 (OH).

He suggested that there is a way to avoid breast cancer, and that is by increasing supplemental use of indole-3-carbinol (e.g., broccoli and cabbage), lowering fat in diets and exercising. (Dr. Kabat G.C. et al. "Urinary estrogen metabolites and breast cancer: A case controlled study." Cancer Epidemiology and Biomarker Prevention, 1997; 6(7):505-509.)

Powerful Protection Info: Low 2/16 ratios are associated with Breast Cancer. *Melilahn, E., Br. J. Cancer 1998; 78(9):1250-1255.*

In the liver, one form of estrogens converts into different estrogens, or they're propelled into the bloodstream. When estrogens are sent to the bloodstream, they circulate throughout the whole body until they make their way towards the kidneys and are eliminated through urination. This is why many pregnancy tests work. Doctors "in the know" monitor or evaluate the health of a placenta by examining the estriol in the urine.

Secret steps you can use to raise 2 Hydroxyestrone to improve 2/16 ratios:

1. Moderate execise. *De Cree, C., Fertil Steril 1997; 67;505-516.*

2. Eat cruciferous vegetables. *Telang, N., J. Clin Ligand Assay, 2000.*

3. Add Flax seeds to your diet. *Haggins, C., Cancer Epid. Biomarkers & Prev 2000; 9:719-725.*

4. Supplement Kudzu and Indole 3-carbinol. (300mg). *Michnovicz, J. Int'l J. Obe. 1998; 22:227-229.*

5. Increase Protein diet and Omega-3-fatty acids. *Osborne, M., Cancer Invest 1988; 8:629-631.*

6. B6, B12, and folic acids. *Bland, J., The Functional Medicine Institute, 2001, pg. 68.*

Separating the three: Studying Estriol

In 1966, The Journal of American Medical Association (JAMA) published a study by the late Dr. Lemon (et al.) on breast cancer patients prior to providing them with endocrine (hormonal) therapy. Dr. Lemon gathered a variety of women with breast cancer and tested each of their estrogen levels (estrone, estradiol and estriol). He found that 26 women showed extremely low estriol levels compared to estrone and estradiol. The estrogen comparison sparked curiosity in researchers. Did lower estriol levels mean greater chances of developing breast cancer? (Lemon, H.M. et al. "Reduced estriol exertions and incretions for breast incretions prior to endocrine therapy." *JAMA, 1966; 196: 1128-1136.*)

Apparently the answer was yes; in 1978, Dr. Follingstad's study was published in JAMA (Journal of the American Medical Association) entitled "Estriol the Forgotten Estrogen?" Dr. Follingstad showed that a majority of study's participants had low estriol levels, and that these very same patients showed a 37 percent decrease in mammary (breast) capacity. (Follingstad, A.H. et al. "Estriol the forgotten estrogen?" *JAMA, 1978; 239:29.*)

Just two years later, in 1980, Dr. Lemon decided to get back to estriol, although this time his experiment was on rats instead of women. Dr. Lemon showed that estriol proved to be non-carcinogenic, and in mice it neutralized the carcinogenic effect of a much stronger estrogen—estradiol. (Lemon, H.M. et al. "Patho-physiological consideration in the treatment of menopausal patients with estrogen; the role of estriol in the prevention of mammary carcinoma." *Acta Endocrinology, 1980; 233: 17-27.*)

The estrogens can be tested separately; it's been proven that of the three estrogens, estriol has the weaker effects. However, it appears to have positive progesterone-like effects by modulating and balancing the more damaging effects of estrone and estradiol excess. Unlike estrone and estradiol, estriol doesn't convert into anything; it is what it is.

Theoretically, a healthy estrogen ratio is one in which there is four to five times more estriol than estrone and estradiol (assuming that both estrone and estradiol are left to combine). Check estriol's level to avoid estrone and estradiol dominance, which will increase the chances of forming cysts, tumors and various cancers.

Three estrogens and the three phases of Eve:
Pregnancy (Postpartum Depression)
Peri-menopause
Menopause

After the "first phase of Eve," pregnancy, hormonal changes in a woman may trigger depression. If you've read the section on the three kinds of estrogen, you would've seen that a form of estrogen referred to as estriol is a 1000 percent greater in a woman when she's pregnant. This massive estrogen drop may cause a depression commonly know as "postpartum blues."

Some women can handle the "after-the-fact" portion of childbirth, while others cannot. Famous actress/model Brooke Shields is the first person who comes to mind. In her book Down Came the Rain: My Journey with Postpartum Depression (Hyperion, 2005), Shields was interviewed by reporter Denise Mann in a March 2005 issue of WebMD: The Magazine.

Shields said, "I really didn't want to live anymore. I just wanted to leap out of my life, but then the rational side of me [would say], 'You're only on the fourth floor. You'll get broken to bits and then you will be even worse.'"

I don't think she could have put it better than by saying, "I really didn't want to live anymore." Along with a serious hormonal drop of estriol (estrogen) and progesterone, a lot of women have a problem with letting go of a tiny body that grew within them for almost a year. Mothers experience feelings of loss— loss of identity, or rather who they were before having the baby. They experience feelings of loss of control, loss of their "figures," and a sense of being less attractive. After the baby is delivered, the principal actress in the entire drama is neglected. All too often, new mommies are left with the "baby blues," because they're left with terribly sore bodies to deal with a baby that everyone else gets sappy over. But what about her?

I'll never know just how traumatic an experience giving birth is, because for one, I'm not a woman. But I've seen it happen. I'm a father and a doctor, and let me just say one thing about childbirth—it's amazing. OK, let me say two things— women are heroines!

Mothers have to go through an extremely painful experience that will render emotional shock that can be potentially dangerous to themselves and their newborns.

Dr. Tai's "Did you know?"

Women are born with nearly five million eggs. By 20, women have 500 and by 50, they'll have fewer than 50 eggs.

Testimonial: Postpartum Blues

"Once—pregnant girlfriends told me about postpartum depression, I really didn't think it was going to be that bad until, at 29, I had my first child, Lindsey-Grace. God bless my little girl 100 times. I love her so much and I feel guilty for feeling the way I did after I had her.

"At nine pounds, when Lindsey-Grace left my body I felt as if I had released a watermelon. Funny as it may seem, it was a very painful experience. For weeks I hid from friends and family. My incredible husband did most of the meeting and greeting as I planted myself in our walk-in closet.

"I was the fattest I'd ever been, and I continued to eat even when I was full. Instead of celebrating my baby's birth I acted like I was at a funeral, a never-ending funeral. And it was fitting, because black was the only color I'd wear for months.

"Most of my time was spent with my wheelchair-bound mother. She, unlike my husband who was always at work, was at home. If it weren't for her loving face and encouraging words, I would have been close to doing something insanely wild to myself, like taking my life. To be completely honest with you, I'm embarrassed to express the feelings I had about birth-giving. It's hard, and it was even harder thinking that I was alone.

"But because of a caring doctor, who was completely devoted to my well-being and my healing process, I realized that I wasn't alone. While a woman is pregnant, her hormones reach their peak, and after she's pregnant, many of them reach their demise. This can cause postpartum depression, or at worst postpartum psychosis, a condition that's characterized by homicidal and suicidal impulses, hallucinations, delusions, disorganized and bizarre thinking.

"I feel like I somewhat touched that point—my impulses were suicidal and I did think of very bizarre and sometimes cruel things. I created arguments with my husband; he was working to support our new little family, while I accused him of cheating on me.

"With my mother, I brought up every single argument we've ever had, like in the eighth grade when she didn't let me sleep at friend's house, or that one time she wouldn't let me take her car to a party. I was looking for arguments and after a few attempts both my mother and husband wouldn't let me have what I wanted. They nodded and responded with, "you're right," "absolutely, honey," or "I don't know what to tell you, sweetheart."

"The reason behind this letter is, unlike many women, I'm blessed with strong family support. I can't imagine how life is for single mothers or women with limited *choices. I had resources like my doctor, and my mother (who had me)—they both were a great help in sharing the experiences other women like myself had, and that my feelings were "of the norm."*

"I'm also blessed for realizing that hormones can make or break you, especially if you're a woman."

—*Jennifer, 33*

Perimenopause

The "second phase of Eve," perimenopause, occurs when the pituitary gland and the hypothalamus produce hormones like GnRH, FSH and LH, but the ovaries produce lesser amounts of estrogen for ovulation. (Like a river that turns into a creek, it never stops running, although less water circulates).* If you'd prefer a direct translation of the word, perimenopause just means "before," or "around" menopause. This period in every woman's life usually lasts 5-7 years. Perimenopause symptoms occur as early as 35 before menopause begins.

As women age, I've heard them discuss the fear they have over menopause. Menopause should be the least of their worries—it's perimenopause that's a disaster. If you've gone through it, you'll know exactly what I'm talking about. If you haven't—please be wary.

During perimenopause, women tend to be erratic, they act lost, and their naturally capricious nature is multiplied to 10th power. I always thought of it like this: women going through perimenopause are like cars, cars that chug alongside emergency lanes. They spit and sputter, taking them longer than all the other cars to get to their intended destination. In the winter, it takes them half the morning just to start and in the summer they go from point A to point B by smoking and over-heating. Overall, the car is completely unreliable.

In my example, one sole entity, the car, is meant to represent many other entities in a woman's body. Glands begin to spit and sputter. During a woman's period, her menstrual cycle become so erratic it's no wonder why their personalities are affected by not bleeding. With perimenopause, women can bleed to point where they're afraid to stand up. I've heard stories of women being afraid to leave their desks and bed due to a fear of experiencing "blood falls." Women can bleed so much blood gushes from their bodies, causing them to change multiple times throughout the course of day. In other cases, periods creep up on women. They don't know what day to mark their calendars—sometimes it's late, sometime it's early and almost always they're never prepared. This marks the transition towards the menopause phase.

Testimonial: Perimenopause

"I know Chicago and Chicago knows me. For 25 years I yearned to go out and party at night, but as a corporate slave I've found myself in my apartment beside a flickering lamp with files, highlighters and week-old Chinese leftover boxes. It's paid off, as I am now a top executive of the electronics firm I once interned at. Now that I'm on top and paid, I can go out as often as I like whenever I like but the problem is, I can't. I can, but I can't.

"I've been twice divorced and I am single. I have someone to clean my loft; I also have someone to cook. I have someone to get me coffee, pick up dry cleaning, walk the dog and I even have a personal shopper. You're probably saying, 'Ah, it must be nice,' but I want you to know that it's definitely not.

"It's taken me five years of therapy to realize that I'm a workaholic that has had an increasingly difficult time establishing interpersonal relationships with people, because of behavior that gives the impression of being nothing short of 'bitchy.'

"I don't want to be a bitch, but I am. With no sleep, an aching body and a nonexistent social life, who can blame me for being one? I know this, but others don't, so they're right to make a claim that I am—they have no other source of information.

"My late mother worshipped Adelle Davis, author of Let's Eat Right to Keep Fit *and* Let's Get Well. *As a child I ate well, slept well and had a daily routine of taking Vitamin As, Bs and Cs. Rarely was I ever sick—as a kid, that is. Today, I can't sleep, I experience night sweats, hot flashes and I'll take a night of decent shut-eye over intimacy any day.*

"I compared my life as a kid and my life currently. The age had a lot to do with the way I felt, but also the way I was taken care of. I revisited some of my mother's ways and I asked myself for the first time in my life, 'What would mother have done?' She would have sought treatment for her ailments the natural way. That, I realized, that was her secret to her glamorous beauty until the age of 85. Bless her soul; she was gorgeous, crazy but gorgeous.

"It wasn't until I visited a client of mine, a woman whom I knew I'd scared away on more than one occasion with my firm handshakes and fixed gaze about 'hormones.' She was the wife of an endocrinologist; she was my peer, but looked fifteen years younger than me. It had to have been her husband I thought (more than a few ways). Indeed it was—she explained that she's been on hormone replacement therapy since the day she turned 35.

"I met with her husband, the doctor, and until this day, I am convinced the man is not of this world. He saved my life and I feel like a new woman. After counting

hormones through a saliva test, I understood that I was low on every single hormone imaginable and both my adrenals and thyroid were exhausted partially because I was perimenopausal. 'That explains it,' I thought. It helped that I was eager to start treatment—psychologically I was motivated and physiologically I was desperate.

What the doctor ordered:

- Cordyceps for energy
- Iodine for thyroid
- Adrenal Modulators—support for years of cortisol overproduction
- Progesterone liposome cream to balance excess estrogen
- Testosterone liposome cream for libido, energy and endurance
- DHEA to help with testosterone maintenance and production
- Estrogen for the perimenopausal symptoms
- Antioxidants with melatonin to help with sleep

"After utilizing the above, I felt like a brand-new woman. Compared to the new me, I'd have to say I was lazy. I do most of my household tasks on my own. I want to get to know the people that work with me. I can go out on Friday nights with my colleagues, I can sleep on Monday evenings and I can be the person I envied, a fabulous woman who can juggle a personal and professional life. The bottom line is—I can."

—Marsha, 49

Menopause

Ahhh, menopause, the third and final "stage of Eve"; tell me, thinning skin, hormonal imbalance, and unreliable personality—where art thou?

Menopause usually occurs anytime after a woman is more than 40, or quite possibly before, as a result of surgical hysterectomy (removal of uterus, or ovaries).

After menopause (the permanent cessation of the menstrual cycle) every woman carries a different risk of imbalanced hormones at different levels. This varies—some women may have an estrogen dominance after menopause where both estrogen and progesterone levels are lower (see aromatization), but estrogen is still relatively higher than progesterone.

Menopause is medically defined as the time when a woman goes through a 12-month period without menstruating (the year-long wait is when a woman knows for sure her have periods have stopped for good). During this time, a monumental change occurs—ovaries shrink! Indeed, all internal organs change drastically, and the body takes a turn for a permanent change; but, once a woman has entered the menopause stage, she's menopausal even after her symptoms have cleared.

Menopausal women experience symptoms that vary, from night sweats that feel like they've been standing in the rain for a good hour and a half to having hair so thin and damaged it looks like a village of toddlers pulled on it for a year, after they dipped their head in a bucket of bleach.

At the supermarket, I bumped into a nurse I used to work with. I always found her very attractive; my patients enjoyed her presence very much. She was a sweetheart and it didn't hurt that she was a gorgeous lady. Every time I saw emeralds I thought of her bright green eyes. She was a brunette who always kept her long locks secured in a loose ponytail. She left my clinic years ago after the birth of her first child.

So there I was, at one of my favorite organic supermarkets, skimming through apples, searching for spoiled spots and feeling the potential product's firmness when I felt a tap on my shoulder. I didn't recognize the woman standing in front of me. Wow, she was different. Imposter! What have you done to the pretty, green-eyed, dark-haired nurse I'd once worked with?

Soon after, I realized menopause had taken over her body. Poor lady looked so old, her hair lacked the shine and luster it once had and it looked as if she'd been plagued by insomnia.

Do you have Symptoms of Menopause?
- Hot flashes
- Night sweats
- Vaginal dryness and odor
- Mood Swings/Irritability
- Insomnia
- Depression
- Loss of sexual libido
- Facial hair
- Painful intercourse
- Panic attacks
- Nightmares
- Urinary tract infections and vaginal itching
- Bloating
- Osteoporosis
- Hair loss
- Frequent urination/leakage
- Loss of Memory
- Night Anxiety

Story time with Dr. Tai:

America's 51st state, Menopause, USA, is an imaginary state where American women (mostly 40 +) go to during perimenopause.

Only women are allowed in Menopause U.S.A., like an Amazon community, no woman is allowed to leave, because perimenopause and menopause involve permanent hormone losses, which makes returning to previous states impossible. Once you're there, you're there forever ladies, and there's no turning back.

She don't get no sleep

Menopause causes not just my former pretty nurse to lose sleep, but lots of other women as well. As a matter of fact, the most difficult time of the day will be the evening for most women going through menopause. Women cry themselves to sleep (if they can actually fall asleep) and their sexual organs will shrink. I'm serious. For many women the only masculine thing they'll want to touch is Fido, their best friend and dog, because their husbands or boyfriends disgust them. Why? Because by this stage, Men-o-pause, most women hate sex, they can't think about sex, they don't want sex, and because husbands and boyfriends are men, women assume they want to have sex.

Dr. Tai asks, "Did you know?"

Because of estrogen, there are more tissues in a woman's body. Balancing and moderating Progesterone plays an important role in cellular growth. When estrogen diminishes, it takes progesterone along with it, leaving the skin, saggy, soft and wrinkly—lacking tone and firmness.

Hair looks ugly, skin looks ugly, sleep is unachievable, sex is undesirable, and, just when you thought the list ended here, women begin to lose their grace! Women who go through menopause develop a loss of balance—they trip more, they forget which words to use, and where they place the grocery bags. (I've seen this. It's amazing. They've assumed they've placed them in their trunks, when really they're on the hoods of their cars!) They walk into rooms and forget why in they're there. Their hearts palpitate and when they sneeze, they wet their knickers!

Why do those things happen?

To sum it all up, menopause is simply a drop in estrogen and progesterone levels with a much larger level drop of progesterone (estrogen's contradiction), which is a protagonist to some of estrogen's antagonistic effects. Progesterone acts as a neutralizer and a hormonal moderator to estrogen. The drop is much larger because the female body encompasses more progesterone than it does estrogen; as abundant as it is, it's weaker than estrogen. However, when both estrogen and progesterone exit the building we call "your body," cells don't work as they once did, due to being off balance. There's no question that after menopause estrogen levels drop dramatically, which can only mean that progesterone drops even more so than the hormone it shields--estrogen. As a matter of fact, progesterone drops precipitously and dramatically, and unfortunately, progesterone isn't a hormone that a lot of doctors make too big of deal about. Most of the horrible menopause symptoms women experience come about due to great shifts in levels of hormones. Symptoms are more prominent when hormone levels change. However, once the hormone drop stabilizes and remains low for good, the symptoms actually become less noticeable and women erroneously think they are *through* with menopause. *Once in menopause, always in menopause.*

Testimonial: Menopause, Urethra Tear

"I've aged impeccably—the older I become, the better I feel. I guess it's because I count my blessings, my successes, I've learned from my failures and I've become my very own best friend. A typical bon vivant, I am a woman who lacks fear and appreciates the finer things in life. As a flower shop owner, my business goes well beyond selling flowers--I sell messages.

"Throughout the years, my clients have sent me pictures of their weddings, christenings, bar mitzvahs and parties with my floral arrangements in the background. I've felt wonderful knowing that I've beautified some of people's fondest memories; however, last year I created a memory for myself that reminded me more of a nightmare than a dreamscape.

"At a client's anniversary party, hours after the event had started, I noticed something terribly wrong with the chandelier placement. Being the perfectionist that I am, I asked one of the caterers to bring me a ladder. As I worked my way up the ladder steps in hopes to pull out a few dead leaves from the African lily and sunflower arrangement, I felt something trickle down my leg. I thought it was water from the centrepiece sponge; upsettingly, it was I. I had urinated on myself after letting out a faint sneeze. I was appalled at myself and I was embarrassed.

"That evening two years ago was a turning point in my life. I told my sister, whom I am very close with, about how I jolted out of the mansion brimming with guests to change my wet dress, stockings and underwear (slip and panties) and she just handed me her gynecologist's number after I finished off three tissue boxes in her living room apartment. The brat in her said, 'I knew it was going to catch up with you,' and I heard it loud and clear!

"Days after, I manage to squeeze an appointment and I visit my sister's OB-GYN; after a few tests, the doctor told me that I had a few small tears on the inner lining of

Dr. Tai's fun facts:
Many Asian women are much less symptomatically affected by menopause than Caucasian women are. Much of this is due to physiological build and diet. In America, menopause will affect over 50 million women a year!

my urethra. The doctor said that the tears were a result of an estrogen deficiency, which explained my shrinking breasts and waistline. He also explained that a weak urethra was the first of many problems that would occur to me because of an estrogen deficiency.

"The doctor offered me liposome creams from his clinic because he claimed, with them, he's seen fabulous results. I gave the bioidentical estriol cream a try and applied to my breasts and inner thighs.

"The first few weeks of treatment I was disappointed, only because I was eager to see results. The doctor assured me that the treatment would work only with patience. He told me it was fine to increase my dosage by using the cream more than twice daily, I did, and two months later I returned the diapers I purchased at the drug store. (They had been on reserve for quite some time, for those "just-in-case moments.")

"I know I'm so thankful that I received treatment before the estrogen deficiency got to my heart and bones.

"Estrogen deficiency is a leading cause in heart attacks and osteoporosis in women. Thanks to my open mind and a great doctor, I can leave the bed-wetting to the toddlers."

Janet, 64

Fear not - help is here!

I believe that in the crisis a woman goes through during menopause is an opportunity to improve herself, and she can improve herself by finding out the exact level of hormones. The first step to re-cooperation is to gently replace natural hormones with bioidentical hormone supplementation.

Get lucky; get evaluated prior to entering the menopause period. Women can delay and stop a number of symptoms that occur to them and suspend or bypass a number of problems. Natural supplementation is crucial! Replacing hormones could potentially save a lot of headaches. Remember, "the tire wouldn't have blown out on the freeway had it been changed in time."

> Many 50-year-old men have more estrogen than women of the same age due to "aromatization"—the transformation of testosterone into estrogen.

Men, beware of estrogen!
No men allowed!

Men, like women, have estrogen. Are you shocked? Well, just so you know, we as people all have the same hormones except that gender dictates how much of a hormone we have. Men have estrogen, but much, much less than women do. This is the reason why estrogen is thought of as "the woman's hormone," and testosterone "the man's." But, again, the world of hormones is like a unisex washroom, in that both sexes are expected to cross the threshold at one time or another.

Once men pass the age of 40, and pass the hormonal "threshold" of testosterone aromatizing into estrogen, they start to look more like women. Men with an estrogen dominance start to gain weight on their hips, develop breasts (called *gynecomastia)* that are larger than some women's chest sizes, and frightfully have a higher likelihood of developing prostate cancer. When estrogen takes an authoritative stance in a man's life, they become increasingly sensitive and have been observed to develop childlike characteristics by becoming increasingly moody and displaying tantrums of all kinds. This is known as Andropause (see testosterone), the process of when men lose testosterone and gain estrogen.

If you, my reader, are a man, you need to do something about declining testosterone levels if you want to reclaim your "manhood." Estrogen is damaging to men and there is a way to retard the process. Certain plants and herbs have bioidentical hormones that'll impede the process of testosterone evolving into estrogen (see aromatization).

Synthetic estrogen—The Troublemaker

"Because of synthetic forms of estrogen, 50 percent of American women suffer from estrogen excess at some point in their lives."

A quarter of American women between the ages of 35-50 will experience benign uterine fibroids, and because of fibroids, endometriosis (severe and lasting bleeding) and tumorous growths can occur. This is all because of an estrogen excess—hormonal imbalances affect 10 percent of perimenopausal women. It's also one of the leading causes of hysterectomies, breast tumors and cancers, affecting 10 percent of America's female population. These percentages upset me. We need our ladies feeling healthy, and ovarian and breast cancer should be something that everyone thinks about. These problems can be avoided, or at least the incidence can be lowered.

The Band-Aid Approach

This is why I stress taking precautions! Problems occur only when health issues are neglected and eventually become too complicated to fix. Don't take what I'd like to call "the Band-Aid approach."

Taking synthetic forms of hormones will probably speed up a few processes (i.e., consuming birth control pills) but, in the meantime, I hope you know that you'll develop more problems, which you'll have to treat before they become out of control.

Among the problems you may have developed from synthetic estrogen pills, you'll need other solutions to remedy the ailments that you've cultivated by taking water pills for excess fluid retention and muscle relaxants for cramps, etc.

Sadly, in some more severe cases, women have developed heart problems, which can turn out to be life-threatening. Excess synthetic estrogen proliferates in the endometrial lining and breast tissues, which increases the chances of provoking tumor development. The imbalance causes the body to shift drastically and disrupt the normal balance of cells dying and new cells forming.

Over 80 percent of the women surveyed by the London Daily Times said their family doctors have been treating PMS complaints with anti-depressants.

I was appalled by the number. Taking anti-depressants for PMS symptoms is probably the most counterproductive thing a woman can do to her body. All of the physical symptoms that are treated with prescriptions carry severe side affects and complications. They couldn't possibly be further away from the target by completely missing the single most important point: She just has an excess of estrogen! Holy Toledo! I find surveys like the one I found in the London Daily Times show just how misguided and misdirected the treatment is for perimenopause and menopausal women.

Synthetic estrogens and cancer: Shhh—the "C" word

Natural estrogens are preferred over synthetic forms as they cause less damage to the liver, they're metabolized and discharged more quickly and correctly, exert weaker estrogenic effects and are less likely to cause problems with long-term use.

Synthetic estrogen and synthetic progesterone hormones don't match our body's cell receptor sites; the body understands them to be foreign substances, but can't get rid of them, which can cause severe side effects. There is a considerable amount of evidence that hormone replacement therapy with synthetic estrogen may cause breast cancer and other fatal complications

I'm the first one to believe that claim, which is the reason why I don't advise women to take synthetic estrogen. Women who are overweight or have a family history of obesity (that's more than half this country) have a family history of breast cancer, diabetes and increased breast density (based on mammograms) should avoid starting synthetic hormone replacement because of increased risks for developing breast cancer while on a synthetic estrogen.

Ovarian cancer, another potential cancer due to "pseudo-synthetic-estrogen-hormone replacement therapy" leads to uterine bleeding and endometrial shrinkage. Fibroids created from endometriosis can be aggravated by synthetic hormone replacement therapy, and bleeding after sex is another frequent complaint.

Isn't it enough that women bleed every month? With synthetic hormones you could be bleeding after sex? That's gotta be scary. Blood pressure can increase after starting synthetic HRT, so repeat doctor visitations are necessary since you must refill and recheck. Synthetic hormone replacement also increases PMS symptoms of breast soreness, pain/swelling, fluid retention, nervousness, and palpitations. However, with bioidentical estrogen and progesterone, you don't have to worry about freakish side effects. You can go as you like, stop as you like, and proceed at your own discretion. It's as easy as 1, 2, 3!

#1) Saliva Test
#2) Bioidentical supplementation;
#3) Dosage adjustment

Fishing for estrogen

If you've been acting funny and you're seeing signs in the way your body is taking shape, do yourself a favor and run a saliva hormone test. Once you find out where your estrogen and progesterone levels are, you'll be able to proceed with life in an intelligent manner.

In fact, if your estrogen levels are giving you trouble, balancing the estrogen effects with natural bioidentical progesterone cream can have excellent and miraculous results, especially women who are having a difficult time dealing with PMS.

Women having problems before the 14th day of their menstrual cycles should run a saliva test and check for a hormone imbalance, due to the possibility of an estrogen excess. However, if most symptoms occur near the end of the menstrual cycle, before bleeding, PMS may be due to an imbalance of too much estrogen and not enough natural progesterone.

ESTROGEN Self-Assessment	
Symptoms of Estrogen Deficiency Note: *If supplementation has already been taken *increase* dosage if following symptoms are experienced:	**Symptoms of: Estrogen Excess** Note: *If supplementation has already been taken *decrease* dosage if following symptoms are experienced:
<ul><li>Sagging breasts</li><li>Lack of libido</li><li>Vaginal dryness</li><li>Urinary incontinence/infection</li><li>Hot flashes</li><li>Night sweats</li><li>Memory problems</li><li>Fuzzy thinking</li><li>Irregular menstrual cycles</li><li>Lack of menstruation</li><li>Thinner skin</li><li>More wrinkles and skin aging</li><li>Increased insulin resistance & Diabetes</li><li>Osteoporosis</li><li>Increased Cholesterol and heart problems</li></ul>	<ul><li>Water retention</li><li>Cervical dysplasia/Fibroids/Cancer</li><li>Hypothyroidism</li><li>Fatigue</li><li>Poor sleep</li><li>Bloating</li><li>Anxiety/ Fear</li><li>Breast swollen/ tender</li><li>Severe headaches</li><li>Excess menstrual bleeding</li><li>Weight gain</li><li>Increased incidence of breast cancer</li></ul>**In Men:**<ul><li>Enlarged breasts</li><li>Prostate enlargement</li><li>Difficulty urinating</li><li>Increased emotionality</li><li>Frequent tearfulness</li></ul>

∽Dr. Tai's Anti-Aging Health Secret∽

As you've read, estrogen is a more complex hormone than you may have thought it was. There are at least 150 different kinds of estrogen, the predominant being Estrone (E1), Estradiol (E2) and Estriol (E3). Each form of estrogen plays a particular role in the three phases of a woman's life (pregnancy, perimenopause and, finally, menopause).

By examining studies, we've seen that estriol has a very important function; it balances the negative effects of various other forms of estrogen. At times perplexing, estrogen is necessary for a woman's health. She loses essential quantities of estrogen well after her menstrual cycle has stopped. The hormone helps her maintain body moisture and fortifies her libido. In men, estrogen does the opposite—it poses the potential threat of causing prostate cancer. Not only can excess estrogen cause cancer in men, it can in women, too. Excess estrogen is known for stimulating cell proliferation and growth, causing benign tumors in the uterus, breasts and ovaries.

Here's another estrogen fact—it's metabolized and broken down into 2 (OH) and 16 (OH). The 2 (OH) is an estrogen protector, but when estrogen metabolizes into 16 (OH), there is a greater likelihood of an occurrence of tumerous growths.

Women need estrogen; men don't need it as much. Bioidentical estrogen does a nice job of leveling how much a person needs by way of a combination of progesterone and estrogen plant extracts. Together, the two have just the right amount to make a woman feel sexier and more energetic. Most men need supplementation in guarding against estrogen formation called aromatization; this is why there are proprietary formulations to safeguard against estrogen dominance. My point: Test your estrogen levels. Guessing how much you have will only complicate the status of your health.

"My favorite estrogen studies"

For additional studies see references.

1) *Archives of Dermatology, December 1997; 133:339-342.*
   - Estrogen therapy decreases skin wrinkling and dryness.
   - Estrogen increases dermal thickness as it preserves skin texture.
   - After menopause, collagen decreases by 30 percent; skin changes are reversible with estrogen replacement therapy.

2) *Biomedicina, 2000; 3(1):5-20.*
   - Estrogen improves memory and prevents against Alzheimer's
   - In women, estrogen decreases hot flashes, night sweats and depression.
   - Estrogen maintains youthful appearance and improves libido.
   - Estrogen keeps bones strong and prevents healthy bones from deteriorating.
   - Estrogen avoids heart problems.
   - Estrogen enhances smoothness, firmness and elasticity.

3) *Chemical Research and Toxicology, 1999; 12(2):204-13.*
   - Bioidentical hormones can eliminate the production of problem causing metabolites, responsible for increased cancer incidence of synthetic hormones.

4) *Hospital Practice, August 1999: 102.*
   - Estrogen has been shown to reduce the risk of macular degeneration by 70 percent.
   - Estrogen reduces the risk of cardiovascular disease in women by approximately 50 percent.
   - Estrogen reduces the chances of women developing urinary infections and vaginal dryness.

5) *Infertility and Reproductive Medicine Clinics of North America, October 1995; 6(4):653-660.*
   - Estrogen therapy maintains premenopausal levels of natural hormones as opposed to using synthetic.
   - It's been reported that women stop hormone therapy due to side effects developed, natural estrogen eliminates these side-effects.

6) *Obstetrics and Gynecology, 1989; 73: 606.*

- Natural estrogen and progesterone decreased cholesterol and increased HDL.
- Natural estrogen protects the uterus.

Estrogen has more than 400 crucial metabolic functions:

1. Improves insulin sensitivity. *Sacks, F., CyrrOpin Lipodol 1995.*

2. Helps elasticity of arteries & dilates small arteries. *Nachtigall, L., Estrogen The Facts can change Your Life. NY:HarperCollins. 1995.*

3. Prevents Alzheimer's disease. *Ahlgrimm, M., The HRT Solution. 1999; NY: Avery Pub.*

4. Prevents platelet stickiness and accumulation of plaque on arteries. *Nachtigall, L., Estrogen The Facts can change Your Life. NY:HarperCollins. 1995.*

5. Improves collagen in skin.

6. Decreases LDL and prevents its oxidation. *Heikkinen, A., Marturitas 1998; 29(2):155-161*

7. Increases HDL. *Sinatra, S., Heart Sense for Women. Washington DC:LifeLine Press, 2000.*

8. Improves memory. Jacobs, D., "Cognitive function in nondeminated older women who took estrogen after menopause," *Neurology 1997.*

9. Improves brain power. *Rice, M. Am J. Med 1997; 103(3A):26S-35S.*

10. Improves water retention, thickness and softness of skin. *Brineat, M., "Long-term effects of the menopause and sex hormones on skin thickness," Br J. Obstet gynaecol 1985; 92(3): 256-259.*

11. Decreases homocysteine. *Van Baal, W.,Curr Med Chem 2000; 7(5):499-517.*

12. Lower Lipoprotein A. *Sinatra, S., Optimum Health, Gatlinbury, TN: The Lincoln Bradley Pub. Group, 1996.*

13. Improves energy and mood. *Vliet, E. Women Weight and Hormones, NY; M.Evans & Co., 2001.*

14. Enhances sexual interest. *Vliet, E. Women Weight and Hormones, NY; M.Evans & Co., 2001.*

15. Lower risk of colon cancer. *Rouzier, N. Longevity and Preventive Medicine Symposium. 2002.*

16. Helps to increase serotonin in brain for depression, irritability, and anxiety. *Vliet, E. Women Weight and Hormones, NY; M.Evans & Co., 2001.*

Chapter 11

Progesterone: *An anti-estrogenic steroid, believed to be the active principle of the corpus luteum. Used to correct abnormalities of the menstrual cycle.*

—Stedman's Medical Dictionary

Progesterone

If progesterone were to mimic a human quality, it would be modesty. Progesterone works alongside estrogen, cleaning up the female super-hormone's messes: relieving PMS, protecting from benign growths (i.e., cysts, fibroids, tumors) and preventing blood clots, all while going unrecognized.

Progesterone takes on just as many roles as a major Broadway production's backstage crew. Progesterone is the one that, if anything were to go wrong with the production, would protect the director. When the press is looking to prop up a bad review, it's progesterone that jumps into the front line and responds to critiques that can be as hurtful and deadly as a sequence of bullets.

Progesterone is a woman's lifesaver; with it, she can avoid a lot of trouble. Women need estrogen, but sometimes they don't need as much as the body produces. Estrogen is physiologically manufactured at a speed where a surplus is probable, and without a balancer called progesterone, there are consequences—bad ones.

Thought I'd tell you which ones?
No, not quite yet; read on and find out.

What to expect

What is progesterone?

How is progesterone produced?

Functions of progesterone

Estrogen and progesterone

Testimonial

Progesterone in women

Progesterone in men

All about PMS

Synthetic vs. natural

Testimonial

Testing of progesterone

Self assessment

Supplementation

Antiaging Health Secret

My favorite progesterone studies

What is it?

In women, progesterone is produced in the ovaries. In men, progesterone is produced from the adrenals. You might not think it to be true, but progesterone is just as necessary for men as it is for women. It doesn't play as significant a role in men as it does in women, nevertheless it's essential in that it stimulates and produces other hormones such as testosterone.

Pro: for
Gesterone: gestation
Progesterone is produced in large amounts by the placenta during pregnancy. If enough progesterone isn't produced, a miscarriage is more than likely to occur.

Women need progesterone because it enhances the actions of estrogen as well as balances its powerful and sometimes overwhelming effects.

Every month, PMS is used as an excuse for arguments, sick days and social bail-outs, partially because progesterone levels aren't as high as estrogen. You can't let progesterone take the back seat in this drive.

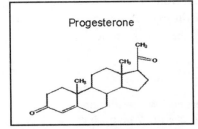

Progesterone

PMS

Almost all women have experienced symptoms of PMS, which occurs most frequently in the second half of the menstrual period. Estrogen dominance has created an imbalance where there isn't enough progesterone available to balance it out. The symptoms of excess estrogen that manifest themselves depend on the individual and include moodiness, abdominal cramps, headaches, etc.

Eighty percent of women suffer from the likes of PMS, and as it increases in severity, increased appetite, food cravings and fatigue are reported. Excess estrogen also interferes with thyroid function, however, progesterone is able to enhance the thyroid hormone. An estrogen interference occurs because it

Women who are recurrently nervous, anxious, fearful and depressed are oftentimes deficient in progesterone.

If this seems like you, try bioidentical progesterone as a natural sedative.

stimulates the production of the thyroid binding globulin, which makes for less free and available thyroid to be used by the body. On a long-term basis, the silent work that progesterone does day in and day out protects a woman's overall health.

During menstrual cycles of excess estrogen and deficient progesterone, women report experiencing painfully tender breasts, water retention, and feeling bloated.

Q: "We want to know why we gain weight before our periods."
—*The Garza sisters: Lucienda, 27; Maria, 22; Carina, 19*

A: Prior to your period, your progesterone level diminishes, leading to the symptoms of excess estrogen. The body's estrogen accumulation causes fluid retention, increasing your body weight by approximately five pounds. Women gain more weight than they think is possible based on their poor eating habits. Balancing progesterone to estrogen will work as a natural diuretic to help you maintain your weight level even while you're on your period.

Water retention solution

One of the little-known super qualities of progesterone is that it has the ability to rid the body of excess water. This wonderful effect is called the *Diuretic Effect*. Progesterone has the ability to remove excess water from tissues, decreasing swelling and bloating effects that most women experience during menstruation. It's also able to lower blood pressure and significantly improve the vascular tone.

Dr. Tai's infomercial:

When you feel bloated, don't reach for a prescription—reach for a transdermal natural bioidentical progesterone cream. Within 24-48 hours, you'll notice significant improvement! Use 20mg of transdermal progesterone at bed time and repeat the same in the morning. Apply to skin and rub vigorously and spreading as much as possible. You may adjust to a higher or lower dosage as needed.

The ups and downs of PMS

Normally, women lose approximately 3-5 ounces of blood during their menstrual cycles. Some months, there is a heavier flow than other months, but it generally alternates. Because of inconsistency, most women have an ambivalent relationship with their periods. If one month is heavier, in most cases the next menstruation cycle will be much lighter. Most women hate experiencing PMS, but when they skip or miss their cycles, they automatically think something's gone terribly wrong with their bodies.

Periods are supposed to be a time of special relief. Not only is a woman releasing ova (eggs), but it's her body's way of eliminating unwanted accumulations. While men have to depend on their urinary system, respiratory system, skin and gastrointenstinal system, women have the natural advantage of having their periods—an extra outlet to release environmental contaminants which have somehow found a way to her body (via food [pesticides] and air [pollutants]). As trees have the remarkable capacity of purifying the air, periods do an awesome job of purifying a woman's body.

After the fact, post-period

From the seventh day to the 15th day after a woman's period, the follicular stimulating hormone, which increases and stimulates estrogen in the body, also matures one of the chosen ovum that's been encapsulated by the corpus luteum (to produce and mature), making the egg ready to be fertilized.

This time of increased estrogen (maturing ovum) culminates on day 14 and day 15 when, finally, the ovum is expelled by the corpus luteum, and then goes down the ovarian tube.

During these same days (day 14 and 15) estrogen is in its premier state, and so is testosterone. Within the next few days, the egg is readily prepared to receive sperm and begin the embryo's journey to full pregnancy.

> **About periods...**
>
> PMS makes women dread having their periods, when in essence periods are supposed to be a great time for women. Instead of repressing this idea, adopt it.
>
> In the early '90s, I had a menopausal patient tell me the one thing she missed most about her younger years were her periods. *Go figure!*

However, during this followup period, estrogen drops quickly as the egg continues to move down the ovarian tube, towards the uterus.

Remember

If you haven't, go back and hit "pause" at day 15. I need to further clarify what happens at that stage before I can go on to other things. From day 15 until day 21, there is a sudden increase in progesterone. Remember, this special hormone supports pregnancy and makes the appropriate changes suitable for the fetus to grow comfortably and without complications. Like a seed in fertile ground, without a plush uterus, the fetus can't develop as it should. By the time progesterone has reached its highest point (day 21), if the ovum isn't fertilized, progesterone falls and the levels decrease precipitously over the following 7 days until menstruation begins.

At the end of the month

From day 22 to day 28, women reach the peak of the luteonizing phase (the second phase of the menstrual period). The sudden drop in progesterone occurs because the body is getting ready for menstruation and because of this drop, the relatively high estrogen is unbalanced, causing PMS symptoms to occur. Some doctors actually see PMS symptoms as caused by a low level of progesterone rater than the stereotypical view of high estrogen. As a practical matter, I think it's both.

At this point, women are likely to experience mood swings, depression, crying spells, a desire for all things sweet (chocolate, cookies, candy, etc.) and headaches that at worst have the potential of turning into migraines.

Periods looking pretty

At day 28, when both estrogen and progesterone have found each other and are both at low levels, this is the finale—menstruation finally begins. Periods are supposed to make women look their best, not their worst. When estrogen and progesterone meet they make a woman look beautiful. They give her bright and tender skin, while keeping her breasts firm and supple.

Extra! Extra! Read all about it!

Dr. Neil Lauersen, author of PMS: Premenstrual Syndrome and You *is a professor of obstetrics and gynecology at the New York Medical College. In his book, Dr. Lauersen said that 90 percent of his patients who used natural progesterone found PMS relief during their menstrual cycles.*

"When nothing works," Dr. Laueresen said, "it's [natural progesterone] that's the treatment of choice. In my practice, hundreds of women who have been severely handicapped by PMS have been completely symptom-free with natural progesterone.

"Synthetic progesterone made the symptoms of PMS much worse due to side effects."

Laueresen said that he thinks that synthetic progesterone competes with natural estrogen to cause imbalances.

Endometriosis

With very high levels of estrogen in the early part of the menstrual period, predominantly in the inner lining of the uterus, a thickening of blood supply is more than likely to occur. A surge in estrogen has resulted in women experiencing endometriosis, a condition that makes women's excess blood flow resemble chocolate syrup.

With endometriosis, blood darkens in color; instead of crimson red, blood turns a dark burgundy, almost brown. Frequently diagnosed by gynecologists worldwide, endometriosis is treated with synthetic progesterone known as progestins. Women with endometriosis have increasing damage to the tubes of their ovaries. Simply by balancing estrogen levels with progesterone, this painful condition, which can become serious (i.e., hemorrhaging), can be avoided.

Usually, during the beginning stages of progesterone supplementation, patients may experience a bleeding surge. This is a normal occurrence—it only means that the progesterone is ridding the body of old blood, or blood that's been left behind from a previous period.

Estrogen and progesterone: Perimenopause

Five to ten years before menopause, women reach the perimenopause stage of their lives. The point in time when women begin discussing "the changes" in their lives, perimenopause denotes a change in rhythmic pattern involving diet, mood, skin, sexual desire, energy, etc.

Today, there are approximately 30 million perimenopausal women because of the population boom after World War II (between 1946 and 1964), which means chances are that if you are a woman, you are a perimenopausal one.

For the duration of the perimenopausal period, women can expect a number of problems to occur because of very erratic and dysfunctional hormonal behavior. And really, we can't blame the hormones (well, the ones that actually still exist), because they're in a "panic state" at what is considered one of the body's most difficult times.

During perimenopause, a woman's body has signaled a red alert, and hormones frantically try to complete the tasks of missing hormones. Attempting to complete more than one task can result in an early retirement for hormones, and in some of the most severe cases, it can result in gland exhaustion and early aging.

What happens to progesterone during perimenopause?

Throughout perimenopause, estrogen diminishes. Because estrogen is a much stronger hormone, progesterone diminishes at a much faster pace and in much larger quantities. As women stop ovulating, progesterone drops even faster than estrogen.

Estrogen and progesterone: Menopause

Q: *"Now that I no longer experience hot flashes or night sweats, does this mean I've overcome menopause?"*

—*Leslie, 51*

A: Menopause means you're not ovulating. Even though you no longer show symptoms of menopause, this doesn't mean that you've wiped your hands clean of it. Once you've stopped ovulating and having your period, you are forever in the menopause stage. This marks the third phase of your life when your hormones diminish. And mind you, they continue to do this for the rest of your life.

Two hormones that decline in full-throttle speed are progesterone and estrogen. When they're down, they're down, and there's no turning back, unless you do something about it.

What happens to progesterone during menopause?

The reason behind estrogen's and progesterone's diminished production during the perimenopausal stage is that the ovaries are nearing their final stage of ovum production. When progesterone decreases severely, this signifies that menopause is right around the corner. During menopause, progesterone loss is at its most dangerous state. I say dangerous because it is—a loss of progesterone can be damaging to a woman's tissues, organs and bones.

Because of progesterone decline, women can lose over 20 percent of bone mass after the first few years of menopause; it's one of the main hormones that stimulate osteoblast (bone-producing) activity. So when there's a deficiency of progesterone, it only makes sense for bones to become weaker and more frail.

Progesterone in perimenopausal and menopausal women

In 1991, researcher J.R. Lee found the best method for replenishing lost levels of progesterone in perimenopausal and menopausal women is via transdermal liposome progesterone cream, which was found to increase osteoblastic activity in women's bones, thereby improving bone deposition and bone mineralization.

Lee and I apparently share a similar philosophy, because, frankly, I couldn't agree more. Bones are living organisms that require constant repair and what better to do it with than with progesterone? (Lee, J. R. "Is natural progesterone the missing link in osteoporosis prevention and treatment?" Medical Hypothesis, 1991; 35: 316-318.)

Progesterone's three stages

Stage 1	Stage II	Stage III*
In a menstrual cycle, estrogen dominates the period from Day 1 to Day 14—or the first day your period begins—until seven days after your period ends. *At approximately 120 minutes for two-hour cycles, progesterone hormones are produced in spurts; they have high peaks and low valleys.	On ovulation Day 14, 2nd phase of menstrual cycle occurs lasting through Day 28. This second phase is known as the *luteonizing phase* of the menstrual period. If by this time the egg isn't fertilized and implanted, then progesterone levels diminish and dramatically drop. This means that a woman has approximately 20-50 pg/ml** of progesterone. At the highest point of the luteonizing phase, it can be as high as 250 pg/ml (as measured on the saliva test).	Progesterone is at its highest during pregnancy. The progesterone count in a pregnant woman's saliva can be as high as 2200 pg/ml. Shortly after the birth of a baby, the level of progesterone will drop to a normal 50 pg/ml. This may not seem like a big deal, but to the body it's a drastic change. Just think, from 2200 pg/ml to 50 pg/ml! The change can create potential problems. At the post-partum stage, mothers can experience depression, anxiety and intolerable headaches.

Progesterone is pregnancy's centerpiece. If the egg isn't fertilized, then the inner lining of the uterine wall gets washed by a new menstrual cycle.

Progesterone's third stage is a very important phase in a woman's menstrual cycle. It can take so many turns that if an ovum isn't fertilized on day 21, then the bleeding begins.

***pg/ml: number of **picograms** per milligram*

Cysts, fibroids and tumors

Estrogen has a tendency to stimulate breast cell growth, thereby leading to possible cystic changes of the breast as well as uterine and ovarian fibroids.

Increasing your intake of bioidentical progesterone will enable you to modulate and decrease the incidence of fibroid, cysts and tumurous growths on soft tissues like your breasts, uterus and ovaries. Estrogen's effects on breast tissues, the ovaries, and the uterus is to create increased cellular multiplication in the breast, fibroid changes in the uterus, and polycystic and multi-cystic changes in the ovaries. All of these are problems that lead women to require therapy. One of the major benefits of progesterone is to monitor and moderate the multiplication of cells. When there is a proper balance of progesterone within the tissues of the breast, it actually prevents and diminishes the occurrence of breast cysts, fibroids and tumors.

Q: *"How do I prevent reoccurring cysts in my breasts?"*

—Nicholette, 24

A: *With increased breast tissue density, X-rays, like mammograms, can't discern whether the tumors are benign or malignant. In many of these cases, patients are left with no choice but to surgically remove these growths (which are most often harmless). Get a saliva test and check your progesterone levels. Progesterone levels should be 10-20 times higher than estrogen. If your levels are lower, you need immediate supplementation.*

Dr Tai's Health Pearl

Breasts full and painful?
   TOO MUCH ESTROGEN
Breasts droop and shrink?
   NEED MORE ESTROGEN
Rings slip on and off fingers?
   ESTROGEN LEVEL **OK**—PROGESTERONE **OK**
Can't sleep—wake up in middle of night?
   NEED MORE PROGESTERONE

Testimonial

"There was nothing I loved more than taking my rumbling hog out for a spin on a summer evening. My brother and I have been assembling and collecting motorcycles since our high school days. Every year, I go to an annual Harley drive with my bike gang down U.S. Highway 395, L.A. to Reno, but last year I missed out because of the terrible pain I experienced in both of my breasts.

"I'm what you'd call one tough cookie and I don't get sick often, but last year I had a scare. I asked myself, 'What if these cysts turn into tumors?' My mother died from breast cancer and so did two of my four aunts on my father's side. Breast cancer runs in my family and I missed the annual motoring tour with friends out of fear and pain that the same would eventually happen to me. When my twin brother left for the tour without me, I spoke to Tiffany, his wife, about the cysts. He was flyin' by the Death Valley desert while I was at home with Tiff sulking over a cup of tea. My sister-in-law is a bookworm whose favorite topic is the human body. She explained to me that my cysts were caused by too much estrogen and not enough progesterone.

"Before seeing a doctor, I used some of her progesterone cream. It was natural so I figured I'd try it before I needed to seek professional attention. In weeks my pain was minimized. In less than a month, the lump—gone! After the lump was completely gone, I saw Tiff's doctor and he saw that the cyst popped. He asked what I was using and I told him natural progesterone. To my surprise he said that he couldn't have given me better instructions. I'm glad to know how cysts form—now I know how to control them. I wish my mom and aunts knew about estrogen—it would have saved them headaches and it would have saved me three heartaches."

—Breightling, 40

Progesterone protecting men

Men produce progesterone in the adrenals, as opposed to women, who produce progesterone in their ovaries. Progesterone's main effect in men is its conversion into testosterone and balancing the negative effects of estrogen. As men age, they lose testosterone in their bodies. Progesterone grabs estrogen receptor sites as they pass throughout a man's body. Therefore, keeping receptor sites busy with a lot of progesterone can prevent estrogen from landing on those sites and causing tissue damage.

Many men have decided to increase their levels of progesterone for 2 reasons:

1) It provides a basis for testosterone conversion.
2) It occupies estrogen receptor sites in the prostate in order to avoid prostate complications like the development of prostate cancer.

Why is this an important issue?

Because, in the past, I've explained to you that estrogen has a propensity to cause the cells of these tissues to reproduce and multiply in an accelerated fashion. It has a tendency to multiply exponentially—if these tissues grab all of the estrogens, then these tissues become hypertrophied (enlarged). This is exactly how benign tumors grow on tissue sites.

Prostate problems

However, if enough progesterone is present, the progesterone hormone occupying the same receptor sites will moderate and diminish the production of the excess tissue created by estrogen. Because of this, men are less likely to experience enlarged prostates, a problem effecting more than 35 million men in the U.S. A lack of progesterone can make urinating painful and can lead to cancer.

As both men and women age, aromatization increases the production of testosterone to estrogen, or the production of estrogen from fat tissue. For men, testosterone is converted into estrogen. If we can use progesterone to occupy the receptor sites in the prostate, we can decrease estrogen's effects on the prostate. If the prostate receptor sites are occupied by progesterone, estrogen can't cause damage. We prefer the progesterone hormone to occupy those receptor sites, because without it, there's a greater likelihood of excess estrogen damage leading to tumorous prostate growths.

Stronger bones

The usage of liposome progesterone has a much higher rate of absorption than that of oral supplements, injections or patches. Until recently, progesterone has only been available in synthetic form. Through advanced technology, bioidentical progesterone can be directly transported through the skin's epidermis and into your dermis, where your blood absorbs it.

Throughout our lives, our bones—living organs—go through a continuous process in which old bone is broken down and new bone is created in its place. This remodeling of the bone is done by osteoblasts (cells that build) and osteoclasts (cells that break). As we age, the osteoclasts outnumber the osteoblasts and create more bone-breaking than bone-building. Estrogen is an essential property in bone production, because it can halt osteoporosis. Estrogen can do this because its sites are located on bones; however, in no way am I saying that men and women who are taking estrogen supplementation can't have osteoporosis. But, with excellent estrogen and progesterone balance the chances of this happening are much less likely.

Studying progesterone's effects on bones

In 1990, a physician from California, Dr. John R. Lee, conducted a three-year study with 100 post-menopausal patients aged 40 to 80. Dr. Lee noted that 63 of his study's participants, who had regular supplementation of progesterone, had an increase of bone mineralization by 15.4 percent. From his study, Dr. Lee concluded that by using transdermal bioidentical progesterone, the osteoporatic rate upon which bones demineralize can be delayed. (Lee, J.R. "Osteoporosis reversal with transdermal progesterone." *Lancet*, 1990; 336:1327.)

That same year, Dr. Jeri Lynn Prior at the University of British Columbia found that progesterone aided in the formation and maintenance of bones, as it was able to speed growth and healing rates.

Five years later, the PEPI trials (Postmenopausal Estrogen Progestin Interventions), one of the largest studies to have ever been conducted on progesterone, tracked 875 women aged 45 to 64 for approximately three years.

The researchers of this major study concluded that bioidentical estrogen, combined with bioidentical progesterone, had the most effect on raising HDL ("good" cholesterol) without producing the pre-cancerous uterine effects that synthetic forms of estrogen and progesterone tend to bring about. The PEPI trials clearly demonstrated that natural progesterone works better than progestin (synthetic progesterone) in protecting the heart and uterus.

Moving up the timeline to 2000, Dr. I.U. Schmidt wrote an article on the effects of estrogen and progesterone on the bones of rats. In his article, Dr. Schmidt demonstrated that estrogen, estradiol and progesterone together were able to remove or reduce the effects of osteoclast (bone removal) activity in rats. (Schmidt, I.U. "Tibia histomorphometry in growing rats." *Calcif Tissue*, 2000; 67: 47-52.)

Bioidentical progesterone can keep osteoporosis from damaging a woman's body. Progesterone stimulates ostoblastic (bone depositing) activities of the bone. Women may not always be too keen on vocalizing their pains, because at 40 (and up), I feel that women have had it with complaining. They realize they do it too often, and they feel that everyone's sick of hearing about their backaches, heads, shoulders, knees and toes, knees and toes. So, they refrain from expressing their displeasures with their current conditions. Sad but true—the worst part of the day for women is the night. I know this—I'm a husband, a doctor, a friend, a brother.

My patients don't need to tell me that they haven't slept in days because they're hurting. A woman who is 40 or older is walking evidence of an irregular sleeping schedule. The under-eye bags, the dark circles, the hunched bodies—all of these images make it apparent that sleep, for many of these women, is nothing more than a daydream.

If women aren't sleeping at night, what do they do?

Well, they aren't practicing the Karma Sutra moves they've read up on, that's for sure. Instead, they wander throughout the house, watch TV or, in worst case scenarios, cry.

I've never understood their emotional outbursts until my interest in endrocrinology and natural medicine grew. I thought that after 40 should be the happiest time for women. Their kids are off to college. They're living their lives. Ahhh, job well done, Mom, you deserve a pat on the back. You're working, your husbands are working. But, no, no—something's missing. Ladies, you're sad, and you're hurting.

During menopause, women suffer mostly at night. This is when they experience severe anxiety, nervousness, depression, fear, hot flashes, headaches, muscle and bone pain, sometimes even spasms. All this because of terribly low levels of progesterone. Women of the world, there is an answer for you! It's progesterone! Doctors can help you. Get a saliva test and start off on a bioidentical form of progesterone. I am sure it will come to you in the form of cream. If and when it does, apply to your upper body. It will take a few days for you to adjust to this new routine, but understand that there is no timeline. Once your hormones are gone, they're gone forever, which means you need to spend as much time as possible replenishing them.

Heartbreaker

Remarkably, progesterone possesses the quality of preventing blood clots that'll cause thrombophlebitis (moving blood clots). Synthetic estrogen excess can create thrombophlebitis. Trust me, the condition is as serious as its name. It occurs when clots form inside your leg's veins (as well as other deep veins), break away and migrate to your heart! Eek—from your legs to your heart?! Yuppers. Watch out—when that happens, it's deadly.

I know these women exist—I've seen them wearing khaki shorts and fanny packs. Some of them are sneaks, hiding their legs in pants or in dark stockings because their legs are crammed with veins that look like giant green spiders. Varicose veins and spider veins are nothing more than oversized veins with possibly dry blood that don't look nice and aren't healthy.

Progesterone is able to moderate the excess effects that cause thrombophlebitis. It also improves the spasticity of the heart's many blood vessels. It's a very interesting phenomenon that women oftentimes have complications of the coronary arteries that go way beyond the typical clot and existence of plaque. Throughout the duration of menopause, many women suffer from severe coronary artery spasms leading to heart disease. Progesterone can relieve the body from producing fatal myocardial infarctions or deadly heart spasms so that your heart can continue beating.

CooCoo without progesterone

Do you want to protect your brain from dementia, Alzheimer's and senility?
No problem! Try dermal liposome progesterone cream before your biological clock gives you trouble!

—*Wendy Liebman*

Higher progesterone levels are actually able to play a significant role in regenerating and protecting the neuron cells of the brain. This allows for a healthier cellular brain as well as improvement to memory and sharpness of thinking. Progesterone not only has a direct effect on neural functions—it also moderates sugar metabolism as it increases oxygenation of the brain and other body tissues. See MaxPerformance Specialist.

Progesterone refill

The healthiest women I know are consistent with a bioidentical progesterone plan. Have you heard of Suzanne Somers? Sure you have! She's gorgeous because she's been balancing her hormones, and she's continuing to balance them. Somers blows some of my daughter's friends out of the water. She's a beautiful woman because she's a smart woman. She's taking care of herself. Why can't you? Why shouldn't you?

Take care of yourself! I feel like I'm yelling, but I'm not—I'm shouting a manifesto that'll hopefully prompt you to rebel against bad habits that you've developed. Knock the habit and balance your hormones naturally. When you're feeling like the sexy woman you know you are, don't thank me—thank yourself.

The case of synthetic vs. natural progesterone

Synthetic progesterone is called medroxy progesterone acetate, or MPA. It's a chemically modified progesterone that isn't at all compatible to the progesterone the body produces. This class of drugs is called progestin, which is nothing close to a bioidentical form of progesterone.

Pharmaceutical companies want you to believe that MPA is similar to natural progesterone (baloney!). It may have only 8% biologic activity similar to a natural progesterone. Over 90% of synthetic progesterone is foreign to the body and its tissue receptor sites.

Studies have shown synthetic progesterone increases the risk of breast cancer by 800% compared to the use of estrogen alone. *Brownstein, D., Overcoming Thyroid Disorders. West Bloomfield, MI:Med. ALtern. Press, 2002.*

The Journal of the American Medical Association published that the risk of breast cancer increases nearly 80% after 10 years of estrogen-progestin (synthetic progesterone) and 160% after 20 years. *Schairer, C., JAMA 2000; 283:485-491.*

Dr. Stephen Sinatra, Cardiologist—"I have found that synthetic progestins can lead to serious cardiac side effects in my patients, including shortness of breath, fatigue, chest pain, and high blood pressure." Sinatra, S. *Heart Sense for Women.* Washington DC: *Lifeline Press, 2000.*

Testimonial

"I've been transformed by the power of bioidentical hormones. I can tell you that I started to grow lumps in my breasts the size of peaches—I am not exaggerating! My lumps were so bad, and my bone density so thin, I wasn't allowed to receive a mammogram scan because my doctor was afraid it would affect my already frail bones.

"I didn't know what to do. I tried going to multiple hospitals looking for help from at least a dozen doctors and they all said the same thing: 'Test results come out normal, you're fine.' Or, 'It's in your head. Maybe if you stop stressing you'll feel better.' The truth was, I was stressing because no one knew what the heck was wrong with me, until a doctor tried a different approach—he checked my saliva.

"From my saliva panel, the doctor concluded that I was producing way too much estrogen, which was the cause of my agonizing periods, painful cysts and tender breasts. I started taking natural progesterone to balance my estrogen levels and within weeks I

Dr. Tai just jokin' around:

"I don't trust my doctor anymore. I saw him giving a mammogram with his Xerox machine."

—David Corrado

understood what the missing link was. I had no idea hormones do so much for the body. There isn't a day that goes by that I don't bless the doctor that told me exactly what my problem was. Every night I rub 20 mg of progesterone, and every morning I rub 10 mg of the cream on my chest. Months ago, my emotional being was at jeopardy because of the way I felt physically. Thank you, progesterone, for helping me smile again!"

—Georgia, 42

The Good Power of Natural Progesterone. Laux, M., Natural Woman, Natural Menopause, NY: HarperCollins, 1997.

1. **Balances estrogen**
2. **Doesn't accumulate in the body**
3. **Improves sleep**
4. **Calms the body naturally**
5. **Improves high blood pressure**
6. **Enhances burning of body fats**
7. **Lowers Cholesterol**
8. **May Protect from breast cancer**
9. **Enhances growth of scalp hair**
10. **Improves libido**
11. **Helps to prevent hardening of the arteries.**

PROGESTERONE Self-Assessment	
Symptoms of Progesterone Deficiency Note: *If supplementation has already been taken *increase* dosage if following symptoms are experienced:	Symptoms of: Progesterone excess Note: *If supplementation has already been taken *decrease* dosage if following symptoms are experienced:
• Premenstrual syndrome • Depression/Mood swings • Anxiety nervousness/irritability • Breast swelling • Bloating/ water retention • Bone loss/Osteoporosis • Uterine fibroids • Excessive menstrual bleeding • Decrease HDL • Insomnia	• Hot flashes made worse • Increases Cortisol • Decreases glucose tolerance • Increases fat storage • Increases appetite / Carbo cravings • Depression • "Drunk" feelings • Water retention caused by progesterone supplementation • Drowsiness

Causes of Low Progesterone

- Low Luteonizing hormone (LH)
- Increased prolactin production
- Stress
- Antidepressants
- Excessive Arginine consumption
- Sugar
- Saturated Fat
- Deficiency of vitamins A, B6, C, zinc
- Decreased Thyroid hormones

Taking Progesterone:

Q: *"Now that I no longer have any of these symptoms, do I still have to take supplementation?"*

—*From no one in particular—this is a frequently asked question*

A: *Of course—supplementation is an extremely important step for prevention. Estrogen and progesterone together protect the heart and prevent tumorous growths from occurring. It preserves the memory and your ability to keep a younger more youthful look. If you want to continue with supplementation, use a balanced estrogen and progesterone. Apply transdermal liposome daily to your skin. You can use bioidentical estrogen cream on your genital area as a preventative for genital atrophy. Use this supplementation from day 7 to day 28 and go 5-7 days without it.*

∽Dr. Tai's Anti-Aging Health Secret∽

When you are having your period and you're having mood swings, anxiety attacks and experiencing depression, look in a saliva sampling for progesterone specifically from the 21st to the 28th day of your cycle. Most PMS symptoms occur near the period and can be helped with supplemental transdermal liposome progesterone when applied throughout the body from day 14-28, or the first day of bleeding, whichever comes first.

For most menopausal women, the optimum plan requires you to follow just two simple instructions. First, test your estrogen and progesterone levels via a saliva hormone test. Second, use supplemental progesterone on the upper torso, around the breasts, all over your chest, making your way down to your tummy and rubbing it in vigorously. Make sure the cream is spread widely across your skin—working the cream vigorously into the skin will generate a good circulation. This will assure the largest spreading of progesterone throughout the body and prevent a concentration of the hormone in one small area. Start the supplementation on day 7 of your cycle, and continue with 20 mg in the evening and 20 mg in the morning from day 7 to day 28. Discontinue supplementation from day 1 to day 7.

It doesn't matter whether you have your menstrual period—you still should discontinue supplementation on day 28 and stop supplementation for 5-7 days. We do have individuals from time to time who choose to use the supplementation every day with no five-day break, but again, that's completely up to doctor's stipulations. I've heard of no harm done to patients that haven't discontinued supplementation, but it's only advised to give your body a break. Follow nature and do what you feel. However, ask your doctor if you have the kind of health where you can just follow nature.

If you are perimenopausal or menopausal, make sure that your diet is in rich in calciferous vegetables. I advise you eat a lot of cauliflower, broccoli and Brussels sprouts. All of these produce a large amount of 1-3 carbonyl; when combined with stomach acid and DI indolylmethane (DIM) (both natural compounds), two kinds of aromatase inhibitors are produced, decreasing the conversion of essential testosterone to estrogen.

"My favorite progesterone studies"
  * For additional studies see references

1) *American Family Physicians, 1999; 16(1): 264.*
  • Side effects of progestin (synthetic progesterone) included bloating, nausea and depression. Natural progesterone eliminated these side effects.
2) *American Family Physicians, 2000; 62(8):1839.*
  • Obtained from plant sources, progesterone has fewer side effects when compared to synthetic progestins.
3) *Mayo Clinic, Women's Health Source, August 1999, p.3.*
  • Surveys show that women prefer the use of natural progesterone over synthetic progestins.
  • Progesterone is not associated with abnormal metabolites found in synthetic progestins.

Progesterone Saliva Reference

Female: Progesterone pg/ml
Test Result Reference

	AGE	REFERENCE RANGE	ASSESSED OPTIMUM RANGE WITH SUPPLEMENT	ASSESSED OPTIMUM RANGE WITH TRANSDERMAL
			100-2500	200-5000
Follicular 1/14 days	FS	28-82		
Luteal 15/28 days	L	127-446		
	Post Menopause	18-51		
Ratio: Progesterone / Estradiol ≥ 20				

Male: Progesterone pg/ml
Test Result Reference

		REFERENCE RANGE	ASSESSED OPTIMUM RANGE WITH SUPPLEMENT	ASSESSED OPTIMUM RANGE WITH TRANSDERMAL
		<51	20-100	200-2500

SECRET VI

"Youth is happy because it has the ability to see beauty. Anyone who keeps the ability to see beauty never grows old."
—Franz Kafka

Chapter 12

Melatonin: *a hormone secreted by the pineal gland in the brain that is important in the regulation of many hormones in the body. Among its key roles, melatonin controls the body's circadian rhythm, an internal 24-hour time-keeping system that plays an important role in when we fall asleep and when we wake up.*

—Stedman's Medical Dictionary

Months ago, I decided to spend some time browsing the Web researching "helpful sleeping tips." During lunch breaks, America was trying to figure out how to sleep better at night. I was surprised—sleep should be simple, yet it's become one of the most difficult things to do, especially as a person ages. This is because of diminishing melatonin levels.

Americans are some of the hardest-working people in the world. This was a disturbing thought; how were such hard-working people experiencing such difficulty sleeping?

Snap out of it! Wake up and pay attention to this chapter. I need you up so we can talk about how you can lie down and stay down for at least six to eight hours.

What to expect

What is melatonin?

How is melatonin produced?

Functions of Melatonin

Melatonin and growth

Sleep

Testimonial

Published research

Jet lag

Self-assessment

Taking melatonin

Anti-aging Health Secret

"It's been a hard day's night, and I've been working like a dog. It's been a hard day's night, and I should be sleeping like a log."
—The Beatles
A Hard Day's Night **(1964)**

Melatonin, made from...?

Created from the pineal (say peen-ee-al) gland, melatonin is the hormone responsible for the "circadian cycle," or the sleep/wake cycle. The pineal gland is a tiny gland in the center of the brain, so tiny it resembles a pea or a kernel of corn. During your first few weeks of growth in your mother's womb, your pineal gland was one of the first organs that grew. It doesn't have access to light, because it is situated deep within the brain, but it does contain light-sensitive cells. When light enters the eyes, it travels to the retina. From the retina, a message is sent through the optic nerve to the hypothalamus (a much bigger gland than the pineal) and that's when the pineal is informed that there is light (or when there is an absence of it). Scientists used to think the pineal was as useless as a person's pinky finger, but without the tiny organ, the body wouldn't have any melatonin, a modulating hormone that relaxes us and processes environmental information, like when it's a good time to get some ZzZs.

Assembling melatonin: the factory line

Light▯ eyes▯ retina▯ cells in retina▯optic nerve▯ hypothalamus▯ pineal gland▯ MELATONIN

Good morning, America!

Allow me to reiterate that hormones go through spurts during different times of the day. Melatonin is a prime example of this because it peaks between 2 and 5 a.m. and then drops as the sun rises; this usually happens at around 7-8 a.m.

Melatonin production

Melatonin is produced by enzymatic conversion from the amino acid tryptophan. Stress depletes tryptophan . You need tryptophan along with vitamin B complex to convert tryptophan into melatonin.

During stressful times, tryptophan depletion leads to a reduction in melatonin, and melatonin is one of the few hormones that actually lowers cortisol levels to help keep you cool, calm and collected when life gets crazy.

Functions of Melatonin

1. Induces sleep
2. Improves mood
3. Helps stress response
4. Assists immune system function
5. Stimulates release of sex hormones
6. Has powerful antioxidant effects *Bland J., "Obesity and endocrine signaling." Health Comm International, Inc. 1999, p.124.*
7. Helps prevent cancer
8. Blocks estrogen binding to receptors. *Lieberman, S., The Real Vitamin and Mineral Book. Avery Publ. 1997.p.216*
9. Stimulates parathyroid bone formation. *Lieberman, S., The Real Vitamin and Mineral Book. Avery Publ. 1997.p.216*
10. Production of growth hormone
11. Decreases and modulates cortisol

Powerful Melatonin Facts

At menopause there is a severe decline in melatonin secretion. *Lieberman, S., The Real Vitamin and Mineral Book. Avery Publ. 1997.p.216*

Research shows that melatonin and testosterone are partners in the synthesis of each other. *Duell, P., "Clin Chem 1998; 44(9):1931-1936.*

Studies have revealed that melatonin is lower in patients with heart disease than healthy patients. *Lieberman, S., The Real Vitamin and Mineral Book. Avery Publ. 1997.p.216*

Helping the world grow

"If each of our hormones were one of the seven dwarves, melatonin would be 'Sleepy.'"

Do you recall your mom ever telling you that if you don't get to bed you won't grow? Well, she was right. Sleeping helps children grow. As a matter of fact, children grow as they sleep. During the adolescent stage, melatonin blood levels reach a new high. These surging levels of melatonin signal the pituitary gland to produce luteinizing hormone (LH) and follicle-stimulating hormone (FSH) when puberty

Study: Melatonin helps fight diseases

Melatonin is rarely thought of as an antioxidant, but D.X. Tan (et al.), a researcher, found that its radical scavenger activities are surprisingly potent. In a lab study conducted on rats, Tan found that melatonin possesses abilities similar to that of glutathione. He saw that over an extended period of time, the rats that had been fed melatonin fought illness much quicker than the rats that hadn't. Tan concluded that melatonin strengthens cell receptors and helps bodies fight diseases (Tan, D.X., et al. "Melatonin: A potent indigenous hydroxyl radical scavenger." *Journal of Endocrinology*,

begins. It's all downhill from there, because after puberty, melatonin production begins to decline. This is the reason your eldest neighbors are up at the break of dawn power-walking. You don't think they'd be sleeping for a few extra minutes if they could? Please…you know it! By age 60, we produce half the amount of melatonin we produced in our 20s. Once we lose the ability to produce proper amounts of melatonin, it is more difficult to fall asleep than it is to wake up.

What are the Causes of Decrease in Melatonin?

Beta blockers	Aspirin
Calcium channel blockers	Caffeine
Alpha adrenergic blockers	Alcohol
Ibuprofen	Tobacco
Tranquilizers	Electromagnetic fields

What are the causes of Increase in Melatonin?

Supplementation	Darkness
Sleep	Exercise

Sleep? Who needs sleep?
You do!

As society continuously becomes more and more competitive, class systems become distinct, the rich become richer, and the poor become poorer. Why sleep for eight hours when you could work for eight hours and make money? Well, because, if you didn't sleep, you would be digging an early grave for yourself. The human body can only go so long without sleep. In a study conducted by researcher Alan Rechtshaffen, rats died after two weeks of sleep deprivation. Although no deaths were reported from sleep deprivation in humans, at most, people can tolerate going 11 days without sleep. Not only will you feel like dying without sleep, but you'll look like death. Rechtshaffen also found that the skin, the body's largest organ, suffers most from sleep deprivation.

Years ago, I had a neighbor who was a lawyer. He was a short, portly man whom we'll call Larry. At that time, Larry was no older than 40, yet he seemed much older, maybe because I rarely saw his face. He had a tendency to walk with his head down; I don't think I've ever seen anyone study their own shoes more than he did. Larry reminded me so much of a pit bull, a tired looking pit bull. He was a few strands away from being bald and his wrinkles were deep. His cheeks drooped and he looked like he'd gotten into one too many messy fights in his life. Larry had bruises around his eyes--two dark circles outlined by a pair of tortoise-shell eyeglasses.

Larry told me that he hadn't slept in days, and because he hadn't slept in days it showed in the courtroom. I'll never forget the expression on Larry's face. Boy, was he sad, I felt guilty for thinking he was a nerd, an anti-social kind of guy who would only talk to people if they'd pay him to talk for them. He wasn't—in fact, Larry was one of the nicest guys you would ever meet.. Nevertheless, he was desperate and had taken all sorts of scrambled routes just to fall asleep, like taking sleeping pills, sedatives and overdosing (on more than one occasion) on Nyquil. I explained to Larry that his melatonin levels were depleting at an above-average rate and that he'd have to replenish his lost hormones somehow. To my surprise, he was a good lawyer and did his research. He replenished his lost melatonin levels using a bioidentical form of melatonin: a supplement which consisted of a whole family of different antioxidants and alpha lipoic acid—called Antioxidant Specialist.

Helping Larry identify his problem prompted the realization of just how much more effective natural medicine is than any sort of pharmaceutically compounded prescription. Months afterward, I saw Larry again, and he told me that he'd been sleeping.

By sleeping more, people lower levels of stress, so for those of you who are passionate about getting ahead, do it by getting a little more "R&R."

Rest and relaxation

With the ability to get better sleep, you'll strengthen your immune system and will decrease your chances of developing obesity. A lack of sleep will generate a host of bodily problems. You'll find that with a few more hours of restful sleep, you'll be more productive and thus much more able to accomplish all of your goals.

Testimonial

"I'm a chef at one of Seattle's top restaurants. It's taken me years to develop a reputation and climb ranks. After a number of excellent restaurant reviews, we've had a great deal of celebrities pop their heads in, expecting me to deliver perfection on a plate. Our menu consists of prime meats and fine wines from all over the world. A number of things make my restaurant a great place: the ambience, the staff and above all, my food. But last year, I was close to losing all of that.

"I had to wake up at 4 a.m. to prep for a party of 250. It was a celebration for a luxocrat's daughter—she was graduating from dental school, and her father, a prominent figure in Seattle, kept a close eye for details. He wanted everything perfect and who could blame him? It was his only child (I too am a father of one, and I know what it's like).

"I woke up at 9 a.m. when I was supposed to be up five hours prior. Nothing could wake me—not my phone, not my alarm clock not even my wife's morning cell-phone wake-up call. Thank goodness for my dependable prep cooks—my absence could have cost my career. I was upset with myself because it could have been prevented somehow. I knew it was because the night before, I went to bed at 3 a.m., and the day before, I fell asleep at 4 or 5 a.m. Before I started taking melatonin, I was sleeping 20 hours a week. Sleeping pills and syrups kept me asleep longer, and when I woke up, I felt drowsy, so I tried an herbal sedative--melatonin. The first few nights it didn't do much for me, but as I adjusted the dosage to fit me, after a week I could fall sleep at around 12 midnight. It's been 30 days since I've used melatonin, and I jump right out of bed. I've lowered my doses because my body has adapted a sleep-wake cycle. Today, instead of being known as the night owl, I'm the morning lark."

—*Michael, 36*

Dr. Tai's fun fact:

About half of America's population age 65 and up suffer from some sort of sleeping disorder.

Goodnight, and good luck
Sleeping pills for people who want to sleep

Temporary sleep relief is habit-forming and can leave you feeling groggy in the morning and unsatisfied at the amount of sleep you received the night before. Sadly, sleep, a physiologically normal function as important as eating, drinking and having sex, is being managed by a multitude of drugs. Sure, sleep sedatives will help for a few nights, but they'll also cause a variety of health problems along the way like raising your blood pressure.

After reviewing a multitude of studies, I've seen that sleeping pills can also produce hangover effects and can be addictive, which means "once you pop, you *won't* stop."

> **Even insomniacs fall asleep in record time while on melatonin. What makes you think you can't?**

Studies: melatonin and sleep

In 1991, Dr. M. Dahlitz (et al.) published "Delayed sleep syndrome response to melatonin" in the *Lancet Journal*. Melatonin was administered to 1,000 study participants, half of them took placebos while the other half took 5 milligrams of melatonin every night, for one month. Researchers recorded that the group, which was treated with melatonin fell asleep faster than the group that didn't. (Dahlitz, M., et al. "Delayed sleep syndrome." *Lancet*, 1991; 337:1121-1124.)

> **It's obvious—melatonin will help you fall asleep faster and stay asleep longer.**

Dr. A. Oldani (et al.) conducted a study with six subjects experiencing insomnia. By taking melatonin, the subjects were able to fall asleep 115 minutes sooner than when they didn't take melatonin. (Oldani, A., et al. "Melatonin: delayed sleep and phase syndrome ambulatory polygraphist evaluation." *Neuro Report*, 1994; 6:132-134.)

What about frequent flyers?

Routinely, I cross three to four time zones, but at least half a dozen times a year I cross 12-14 time zones. I travel frequently due to my teaching schedule. I travel for conventions, seminars, conferences and lectures. I wish I'd have the time to travel more for pleasure, but it's usually for professional purposes. This is what makes the task of going somewhere a bit more tedious, but I realize that I must. Instead of thinking, "I want to," I tell myself, "I have to." I don't mind it as much as I used to, because, finally, I can sleep!

Jet lag used to torture me. It never failed—I learned the routine. I'd get off the plane, find a hotel and wake up completely lost. Days after, I couldn't help but feel groggy. Depending on the time zone, I'd get sleepy either too early or not early enough. The worst trips used to be traveling to Asia. Even now, I don't care too much for traveling so many hours.

Flights to Japan usually last up to 12 hours, which means for 12 hours I'm confined to 24 inches of space, having no choice but to breathe the same air everyone else passes gas in, while sitting next to an annoying person that makes jumping off the plane seem like a fabulous idea.

Sitting for such a long period of time will clog veins and make muscles tense. You'll become anxious and grow frustrated if you don't try to get some sleep or do something that holds your interest like writing or reading to calm your nerves and help you think happy thoughts.

Personally, I manage to get some work done on flights. I prep for my lectures or work on tweaking speeches. But what I found most difficult about the whole ordeal of just getting there was adjusting to the new time zone.

The days that followed led me feeling so heavy! I felt like I was carrying all the pilots and flight attendants on my back. My speech was affected, I was dazed and confused, and I became constipated. There is nothing worse than having a five-course meal with challenging doctors and not being able to produce some sort of a bowel movement...

Practice what'cha preach, docta

I finally started taking my own advice—I started taking melatonin. By regulating my sleeping schedule, I'm able to go on with my life. I eat regularly and attempt to visit the restroom at normal schedule. Anyway, I love melatonin. Without it, my lectures aren't as entertaining.

Now, because I get adequate amounts of sleep, I can tell people enjoy my presence a lot more. I'm more confident even when I'm out of my element, far away from home, because with melatonin, I feel very much at home. I personally take, on average, 2 mg at bedtime. For every time zone I cross, it takes 3-4 days to get completely adjusted. Melatonin is a very powerful antioxidant and you need it when traveling and changing time zones.

Study: Jet lag's a drag!

A clinical study conducted by Dr. K. Petrie (et al.) showed that by taking a melatonin supplement one can minimize subjective feelings of jet lag from a 4.5-day recovery period to a 2.85-day recovery period.

It's been proven that melatonin will save at least two days of your trip. With a quicker recovery period, you can devote more time to shopping and sightseeing instead of moping around your hotel room.

MELATONIN Self-Assessment	
Symptoms of Melatonin Deficiency Note: *If supplementation has already been taken *increase* dosage if following symptoms are experienced:	**Symptoms of: Melatonin Excess** Note: *If supplementation has already been taken *decrease* dosage if following symptoms are experienced:
• Insomnia • The inability to stay asleep • Waking periodically throughout the night • Jet lag • Difficulty adjusting to time zones	• Sleepy/ groggy after waking • The inability to wake • Reoccurring nightmares, or unpleasant dreams • Daytime sleepiness / Fatigue • Suppressed serotonin • Suppressed craving for sugar • Increased cortisol and fat • Headache

Dosage:
Minimum: 0.5 mg
Maximum: 50 mg

On melatonin, you're supposed to fall asleep in hour. If you don't fall asleep minutes before or after an hour, you should increase your dosage. These are my guidelines; however, you have to do what is right for you. If you feel that 0.5 mg isn't helping in any way, make sure to increase your dosage to adjust to your needs. *There are no long term negative side effects.*

⇜Dr. Tai's Anti-Aging Health Secret⇝

I only wish you good nights and even better mornings. This is why I want to assure you that by taking bioidentical melatonin, I am confident that you will fall asleep quicker. I'm also sure that when you begin to use melatonin, you'll feel much more rested in the morning. I had a terrible time falling asleep, and out of all the supplements I've used, melatonin has never failed me. It's been two years since I've started taking melatonin and I've developed so much energy because I sleep straight through the night instead of waking up at irregular intervals as I once used to. When I travel, I make sure to bump up my dosage, only because it strengthens my immunities and helps me fight jet lag. I take melatonin on a nightly basis, and ever since, my dreams and days have become sweeter than ever!

Chapter 13

Thyroid: *one of the larger endocrine glands in the body. It is a double-lobed structure located in the neck that produces hormones, principally thyroxin (T4) and triiodothyronine (T3) that regulate the rate of metabolism and affect the growth and rate of function of many other systems in the body.*

—Stedman's Medical Dictionary

"**Shaped like a butterfly, stings like a bee (if you don't treat it when need be).**" I've added a twist to Muhammad Ali's aphorism to describe the gland too many people all too often underestimate. More than 10 million people worldwide are diagnosed with hypothyroidism, or underactive thyroid and many more go undiagnosed. Hypothyroidism develops when the thyroid gland (butterfly-shaped gland just below the Adam's apple) fails to produce or secrete as much thyroxin (T4) as the body needs. Conversely, hyperthyroidism is an *overactive* thyroid. An overproduction of thyroid can be just as bad, or worse than underproduction. The body is a machine, and with proper thyroid care, your machine has enough fuel to function at its best.

What to expect

Thyroid functions

Thyroid and the pituitary gland

T3 and T4

Hypothyroid

Iodine / Iodide

Hyperthyroid

Thyroid's effects on:
Metabolism
Hair
Skin
Nails
Libido

Thyroid support diet plan

Self-assessment

Synthetic vs. natural

Anti-aging Health Secret

"My favorite thyroid studies"

Thyroid 101

The thyroid gland secretes thyroid hormones, which control how fast or how slow the body's chemical functions proceed (metabolic rate). Thyroid hormones influence the metabolic rate in two ways: by stimulating almost every tissue in the body to produce proteins, and by increasing the amount of oxygen that cells use. Thyroid hormones affect many vital body functions: the heart rate, the respiratory rate, the rate at which calories are burned, skin maintenance, growth, heat production, fertility and digestion.

The two thyroid hormones are T4 (thyroxin) and T3 (triiodothyronine). T4, the major hormone produced by the thyroid gland, has only a slight, if any, effect on speeding up the body's metabolic rate. Instead, T4 is converted into T3, the more active hormone. The conversion of T4 to T3 occurs in the liver and other tissues. Many factors control the conversion of T4 to T3, including the body's needs from moment to moment and the presence or absence of other illnesses.

To produce thyroid hormones, the thyroid gland needs iodine, an element contained in food and water (more on iodine later). The thyroid gland traps iodine and processes it into thyroid hormones. As thyroid hormones are used, a small amount of the iodine contained in the hormones is released, returns to the thyroid gland, and is recycled to produce more thyroid hormones.

T4 / Thyroxine

Eighty percent of the body's thyroid is made of T4 which regulates such essential functions as heart rate, digestion, physical growth, and mental development. An insufficient supply of T4 can slow life-sustaining processes, damage organs and tissues in every part of the body, and lead to life-threatening complications. And when I say life-threatening complications, I mean it in every sense—a weak thyroid can tear your world apart, affecting your personal, professional, romantic and social life. T4 turns into T3 in the liver or kidneys. T4 can also convert into an inactive reverse T4.

Let's play a game: Read the following paragraph and then close your eyes and visualize it. If you're able to visualize while reading, don't worry about closing your eyes.

Imagine

Imagine yourself 10, 15, OK, let's bump it up to 50 pounds heavier. You've become a nightmare, a slob! All day you schlep around the house, up and down the stairs, proceeding at insect speed while wearing sweat pants you haven't washed in a month! The only thing you do quickly is snap at pitiable souls that are too scared to debate with you. You're snappy and anxious to start the most random arguments, and really, who could blame you? You're fat and you haven't eaten in days (if not, weeks). In one week, you've had, oh, let's say, four to five meals at most. Your refrigerator, cabinets and pantry are empty on purpose. You think the less you eat, the more weight you'll lose, and you've held this philosophy all your life. Sure, it worked when you were 20, but I highly doubt that you're 20. (If you are, why are you reading this? Go enjoy life!) You've rid your secret hiding spot (your underwear drawer) of candy bars, packaged bon-bons, chocolate and gummy bears from four Halloweens ago; you know—the stash you keep aside for a "rainy day."

Exaggerations aside, if you feel like you're similar to the made-up version I've created for you, than you're one of the millions of people I've described who experience hypothyroidism.

Interesting Facts about Thyroid

1. No thyroid—no increase in muscle. Thyroid hormones influence muscle metabolism. Low thyroid does not build muscle.
2. Low thyroid directly causes low pregnenolone. *Tagawa, N., Clinc Chem 2000; 46:523-528.*
3. Thyroid dysfunction is associated with heart disease. *Rouzier, N., Longevity and Preventive Medicine Symposium. 2002.*
4. Decreased T3 hormone causes increase of cholesterol up to 50% and LDL. *Brownsten, D. Overcoming Thyroid Disorders. Medical Alt. Press, 2002. p.8*
5. Low thyroid hormones associated with chronic fibromyalgia. *Brownsten, D. Overcoming Thyroid Disorders. Medical Alt. Press, 2002. p.8*

Functions of Thyroid

1. Modulates carboydrates, protein, and fat metabolism.
2. Directs proper utilization of vitamin
3. Improves digestion
4. Affects function of mitochondria (energy of the cells)
5. Stimulates muscle growth and repairs metabolism
6. Controls electrical transaction of nerve activities
7. Increases blood flow
8. Improves overall bodily hormone excretion
9. Improves utilization of oxygen
10. Modulates sexual function

Thyroid and the body

Well, who cares about the thyroid when you have your heart, lungs, kidneys and liver to worry about? The thyroid is small, split into two and you can live without it if you're on the right meds. This is true if you don't care about your appearance, sex drive, body temperature, sleep patterns, and mental and emotional characteristics.

Your thyroid affects all of your organs. One chapter on the thyroid gland is far too small for such an important gland. Due to the other topics I must discuss, I have a limited amount of space so a lot of information is packed here.

> The ovaries have thyroid receptors. Thyroid glands have ovarian receptors. Therefore, loss of testosterone and estradiol during menopause can cause lower thyroid function and production.
>
> -Pamela, S. HRT, The Answers. *Healthy Living Books.* 2003.

"I get no respect."
—Rodney Dangerfield

Public attention rarely focuses on the thyroid, a gland that doesn't receive nearly as much attention as the body's other organs and glands. Instead, throughout the years, much focus has been placed on America's most common problems (rarely examined at the root) such as obesity, memory loss and anxiety issues.

As a fast-paced nation, we love statistics. We like to know what the problem is and how many people like us have it, and that's how we've been conditioned to draw conclusions. Obesity is a common problem, so collectively we try to lose weight. Fast-food restaurants expand on healthier menus, people turn to sugar-free delights, gyms are exploding with memberships, and schools are banning vending machines. Memory loss is another common problem many have, as I, experienced on a first-hand basis. As a solution, companies are producing more herbal formulations to aid in brain-cell communication and information retention, while publications insert brain-teasers and puzzles into their pages. But did you ever for a moment, just stop and think, "Maybe it *isn't* my eating habits," or perhaps "Maybe it's *not* my age?"

Maybe... you're right.

I really do believe that more physicians should make a much bigger deal about the thyroid than they actually do. I'm convinced that nearly everyone has a thyroid problem. It'll probably be more often underactive than overactive, but nonetheless, your thyroid is abnormal. Though this may seem to be a sharp statement, it's true. If you've spent your days away from stress, in a meditative state and eating nothing but fiber-enriched foods and iodine-packed fish from undiscovered lands and waters since the coming of your baby teeth, then thyroid problems should be of no concern to you. But if you're living in the USA like me, where stress and fast food have become facts of life, then you, my friend, most definitely have a thyroid problem.

Thyroid problems: Consider this

The thyroid is a gland that produces hormones vital for the upkeep of your body. It's essential for the metabolism and performance of almost every single organ and system in the body and has an effect on your metabolism, body composition, energy levels, mood, hair and skin.

Let me put it this way:

The thyroid is an annoying gland. Like a silent cry-baby, the thyroid requires attention. Unlike babies who cry to announce their hunger or other discomforts to the world, you won't know what your thyroid needs until you find out what's wrong with it, and finding out what's wrong with your thyroid is a "pain in the neck" (pardon the pun).

Signs of hypothyroidism

Clinical signs of hypothyroidism (underactivity) and hyperthyroidism (overactivity) are confusing. Tests may not always confirm the diagnosis, since blood tests TSH, T4 and T3 alone give you inadequate information for complete diagnosis. Clinical symptoms are especially important in determining thyroid function/dysfunction. Auto-antibodies in the blood almost always test negative, and thyroid ultrasound studies are rare and uncommon (most clinics aren't equipped with this piece of equipment). All of these factors can make testing the thyroid a complicated process.

What causes Low Thyroid Hormone?

Low T4 and T3 is caused by deficiency in iodine and iodide, zinc, copper, Vitamin A, B2, B3, B6, C and Selenium.

So, what do I do?

Proteins in the blood carry thyroid hormones to targets: lungs, stomach, intestines, skin, hair, nails, the brain, the heart and the bones. Because thyroid hormones are attached to proteins, less than one percent floats freely in a person's bloodstream.

If your doctor knows the total TSH and T4 amount in your blood, he or she needs to order a second test to determine the unbound T3 (the active hormones). Also, please note that excessive levels of different hormones (e.g., testosterone) can give you false thyroid hormone results. Synthetic estrogens increase the amount of thyroxin-binding proteins in your body, creating a smaller number of unbound thyroid hormones.

What causes inadequate T4 conversion to active T3?

Selenium Deficiency	High carbohydrate diet
Stress	Elevated cortisol
Cadmium, mercury, or lead toxicity	Chronic illness
Starvation	Decreased kidney or liver
Inadequate protein intake	function

What Factors increase the conversion of T4 to active T3?

Supplementation of Selenium	Vitamin A, B2, E
Potassium	Growth hormone
Adequate Iodine/Iodide	Testosterone
Iron	Insulin
Zinc	Glucagons
Ashwaganda	Melatonin
High protein diet	Tyrosine

-Nishiyama, S., J. Am. Coll. Nut. 1994; 13:62-7.
-Meinhold, H. JAMA 1992; 19:8-12.
-Berry, M. Endocrine Rev 1992; 13"207-20
-Kohrle, J., Cell Mol. Life Sci 2000, 57:1853-63

Everyone has someone to answer to—the thyroid and the pituitary

The thyroid gland is under the control of the pituitary gland. When the level of thyroid hormones (T3 and T4) drops too low, the pituitary gland produces thyroid stimulating hormone (TSH), which stimulates the thyroid gland to produce more hormones. Under the influence of TSH, the thyroid will manufacture and secrete T3 and T4, thereby raising their levels in the blood. The pituitary senses this and responds by decreasing its TSH production.

Furnace and thermostat

The thyroid gland is like a furnace and the pituitary gland is like a thermostat. Thyroid hormones are like heat. When the heat gets back to the thermostat, it turns the thermostat off. As the room cools (the thyroid hormone levels drop), the thermostat turns back on (TSH increases) and the furnace produces more heat (thyroid hormones). The pituitary gland itself is regulated by another gland, known as the hypothalamus. The hypothalamus is part of the brain and produces TSH-releasing hormone (TRH), which tells the pituitary gland to stimulate the thyroid gland (release TSH). One might imagine the hypothalamus as the person who regulates the thermostat, since it tells the pituitary gland at what level the thyroid should be set.

Hypothalamus

The hypothalamus, located just above the pituitary gland in the brain, secretes thyrotropin, the releasing hormone, which causes the pituitary gland to produce TSH. The pituitary gland slows or speeds the release of TSH, depending on whether the levels of thyroid hormones circulating in the blood are getting too high or too low. The thyroid gland also produces the hormone calcitonin, which may contribute to bone strength by helping calcium to be incorporated into bone.

For those of you who love stats:

The thyroid gland makes approximately 80 percent of T4 and 20 percent of T3. However, the thyroid can only use so much of the T4 it produces, which is why it doesn't use much of it. In order for it to be a hormone that actually does something, it has to be activated by *enzymes to convert T4 to T3 (active thyroid hormone), which are then released into the bloodstream and are transported throughout the

Power of iodine

In a 1994 issue of the *Journal for Clinical Investigation*, researcher A.A.S. Berson (et al.) published an article examining the effects of iodine on rat thyroids. Based on his observations, iodine is broken into two organic component pools: thyroidal and extrathyroidal. In female rats, both pools concentrated in breast tissues more so than in male rats. In animal studies, both pools had approximately 7-13 milligrams (mg) of iodine. (Berson A.A.S. et al. "The effects of iodine on rat thyroids." *Journal of Clinical Investigations,* 1994; 33: 1533-1552.)

Iodine/Iodide & Fibroids

The following year, Erskin, another researcher, concluded thatdifferent issues respond in other ways to iodine. In iodine-deficient female rats, it was observed that iodine traveled into the chest cavity and rested within the breast tissues. When iodine and iodide were combined, benign growths in the rats decreased in size. It was concluded that iodine improves ovarian and breast fibroids and cysts while sidestepping abnormal metabolisms and breast cancer. (Erskin et al. "Iodine response in rates." *Biological Trace Element Research,* 1995; 49;209-219.)

body where they control metabolism (conversion of oxygen and calories to energy). Every cell in the body depends upon thyroid hormones for metabolism regulation.

Enzymes? What kind of enzymes?
The thyroid and iodine

The thyroid gland needs iodine in order to make thyroid hormones. Just to recap: The thyroid makes *two* hormones that it secretes into the blood stream. One is called thyroxine, which contains four atoms of iodine and is often called T4 for short. The other is called triiodothyronine, which contains three atoms of iodine and is often called T3.

Iodine

Iodine is vital for good thyroid function, which in turn is essential for health. Iodine deficiency during pregnancy and early infancy can result in cretinism (irreversible mental retardation and severe motor impairments). In adults, low iodine intake (or very high intake) can cause hypothyroidism. Hypothyroidism can manifest as low energy levels, dry or scaly or yellowish skin, tingling and numbness in extremities, weight gain, forgetfulness, personality changes, depression, anemia, prolonged and heavy periods in women, and loss of hair.

Where can I find iodine?
Concentration in humans

Iodine constitutes most of your T4 and T3 cell's weight; therefore, you can find iodine right below your Adam's apple in your thyroid. However, with a thyroid deficiency, you are most likely also lacking in iodide. However, iodide concentrates in breast tissues, ovaries and the uterus, where it helps regulate and prevent excess cell multiplication and growth.

America's bread basket

Most middle Americans who depend on the bread basket for most of their caloric intake have a minimal food source of iodine, known as "Goiter belt." People who live on coastal regions have a greater advantage due to the multiple sources of iodine found in seaweed and seafood.

Because iodine is found in oceanic flora and fauna, Asians, whose cultural diet is rich in seafood and seaweed, have significantly fewer thyroid problems than any other geographic group. Throughout my family history, we've depended on fish for sustenance, but because of my ever-increasing frenzied schedule, I have eaten whatever I could find for now almost half of my life. As a result of this, I suffered from hypothyroid in my later years. I'm still on thyroid supplementation.

Iodine is found mostly in fish, and to a lesser extent, in milk, eggs, fruits and meat. 200 to 300 micrograms of iodine a day are necessary to avoid severe thyroid problems, or iodine deficiencies, which have caused millions of people throughout the world to experience the weakening pain of goiters leading to hearing and speech defects and, in more severe cases, contributing to brain damage called cretinism.

Thyroid advice

For starters, try to take a pinch of iodized salt daily with your nutritious meal. You know, the one you eat three times a day packed full of nutrients—vegetables, fruits, proteins and active vitamins, minerals and active enzymes. This is the first step to nourishing the body and supporting your thyroid. Secondly, you could take supplemental seaweed or concentrated sources of iodine or iodide supplement. BEWARE: Industrial and restaurant salts are not iodized, therefore they contain no source of iodine.

Q: "I love salt. I'm of Mediterranean descent and my family members have always used a lot of salt in their cooking. Wouldn't I be a good candidate for hyperthyroid instead of hypothyroid?"

—Olivia, 28

A: Great question! Only specially iodized salt has supplemental iodine with increased salt intake. Even so, it has very small amount of iodine—200 micrograms. According to Dr. Abrahms and the United National Research Study, Chinese and Japanese people living in coastal regions have an average consumption of 15 milligrams of iodine and iodide, which is more than 1000 percent more than table salt. So go for it, but salt may cause water retention which can lead to hypertension and weight gain.

Besides testing my thyroid and getting iodine from a healthy diet, what else can I do?

Selenium and Exercise

Selenium is a mineral, meaning it is not of animal or vegetable origin. Like iodine, it is essential for the thyroid to create the enzyme that turns T4 to T3 thyroid hormones. As I've stated before, T3 is a much more active thyroid hormone than T4 in that when the thyroid releases these cells, only 10 percent of T3 is released, making lesser amounts of T3 more effective than larger amounts of T4. Selenium helps with the production of T3 and can ultimately lead to thyroid gland support.

Exercise is another aspect of the healthy thyroid protocol. It's possible to maintain a healthy thyroid without going to the gym every day. As a matter of fact, overexercising can exhaust the adrenals, which can in turn negatively affect the thyroid. Overexercise will exhaust the adrenals and exhaust the thyroid by causing weight to fluctuate (more on metabolism later). I suggest moderate exercise—a 20-minute jog in your neighborhood or a 30-minute walk in the park. Instead of driving, ride a bike; try to substitute convenience with body movement. The more activity, the better you'll feel. Exercise promotes a healthy self by improving heart and lung function while raising good cholesterol and strengthening muscles.

If you're trying to lose weight, you may want to increase mini-meals throughout your day, or graze so you don't overeat at mealtimes. Exercise four to five times a week instead of three. If you've been diagnosed with hypothyroid, your energy levels may be lower than everyone else's. This should be considered in your workout and serves as no excuse for you to not get moving.

Studying selenium

Lab tests done on rabbits, mice and guinea pigs show that selenium protected the warm blooded creatures against diabetes by exhibiting insulin-like effects; selenium not only supports the thyroid, but it works as an antioxidant by enhancing immune function.

In 1974, Dr. J.P Isaacs (et al.) delivered a speech at the Texas Heart Institute for coronary surgery and medicine on "Trace minerals, vitamins, hormones in treatment of heart disease." During his speech, Dr. Isaacs said half a thyroid grain along with vitamins (I'm assuming he spoke of antioxidants vitamin A, E and K, along with B vitamins) over a ten week period improved cardiovascular functions in patients, avoiding the problems of experiencing hypo- and hyperthyroid and heart problems.

Dr. Isaacs also stated that mothers who have sufficient amounts of iodine while pregnant can be a major predictor of their child's thyroid destiny. Sufficient iodine consumption is necessary early in a person's life in order to avoid future thyroid, and thus body, problems.

Since the heart is positively affected by exercise, hypothyroid can pose problems. Therefore, you need to make an extra effort throughout your supplementation period to be as active as possible, especially under circumstances when sleeping is something you can do all day and all night. Whatever you do, you need to get your heart pumping enough blood for a healthy respiratory and nervous system.

I would advise hyperthyroid patients to relax and exercise moderation until they've treated their thyroid problem. Hyperthyroid patients have above-average heartbeats, and exercising may be the basis for abnormally high heartbeats. I don't want anyone having a heart attack, so please proceed with caution; treat your thyroid and then get moving!

Metabolism

Hyperthyroid and hypothyroid can both be distinguished by how fast or how slow a person loses weight. Most people with hypothyroid have trouble losing weight, while most people who have a hyperthyroid experience trouble gaining weight.

T4 is required for the muscles of the stomach and intestines to push food along for digestion and excretion. When there isn't enough T4 present, food absorption is slow, which can result in delayed bowel movements. This is different from hyperthyroid, which usually results in diarrhea.

The heart plays a special role in metabolism. Thyroid hormone makes the heart beat faster, and when the heart beats faster, body temperature is raised. When the heart beats faster and body temperature is higher, the body increases the rate at which metabolism moves. The body doesn't have to be in motion to set internal signals of motion —if basal temperatures are warm and the heart beats at an accelerated rate, the body will need to use energy by burning calories. Because hypothyroid patients experience feeling cold frequently and have slower heartbeats, their bodies metabolize less calories, which makes losing weight seem like an impossible task.

Seeing that we Americans struggle endlessly to lose that last 5-25 pounds, you're probably asking yourself why anyone would want to complain about having an overactive thyroid. As a matter of fact, I bet you're wishing for hyperthyroid to happen to you, but based on my observations and experience, I can tell you that hyperthyroidism is no pretty sight and I wouldn't wish it upon the worst of my enemies.

Less common than hypothyroidism, hyperthyroidism is an illness that affects a few hundred thousand Americans each year and the consequences are monstrous.

Years ago in med school, I envied one of my classmates. I remember observing Terry in a molecular biology class. He seemed so sharp. Any time my professor would ask a question that required contemplation or intense problem-solving, Terry would answer on the spot. Terry was a genius. He looked like he was studying more than my other classmates because he appeared to look the worst. His eyelashes looked like they'd been glued to his eyebrows. He had these big, bulgy brown eyes, in which you could see infinitesimal red blood vessels, which seemed to congregate around the spherical border of both his pupils.

Terry agreed to help me study for the next exam. I observed him while we studied. He didn't drink coffee, yet he was so antsy. He ate massive amounts of food, all the time, every day. He professed that sometimes late in the evening he'd raid the refrigerator for food. Along with faint tremors, the inability to sit still, bulgy eyes and the unsatisfying desire to eat, he took excessive amounts of bathroom breaks.

Terry suffered from a hyperactive thyroid. Patients with hyperthyroidism have such elevated sugar and accelerated basal metabolism that their bodies absorb food at a hastened pace, which in turn creates a never-ending craving for sugar. This almost always leads to diabetes.

The skin, hair and nails

Hyperthyroid patients sweat more than hypothyroid patients because their bodies constantly have the heat on. The increased blood flow from an increase in thyroid hormone will make the hair greasy, the hands clammy, and the skin moist, wet and dewy.

In hypothyroid patients, the opposite occurs—instead of having moist skin, their skin is dry, their nails brittle, and their hair fragile and falling out.

Testimonial

"Graduating college early at 20, I became a laboratory technician. Subconsciously, I think I competed with my boyfriend of three years who is an overachiever. He obtained his bachelor's in two years while teaching swimming lessons to four-year-olds. Today, he is in law school, soon to graduate. I am contemplating my next move. He motivates me to push myself but I feel as if I have overdone it.

"I have not seen the doctor in months, yet I am fairly certain that something is gravely wrong with me. I abandoned my partner and saw my physician after experiencing a series of mentally and emotionally paralyzing symptoms. Sniffling away to the doctor's office, I told her I had not recovered from a cold I had developed two months ago. A kindred spirit, she was concerned at my neglect and conducted the works.

"After checking my temperature and advising me to check my own temperature in the morning for the whole week, she told me what the problem was—it was my thyroid. My doctor convinced me that complete recovery would occur to me maybe within days, but surely within weeks.

"I was eager to commence treatment. The assessment made me realize how delicate the thyroid is, and that it can be triggered by an array of factors like stress, a lack of iodine and periods of dieting and self-starvation. I had done all of those things to myself, and as a result experienced painful PMS symptoms, on-again, off-again cramps, dizzy spells and unending nausea.

"My doctor refused to aimlessly lure me into the world of pharmaceuticals. She had me take a natural iodine supplement and suggested I take up yoga or tai-chi. I did so. After nine hours in the lab, yoga seemed relieving and refreshing.

"I get along well with the iodine supplement I was prescribed, and because I've followed instructions exactly as they were given to me, I feel less cold. I leave my pullovers and knit-wear at home in the winter drawer where they belong.

Most of PMS symptoms have been alleviated, and finally, I am thankful to have taken my own path instead of continuing [to] side [with] my boyfriend with his self-negligent itinerary."

—*Yasmina, 24*

Libido

The thyroid plays such a significant role in the body (e.g., metabolism, basal temperature, etc.). So, when it experiences a dysfunction by overproducing or underproducing thyroid hormones, the body enters a state of trauma.

Experiencing such burdening internal stressors can make you anxious, nervous and tense. These are all normal feelings (especially when you look in the mirror and are highly disappointed in the person you see). When weight-loss or weight-gain attempts have been unsuccessful, your hair falls easily and your heart beats at an uncomfortable pace, it's no wonder the libido is affected. Besides sex being psychologically undesirable, sex will be physiologically undesirable as well for three reasons: your body is producing irregular amounts of T4 (and predictably T3); in women, menstruation cycles are skipped, thus stopping the production and ovulation of eggs; and the body experiences a discomfort where it becomes confused as to how it should act. All that confusion results in an indifference towards pleasurable acts, like sex, for instance. Thyroid dysfunction can impair people's social lives; they become too jittery for anyone to tolerate, or too fatigued to want to be social.

The heart

The less blood your heart pumps, the weaker it is. Low blood pressure can result in low energy and muscle wasting. In hypothyroid patients, the heart doesn't pump proper amounts of blood for efficient coronary circulation, which can result in heart failure. If the heart pumps out more blood than it's used to, the body

Study: When the heart skips a beat: The heart and hypothyroidism

Dr. Ahak et al. showed hypothyroidism can cause myocardial infarctions in elderly women. This just confirms what the researchers at Erasmus University's medical school found—menopausal and post-menopausal women who've been diagnosed with hypothyroid have a much greater likelihood of developing cardiovascular diseases than women who have a normal functioning thyroid. This is a scary stat, especially since we know that "20 percent of American women have been diagnosed with sub-clinical hypothyroid."* (Ahak, A.E. et al. "Hypothyroids and myocardial infractions." D. Rotterdam. Netherlands. *Annals of International Medicine*, 2000; 132: 270-8.)

*Data shows 20 percent, but I'm convinced this number is much higher.

—Dr. Tai

responds as if it's relentlessly running—this can also lead to other problems like adrenal exhaustion.

Beyond hypo- and hyper-thyroidism: serious illnesses
Hashimoto's thyroiditis and Graves' disease

Hashimoto's disease is named after Dr. Hakaru Hashimoto, who first described the symptoms in 1912. This disorder is believed to be the most common cause of primary hypothyroidism in the U.S. and is more prevalent in women than in men by an 8:1 ratio.

If you're experiencing signs of low thyroid function, you must treat it before it has long-term effects. Herbal thyroid medicine can replace the hormones your thyroid gland usually makes. How long you need to take the medicine will depend on your body's repair rate. For most people, natural thyroid hormone medicine causes no problems. Taking natural supplements can help prevent symptoms like tiredness, weight gain and constipation.

---

*Dr. Tai's backtrack—

In the July 1996 issue of the *Journal of American Medicine Association* (JAMA), medical professors at Johns Hopkins University published an article persuading physicians to include more testing of hypoactive thyroid before it tailspins into Hashimoto's hypothyroidism in patients as young as 35. The argument was made that too many cases of gone undiagnosed. This is not only dangerous but an embarrassment to the medical community's aptitude.

As a more serious form of hypothyroid, Hashimoto's thyroiditis (HT) rears its ugly head from people's necks and collar bones. HT can usually be detected through a goiter, a lump on a person's neck.

Hypothyroidism can be a silent killer since the immune system fails to recognize that the thyroid gland is a part of the body's own tissues and attacks as if it were posing a threat on the body. The disease is common among those aged 50 and up.

If you have or have had family members with HT you're at even greater risk, as you may have a genetic predisposition to it.

The other extreme is Graves' Disease, a *hyper*thyroid disorder. Instead of feeling cold, individuals with Graves' Disease feel exceedingly warm and their body temperatures are persistently high, causing them to lose weight despite increased appetite. The heart beats at an abnormal pace, causing the pulse to move irregularly, and the eyes pull high up so more white is seen in the area above the pupil, producing a cartoon-like appearance. Many have said that the eyes are the windows to the soul, and if you, like me, try to sustain eye contact when speaking with people, it becomes difficult to look at a person with Graves' disease. An ultrasound of the eye is mandatory when experiencing this symptom, as blindness can result. Autoimmune diseases like Hashimoto's thyroiditis are more common among older populations (*60+) as immune systems become weakened because the hormones that serve as the body's natural antioxidants and immune builders become depleted. Among these hormones are DHEA and melatonin. By replenishing both hormones via bioidentical hormone therapy, you can support the thyroid.

Dr. Broda Barnes

Dr. Broda Barnes, author of *Hypothyroidism: The Unsuspected Illness,* devoted much of her whole life to the thyroid. Her research started as an extensive analysis of the medical records of people who died in Graz, Austria during World War II. After reviewing records from the city's National Hospital, she found that after the war, people began to die from infectious diseases. When antibiotics were finally administered, people began to die from coronary artery diseases. This led her to make the correlation between infections and the heart, but "what…," she wondered, "…could trigger both?" It took until the mid-1970s for Dr. Barnes to expose the relationship between the two—it was the thyroid gland that was causing infections and cardiac-related deaths in these people.

Well ahead of her time, Dr. Barnes demonstrated that an excellent indicator of a thyroid status is basal body temperature. Body temperature is a great way to clinically test your thyroid, and the best part is that you can conduct the simple test at home, before you visit your doctor or get your blood tested.

Testing your thyroid at home

Materials needed:

- *Glass mercury thermometer*
- *15 minutes*
- *Diligent attention to instructions*

Instructions:

- *Keep the thermometer beside your bed. Immediately after waking, tuck the thermometer snugly in your armpit and keep it in place for 15 minutes. Keep as still as possible. Then, remove the thermometer, take a reading, and record the results.*

- *Follow the procedure for three days. Then, determine an average reading by adding all three readings together and dividing by three. If your average temperature is below 97.5 degrees F, in all probability you are suffering from sub-clinical hypothyroidism and should discuss your findings with your doctor.*

Dr. Barnes's advice to you is to take your morning basal temperature and determine if you are one of many people who need to be on thyroid support or, under the worst circumstances, be on thyroid hormone replacement.

THYROID Self-Assessment	
Symptoms of Thyroid Deficiency Note: *If supplementation has already been taken *increase* dosage if following symptoms are experienced:	**Symptoms of: Thyroid Excess** Note: *If supplementation has already been taken *decrease* dosage if following symptoms are experienced:
• Excessive coldness • Morning fatigue • Thinning skin • Weight gain • Dry skin and hair • Regular constipation • Thinning hair	• Anxiousness • Weight loss despite increased hunger and thirst • Shaky hands and fingers • Intense sweating

Synthetic vs. natural

When it comes to the thyroid, the hands-down best way to treat it is naturally. Again, the thyroid is an extremely sensitive gland—too much will effect the way you feel, and too less of the thyroid hormone will also affect you, both in very negative ways. Thyroid functions must be in balance for you to feel yourself. It's a sensitive gland that, if out of balance, can cause eye problems, breathing problems, psychotic disorders and take your metabolism beyond the point of no return.

If you're experiencing minor thyroid symptoms, the worst thing you can do to yourself is pick up your prescription at the drug store. It's almost guaranteed that you will experience further problems in the future. However, if you're showing major signs of severe thyroid dysfunction, you'll have no choice but take extreme measures. Follow doctor's orders, but if you can avoid taking synthetic thyroid support, it would be wise to do so because many synthetic forms of thyroids are known for promoting brutal side affects like weight gain, anemia, elevated fats, disturbances in heart rhythm, convulsions, mild to severe forms of anxieties and so on.

Natural way of doing it...

- Exercise moderately
- Eat foods rich in iodine
- Natural supplements of iodide/Iodine
- Natural thyroid glandular powder
- Take a supplement with selenium and iodine extracts from seaweed and seafood. *See Thyroid Specialist.*
- Don't you dare attempt a binge diet—no yo-yo dieting. Do it the right way or don't do it all! Starving yourself will only hurt your thyroid and you'll accomplish only gaining the pounds lost the following month.
- Breathe deeply. Deep breathing exercises increase ATP Adenosine Triphosphate; ATP fuels the cells within our body with oxygen. ATP is the source of all your energy. *See MaxPerformance.*
- To be comfortable is to be sexy. Don't attempt to sex up your image by wearing nearly nothing during cold months. Throwing basal temperatures off can "tinker wit' de t'yroid, mon." For Pete's sake, if you're cold, put on a sweater! *See MaxThyroid Specialist.*

⋙Dr. Tai's Anti-Aging Health Secret⋘

I can't say enough about the thyroid since it's the cause of so many problems. There are new developments all the time in the world of health especially with regard to the thyroid. People born without a thyroid have to depend on a lifetime of thyroid replacing hormones. Those of us blessed with a thyroid gland need to do a good job of taking care of it before we are without one. A healthy thyroid is a real gift for the body, as it helps us gain and lose weight while moderating our basal temperatures, keeping our heartbeats steady and maintaining the suppleness, moistness, and firmness of our skin. Excessive thyroid secretions can leave a person sweaty and greasy, while inadequate amounts of thyroid hormone will leave the skin wrinkled and dry and the hair brittle and fine.

Women experience more complications from the lack of iodine than do men, since their bodies are more abundant with estrogens, which can cause abnormal growths in the body. This is the reason that if you're a pre-menopausal woman, it's especially important that you regulate adequate intake and level of iodine/iodide. Low levels of iodine/iodide amidst excessive estrogen levels not in balance with progesterone can cause benign growths in soft tissues, i.e. cysts and fibroids in breast tissues, ovaries, etc.

If you're menopausal, hypothyroidism may be an issue. Women who have lower estrogen levels have a more difficult time producing sufficient amounts of the thyroid hormone without iodine in their diet. However, both men and women need to concern themselves with the thyroid regardless of the life stage they're in. Consider taking iodine from Mozuko seaweed or angel hair seaweed, the highly regarded seaweeds from the Pacific Ocean off the coast of Japan. This product is called Thryoid Specialist.

A vitamin B complex will allow necessary minerals (zinc, selenium and iodine) to be absorbed more quickly, increasing cell proliferation and aiding the nervous system in producing rapid communiqués amongst cells, so each little guy is completely aware of what his task is. B vitamins turn your cells into busy bodies in quite possibly the only place where busy bodies are appreciated—in your body. B vitamins also maintain the skin and eyes—this is especially important for people who are experiencing hyperthyroidism, since symptoms are most apparent on eyes and skin.

Cordyceps sinensis is another favorite of mine. The fungus (mushroom, if you prefer) increases oxygen in cells by 40 percent. This, along with deep breathing exercises, moderate exercise, vitamin B complexes and most importantly iodine, is a winning formula for maintaining a fully functioning thyroid, great skin, a normal metabolism, healthy hair (including the eyebrows and eyelashes) and increased libido. Consider Max Thyroid Specialist from Health Secrets USA.

By regaining all of these youth-related characteristics, a return to optimism and enthusiasm is guaranteed. So go ahead and grab your rose-colored glasses, because there's a brilliantly gleaming world outside!

"My favorite thyroid studies"
    * For additional studies see references

1) *American Journal of Cardiology,* 1998; 81: 443-447.
- Patients with advanced congestive heart failure have altered thyroid hormone metabolism.

2) Annals of Internal Medicine, 2000; 132: 270-8.
- Hypothyroidism is linked to heart attack risk among women aged 55 and older.
- Hypothyroidism is an indicator of atherosclerosis and myocardial infarction in elderly women.

3) *Journal of Gerontology: Medical Sciences,* 1999; 54A (3): M111-M116.
- Older subjects may require circulating thyroid hormones in middle to high levels in order to maintain optimal brain functioning.
- Hypothyroid patients may suffer subtle cognitive deficits.

Chapter 14

Adrenals: *Endocrine glands located above each kidney, which secrete stress-releasing hormones.*

—Stedman's Medical Dictionary

If the adrenals were a planet, it would be the Mars of the solar system, the red, volcanic, fiery planet. If the adrenals produced a sound, it would be synthesized and high-tech kind of sound. If the adrenals were a car, it would be an Indy 500 dragster. The adrenals are the body's power-players. They're considered two of the hardest working organs that produce the hormones that get you going—cortisol, and adrenaline.

Cortisol, a hormone essential to our survival. Produced under stress, cortisol is responsible for maintaining the ability to process sugars, sustain blood pressure and react to stressors that set off illness-- or conversely--illness that causes stress. As an antagonist to insulin, cortisol metabolizes carbohydrates and proteins, relieves inflammation, and allows the body to adapt to a broad range of circumstances. However, a high level of cortisol for prolonged periods leads to obesity, high blood pressure and adrenal fatigue. In contrast, low cortisol has been observed in patients with chronic fatigue and stress-related disorders. Cortisol is a sensitive hormone and it's produced by a glands that aren't as "tough" as they're depicted to be.

What to expect

Adrenal glands

Adrenal gland production

Cortisol

Functions of Cortisol

Hypoadrenal

Adrenals and stress

Self-assessment

Anti-aging Health Secret

Adrenal glands

As small as walnuts, each adrenal gland is located above a kidney. The adrenal gland secretes catecholamine adrenaline (epinephrine), a hormone that pushes a person to react to stress. The cortex (the outer part) affects blood pressure and balances salt levels. It also secretes cortisol and androgen (male) hormones and produces an aldosterone electrolyte balance.

The adrenals produce adrenaline and noradrenalin, two hormones which are directly related to "fight or flight."

Adrenaline and cortisol

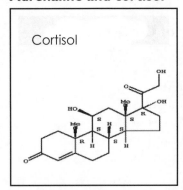

Cortisol

Adrenaline, which is named for the grand that produces it, is known as the "athlete's hormone." Athletes take a variety of supplements that promise to raise adrenaline and cortisol levels, both needed for damaged tissue repair and immediate energy boosts.

Adrenaline is a hormone that excites you. It leaves you energized and makes you hyper, jumpy, happy and feeling a little crazy. But it's the good crazy—the kind that makes you feel like you can take on the world. It's a godly feeling, the kind that makes you feel like you're capable of anything and everything.

Contrary to adrenaline, cortisol is triggered primarily from "good" and "bad" stress. "Bad" stress is whatever makes you cringe— unrealistic goals, deadlines, noise, being too self-critical and shifting body temperatures (from hot to cold and vice versa).

"Good" stress is derived from accomplishing goals and anything happily beyond a person's neutral state of existing, like feeling especially exultant, joyful, etc. The adrenal cortex produces corticosteroid hormone, dubbed cortisol, during the adaptation and repair phase of the stress response.

Cortisol's foremost job is to get along with invaders and inhibit excessive inflammation they may produce, and by invaders I mean stress. These stressors can be physical, environmental, mental or emotional. An example of environmental stress is being too hot or too cold. Other examples are being frequently exposed to loud noise, people arguing in your presence, or even working or living in a messy, unorganized or polluted environment.

Dr. Tai asks "Did you know?"

Adrenaline protects us by making more blood sugar and oxygen available to our legs so we can run from danger. It also provides more blood to the muscles of the arms and legs just in case one chooses to fight, instead of flee. Blood surges to the heart and muscles, the heart beats faster, breathing increases, the pupils in a person's eyes dilate and the stomach begins to tighten.

Various forms of stress provoke aggressive behavior—excess cortisol is released from your adrenal cortex. After enough cortisol production, glucose and glycogen (sugar) reserves are used to produce energy reactions (e.g., outbursts, verbal or physical gestures).

Causes of Abnormal Levels of Cortisol

Menopause	Panic disorder
Chronic fatigue syndrome	PMS
Fibromyalgia	Infertility
Depression	Sleep disorders
Impotence	Osteoporosis
Anorexia nervosa	Heart disease

—Heller, L.., *The essentials of Herbal Care Part II. Metagenics, Inc., 2000, p. 1144*

The correlation between cortisol and the adrenal glands

When the body feels it's under attack, it releases adrenaline in preparation for the cortisol carrier to either put up its dukes or attempt a great escape. This is where adrenaline gets the name "fight-or-flight hormone." Cortisol comes right afterwards and repairs, soothes, and protects.

Right place and time

The pituitary gland sends adrenocorticotropic hormone, abbreviated and more commonly known as *ACTH*, to stimulate the adrenal glands to produce cortisol. ACTH shows in the blood 30 minutes before cortisol does.

The outer layer of the adrenal glands produce *aldosterone*, a mineral hormone that balances water retention by controlling the volume of sodium in the body.

Cortisol production, in amounts produced at the "right time," helps heal tissues as well as protect the body by moving available sugars for proper nutrition meant for healing. Cortisol in minimal amounts can assist in retarding the aging process and fighting fatigue.

Functions of Cortisol

Balances blood sugar	Influences mood and thinking
Helps weight control	Affects testosterone/estrogen ratio
Improves immune response	Affects DHEA/Insulin ratio
Helps bone metabolism	Affects pituitary/thyroid/adrenal system
Balances stress response	Helps protein metabolism
Improves sleep	

—Heller, L. The Essentials of Herbal Care Part II. San Clement, CA:Metagenics, Inc. 2000, p.1144

Cortisol and the skin

Depleted cortisol and adrenaline levels will have the most effect on a person's nervous system, which will eventually affect the skin.

As I mentioned in the adrenal glands and cortisol section, the inner gland of the adrenal produces epinephrine and norepinephrane, which also produce pregnenolone and progesterone, anabolic tissue builders. The excess of cortisol production thins the skin, making one look old prematurely. However, cortisol at correct levels acts as an anti-inflammatory agent and an allergy reliever that controls the swelling of tissues and organs.

Cortisol overload

Excessive cortisol release can and will burn out the adrenals. Exhausted adrenals will cause people to age biologically sooner than normal by suppressing their immune systems and thinning their skin. Excessive cortisol production will eventually cause deep lines and excessive wrinkles.

Within such a competitive and capitalistic society like the US, things get intense. Increasingly, people are confronted with obstacles they are expected to overcome. Our bodies have adapted by producing more and more cortisol. Cortisol is continuously released when we get inadequate amounts of sleep. Unfortunately, due to a lack of proper nutrients, exercise and yo-yo diet-plans, many people run solely on cortisol; it is often the only thing that keeps many people awake at the office, during meetings and at social functions. The reserves of the hormone are used up by the body, causing depletion to occur sooner than expected, and adrenal fatigue sets in. Danger ahead!

Bad to the bone:
The negative effects of excess cortisol

Cortisol can negatively impact bone mass, causing greater likelihood of osteoporosis development in younger people.

Excessive cortisol production increases the chances of developing diabetes.

Cortisol increases fat deposits around the abdomen and waist.

Cortisol also increases the chances of early memory loss, hypertension and cardiovascular disease.

Excessive cortisol production exhausts adrenals to the point where cups of the darkest Columbian roast coffee won't be enough to keep a person awake. This is dangerous, especially when we operate two-ton machinery such as automobiles. Every year in the U.S., thousands of car accidents occur because people fall asleep at the wheel. Sadly, half of these car accidents are fatal; the others end in severe injury.

Cortisol, Sugar, and Fat

When stress causes excess production of cortisol and epinephrine, more sugar is rapidly mobilized into the blood stream in a process called Gluconeogenesis. But because we are sitting behind the desk stressing out, and our bodies cannot use the extra sugar energy to fight off or run away from some "man-eating" animal, the excess sugar turns into fat cells as stored energy. These fat cells accumulate around our waists and all over our bodies, making us fat and eventually obese.

Hypo-adrenal

The term functional hypo-adrenal means slow adrenal (low cortisol). As I said, adrenals become exhausted and struggle to produce enough cortisol and adrenaline to keep a person strong in stressful situations and up on their toes when they need to be the most alert.

The most severe case of hypo-adrenal syndrome can develop into Addison's disease, where the gland is badly broken down. Addison's disease patients display day-long signs of fatigue. Sufferers are tired all time, their speech tends to be slow and their voices are generally very soft because they lack the energy for an upbeat delivery, which makes the way they move slow-motion-like. In extremely severe cases, Addison's disease is deadly.

Women with High Cortisol

Decreased progesterone and its activity. *Bland, J. Functioinal Medicine Institute, 2001; p121*
Decreased thyroid activity due to higher thyroid binding. *Vliet, E. Women Wt. & Hormone, 2001,p129*

Adrenal advice

People relentlessly attempt to fight fatigue for no good purpose. Give in! If you feel tired, try some deep breathing exercises, close your eyes for a few minutes or splash some cold water on the back of your neck and wrists. Do something to calm down during moments of stress. Remember, short-term stressors can have very negative long-term effects. The body's response tells you it needs rest, quiet repair and sleep.

Getting personal

If anyone understands how important responsibilities are, I think I do. I constantly juggle a dozen things at once. At a family gathering last spring, one of my cousin's younger children asked me what I'd wish for if I could wish for anything. I told the six-year-old I'd wish for another set of hands like Vishnu, the Hindu god of reincarnation, so that I had the ability to complete twice as many tasks as I do. Everyone in my social sphere shares an almost identical work ethic. Most of my friends, family members and colleagues work themselves to the very core. We are overwhelmed and often suffer from adrenal fatigue. I am personally very strict about eating a proper diet, getting adequate sleep, and I take supplementation (support adrenal) such as Cordyceps sienesis in Max-Performance Specialist.

BEWARE! In Adrenal Fatigue, Adrenal Weakness, or Adrenal "Burnout," your Cortisol & DHEA levels will drop critically.

Overwhelmed? I understand.

Feeling overwhelmed is probably one of the most terrible sensations a person can experience these days. Aging baby-boomers have to worry about their aging parents. People are going back to grad school to seek master's degrees and doctorates, which can be expensive, especially if a person is trying to pay for his children's education as well. Employment interviews have become more rigorous, and everything requires a 360-

Studies: Cortisol makes people go CrAzY!

1) A recent study was conducted in Geneva, Italy by researcher Dr. Murialdo and his group of chemistry lab students. The group found that high cortisol levels effect dementia! (Murialdo, G., et al. "Endocrinology alterations in the aging male." *Clinical Chemistry Laboratory Medical Journal, 2003;* 41(7):934-941.)

2) Renowned German endocrinologist Dr. Elmlinger tested a group of 21-31 year-olds in Berlin. By testing their cortisol levels, he found that more than half the group (54 percent) were closer to age 70!

degree background check. People have less and less time to establish relationships of any sort because they're so busy advancing their careers. Unhappy marriages, death, divorce, bills, surgeries and constantly worrying about your position in the workplace can all lead to overwhelming stress. Before you realize it, your body exists in an everlasting distressed mode and like the Hollywood gangsters who keep handguns under their pillows while they sleep in case one of their many foes decides to raid their home, one can become so precautious that they're a complete wreck.

Just breathe...

Try to break the stress cycle. I'm not sure what the correlation is between stress and the mouth, but all too often I notice people stuff their mouths with food, drinks or cigarettes when they get upset. Physiologically, all it takes for the body to leave a panic episode is a few deep breaths. By breathing, one has more control over situations. Inhaling and exhaling promotes bodily oxygen entrance and calms nerves.

Relax when things seem overwhelming.

Get a saliva test to check your cortisol and depleted levels of other hormones (e.g., DHEA) the adrenal glands make. Eating the right foods, controlling stress and deep breathing exercises alone aren't going to do the trick. People need nutrients from natural foods—this goes without dispute. However, a saliva test is mandatory in establishing a proper baseline for additional supplementation and evaluating whether you are in serious danger zone.

Adrenal exhaustion

World-class athletes are not solely focused on surpassing already broken records but also on prolonging the length of their professional lives. Regardless of whether he is a World class soccer player or a swimmer, an athlete depends on putting on a great show for critical audiences and coaches.

Day in and day out, athletes train twice, sometimes three times a day, for hours on end under scrutiny. Winning the Olympics and other such championships are the goals of athletes and coaches world-wide. They hope to make a name for themselves and the people and places they represent. But after training for months and years for one particular event, what happens when it's all over? One would be surprised to note that despite presenting such physically powerful sides of themselves, athletes are very weak. From formidably fit to frail is a very thin line—many athletes suffer from adrenal and thyroid exhaustion, which leads to immune weakness and colds that can last for months. It destroys lives, ends brilliant careers, and dashes lifelong dreams.

Unique capabilities

Ambition and determination can drive athletes to their demise both personally and professionally. What separates superstar athletes from the rest of their world is the controversial talent they possess. Some hold firm the belief that superstars like Babe Ruth and Michael Jordan were born with talent. Others beg to differ and claim that their talents are due to unremitting practice and careful physical training. Whatever the case, practice is necessary for jaw-dropping performances.

Besides talent, ambition and determination, another astounding characteristic that sets superstars apart is their ability to heal. Athletes like Lance Armstrong (a seven-time Tour de France-winning road racing cyclist) have overcome physical limitations to surpass some of their own expectations. Practitioners in most medical arenas are flabbergasted at the uncommon ability these people possess to overcome obstacles in health. People who haven't trained their bodies to adapt to rigorous training routines will most likely suffer the likes of glandular exhaustion and surges of catabolic hormones, while anabolic hormones precipitously fall. It is the end of a promising athlete.

Adrenals: Tiko's story
Finding exhaustion at the finish line

"Ever since I was kid, my role models were athletes. My dad, a stout man from Guadalajara, Mexico, was known for his speed and strength. Unable to focus his interest on playing football [soccer] because he had to help support his aged parents, he worked stringing tobacco in a factory an hour away from his village. At 24, he moved to New Jersey with abuelo and abuela [grandpa and grandma]. A few months after his move, he met my mother, a soft-spoken girl from a village miles away from where my father once lived. Years later, I was born: Tiko, the only child, and probably, at times, more than they could handle. Everything my parents have done, they've done for me, and everything I've done, I've done to make them proud. Between school and my father's lock-smith and shoe repairing business, I ran. A high-school state champion, I brought medals to the school and gave our school district a reputable name.

"At 5-foot-10, I was told by past coaches that I was built to run—strong legs, upright and aligned posture with long, lean arms. I had enough muscle strength to carry me through the nastiest weather conditions and roughest terrain. Against high winds, traffic, bucketing rain and feet-tall snow, I made sure to get an early-morning run before school and a late-evening run after working or studying. My dad encouraged me to train more than I worked at the shop because he knew how much running meant to me. So I did and I devoted my senior year to burning my adrenals.

"As a high-school senior, different universities were looking to recruit students for their team. I had my heart set on Syracuse University. If there was anything I'd wanted was a full-ride scholarship to a highly regarded school like Syracuse. I planned on going pre-med and to be known as campus' Jersey boy who shattered records."

"I made the mistake of over-training. I trained to the point of exhaustion. My routine consisted of back strengthening, biceps curls, chest strengthening, leg strengthening, curls, shoulder presses, a five-mile morning run and a three-mile evening run.

"In March, I developed a deadly cold which I couldn't recover from. As soon as I thought I recovered, I got worse. Finally, when Syracuse came to visit the school, they weren't impressed by me. My performance was poor and I had made running look painful. I blew my chances of making the team because I over-trained. It took me months to recover from an exhausted body and depression. I was really hard on myself; I got accepted to Syracuse, but not on a sports scholarship.

"Currently, I'm a junior at the university and I've learned not to be so hard on myself. It was unfortunate that I had to learn the hard way. This year, I'm taking it easy. I'm worrying about my G.P.A. and training lightly. If I make the team when the season arrives, I make the team—if I don't, then that too will be OK. Right now, my health has become my top priority."

—Tiko, 22

Overachievers, perfectionists and workaholics

Bless their brave hearts for attempting to achieve the impossible. They break records, they're detail-oriented, and they come in a variety of species. Like athletes, workaholics are all about achieving their goals in an all-or-nothing way. They savor their workload, they're relentless, and they have trouble stopping what they're doing only to make careless mistakes along the way, which end up working against them. Obsessing over details to the point of paralysis, perfectionists and overachievers have what I like to call a "hero complex." They get kudos from their professional superiors and they give the impression that they are capable of things above and beyond the call of duty. They're slaves in their own offices, attached to their desks or, in an athlete's case, the gym, track, court or field. This can be because they try to avoid going home, or maybe don't have much of a social life. As with everything, cases vary and everything is relative, but one thing remains absolute—workaholics and athletes have higher than normal cortisol levels that will only lead to their demises.

If you're one of these…You're walking on thin ice.

> **No pain, no gain:**
>
> Recovery periods for athletes typically last around 48 hours. After an intense workout, if they don't allow ample time for their muscles to repair, the body's immune system is sure to be weakened. During the 48-hour healing period, DHEA and cortisol are released in the blood as a mending mechanism for damaged tissues. At the end of this period, cortisol slows in production to relieve the body of feeling overwhelmed or over-burdened, replenishing and preparing the body for additional activity.
>
> *Die-hard athletes are more susceptible to allergies, colds and injuries, more so than people who exercise reasonably. This is why it's especially important for athletes to take a day or two off after intense training to allow their bodies to repair muscles and foster immunities. *Overtraining*, not under-training, is the athlete's worst enemy.

Untrained, trained and over-trained

After researching untrained and trained athletes and athletes who are over-trained, I noticed that the cortisol response to the exercise training is minimal in an untrained athlete as compared to a well-trained athlete, who has a much higher level response relative to his training. This marker has the major effect in terms of those weekend-warrior athletes who are not well-trained—they overdo it. For only a weekend endeavor, they do not heal because they do not have the high cortisol response that is required for tissue repair.

I can certainly see a similar pattern in our over-trained athletes with adrenal fatigue. Their cortisol levels are very low relative to their training activities. They experience inflammatory reactions, muscle protein and tissue breakdown, pain and discomfort post-training, and delayed healing and recovery time. These fatigued, over-trained athletes require greater rest and more time to recuperate and heal. Pushing and going back to training before the body is ready only exacerbates the situation, making already broken tissues even worse, and ultimately causing permanent damage or injury.

Robbing the "bank"

While in Paris for an anti-aging conference, I had the pleasure of meeting a variety of doctors from all over the world. It was raining, and many of the conference attendees were restricted from probing the Parisian streets that particular Sunday afternoon.

With newspapers over our heads, we fled the conference hall and headed to the nearest café for tea and coffee. A doctor from Florida, who had one of the largest practices in the country, told a story about a Miami police officer, whose name was Will.

A religious family man in his early thirties, Will turned into a martyr for the city of Miami. In a year, he transformed from one to be envied into a graying, chubby, hackneyed version of a has-been superhero.

The doctor, concerned about Will's appearance, spoke to him briefly about what he had observed. The officer promised to make an appointment and did..

After a saliva panel was taken, Will was diagnosed as having exhausted adrenals. He was producing massive amounts of cortisol for years, "burning out" his adrenals, which in turn had resulted in adrenal fatigue. Though Will realized that it was lucrative for him to stay awake during the midnight hours, he wasn't able to. He confessed that he'd actually fallen asleep in his patrol car while robberies and drug dealing were taking place right before the eyes he couldn't help but shut. The officer could have risked his job and his life.

ADRENAL Self-Assessment	
Symptoms of Cortisol Deficiency Note: *If supplementation has already been taken *increase* dosage if following symptoms are experienced:	**Symptoms of: Cortisol Excess** Note: *If supplementation has already been taken *decrease* dosage if following symptoms are experienced:
• Insomnia • Fatigue • Digestion problems • Emotional inbalances • Loss of sexual interest • Low blood pressure • Low blood sugar • Slow heartbeat • Severe fatigue • Sugar cravings • Feeling stressed • Lightheadedness when sitting or standing	• Sleep problems • Sugar cravings • Decreased effciency • Fat deposits • Osteoporosis • Lack of energy • Increased blood pressure • Increased Cholesterol & Triglycerides • Water retention • Increased blood sugar • High blood pressure • Thinning skin • Loss of muscle mass • Anxiousness, irritability and nervousness • Feelings of stress • Trunkal weight gain • Arthritis and muscle pain • Hair loss

∾Dr. Tai's Anti-Aging Health Secret∾

The adrenal glands play an important role in producing a variety of hormones, specifically cortisol. However, cortisol production is like a double-edged sword. If the body doesn't produce enough cortisol, a person is fatigued and isn't as alert as he should be. But if the body produces too much cortisol, a person's chances of being overweight and of developing into a tired sugar junkie are more than likely.

High cortisol levels can lead to dementia, insomnia and obesity because the hormone acts as a metabolic inhibitor, affecting the receptors in the body by pushing sugar to deposit into fat at great speeds. Invariably, this affects your appearance, causing weight to congregate at the waist, as in apple-shaped bodies (wide hips and thin legs).

Health and appearance are in sync with one another and, as stated in the beginning of my chapter, the adrenals are extremely sensitive power players. This is why I recommend saliva tests, because the slightest amount of an adrenal hormone excess can throw a person off balance, placing them into a neverending lose-lose situation, where for a short time the rush is felt but is paid for in the long run.

Through saliva testing, the biomarkers of people who lead active, stressful lifestyles can be helped. Hormones mark how much energy a person possesses and how healthy he is. By measuring saliva hormones, we can evaluate cortisol, testosterone and DHEA and help people maximize energy potential.

By making the right lifestyle choices relating to dieting, bioidentical hormone replacement and moderate exercise, you'll be able to avoid the mental and emotional havoc that excess cortisol produces.For added relief, use Max-Performanes and Glucose Specialist as a supplement for high cortisol. Glucose Specialist mobilizes sugar in our bloodstream, helping to avoid sugar accumulation that can result in diabetes, heart disease and hypertension. Max Adrenal helps restore adrenal function and energy in very severe adrenal fatigue.

SECRET VII

"I may not be totally perfect,
but parts of me are excellent."
—Ashleigh Brilliant

Chapter 15

Hormones and Our Skin

Our skin is a multilayered meticulously complex organ. It covers every inch of our entire body. It's what protects us from an environment that has increasingly become more and more unpredictable. With pollution taking a more prevalent role in our lives, it's difficult to preserve our skin's condition, which serves as visible evidence for our age and health. There is no specific age at which a person becomes "elderly," but because our skin is visible, we place an emphasis on its appearance. Even while wearing makeup, most women attempt to look natural. *Your skin can't lie—it doesn't and it won't.*

Cosmetic surgery is one of many artificial extremes to which women are willing to go to fight aging, and it is both painful and expensive. There has been many a time I've examined the problem of aging, and I use the term "problem" loosely because throughout the years, aging has developed into a problem. It's affected self-esteem, confidence and finances. America spends billions of dollars annually on products they think will help them look and feel younger.

Age Gracefully

You've heard the phrase "to age gracefully." What the heck does that mean? What's graceful about crow's feet and wrinkles that resemble desiccated rivers? Can somebody please tell me what's graceful about bags under the eyes, liver spots and turkey necks? What's so graceful about no energy, no libido, no memory, and hurting from everywhere in the body? I'm sorry, but I don't find any of that graceful or healthy. Nothing will get me to consider old folks in nursing homes, shadows of their former selves, as attractive. Society has tried to justify wrinkles, and this is all thanks to phenomenal writers who do a nice job of finding beauty in the ugliest of things.

Motivating people to be as optimistic as possible, writers state that wrinkles are "lines of wisdom." Oh, how lovely! But look here, Shakespeare, I know some people with wrinkles, but that doesn't mean they're wise. I know people in their late 20s and 30s who have wrinkles worse than some of my friends in their 60s. Do the wrinkles on their faces denote any sort of wisdom? No, it denotes neglect and sun damage.

Based on my anti-aging theories, many cosmetic companies would resort to name-calling. They'd label me a heretic, but I've seen enough to understand why we develop faces that add years to our actual age. I've finally figured it out: The trick to treating wrinkles is treating all that lies beneath the surface, it starts with prevention and finishes with deep repair.

> "To treat wrinkles, treat what's below the surface."
> —Dr. Paul Ling Tai

15 years old +

The skin and hair have been referred to as the "windows of age." For thousands of years, many have tried to reverse the effects of aging in order to appear as youthful as possible for as long as possible, so they target the skin. But worrying about the skin is also worrying about the hair and nails. How many 20-year-olds have you seen with yellow, brittle nails? How many 20-year-olds have you seen with dry, brittle hair? Some guys bald at a much younger age, but this normally doesn't occur until their late 20s or 30s.

25 years old +

One thing is certain—the only place I've seen a balding 20-year-old woman is in a medical text book. That's because within that age range, hormones are keyed up. Like buzzing little bees at work, they travel in the blood throughout the body. After 25, hormones start to deplete at a snail's pace.

35 years old +

After 35, depletion begins to pick up momentum and during the stages of periandropause and andropause, or perimenopause and menopause, hormone depletion continues incessantly. Without interruption, like a tear in a shirt, hormone depletions goes straight through the body without stopping. And, as I've mentioned in the "What is a hormone?" chapter, levels of hormones such as human growth hormone (HGH), estrogen, progesterone, testosterone, DHEA, thyroid hormone, melatonin and pregnenolone all decline. The hormones we could do with less of, cortisol and insulin, go up as a result of added life stressors and appalling eating habits.

The "skinny" on the skin

Epidermis (statum corneum): The layer that meets the eyes. The epidermis is the outermost horny (dead) layer, comprised of dead skin cells that protect our interior from external toxins, infections and free radicals found in the air and water. It's thick and takes a variety of shades, hues and pigments. (Every person, or group of people from various geographic locations have a particular shade due to their environmental conditions, diet and lifestyle.) The epidermis is the most important layer as far as looks are concerned, but when it comes to treating the skin, it's the least important.

Dermis: The middle section of the skin between the top layer, and the sub-dermis. It's living skin that produces cells for the epidermis. The dermis serves as supportive nutrient base for the epidermis. This is where most skin care ingredients must reach in order to actively change the top layer's appearance.

Sub-dermis: The subcutaneous layer that contains fat, blood vessels, sweat glands and some hair follicles. Supports our *muscles, tendons and bones.* Without blood vessels from the sub-dermis, the dermis and epidermis won't have an adequate amount of blood supply to repair damages on our epidermis.

Fibroblasts: The dermal cells that make collagen.

Collagen: The main protein in the connective tissues of the body. It's responsible for skin thickness. The most common forms of collagen are collagen 1 and collagen 3 (a collagen form prevalent in our youth). *When you think of collagen, think of steal rods that fasten concrete blocks together.*

Elastin: Gives the skin elasticity and the ability to rebound. It makes up two percent of the skin. Elastin is abundant underneath the dermis, along with the fat cells from fatty tissues that act much like shock absorbers. These cells give the skin certain bounce without allowing it to droop. Once collagen elastin diminishes, the subcutaneous tissues release their hold on fat cells. This is when the skin loses its moisture content and firmness and begins to droop and sag—much like a deflated balloon.

To sum it all up

The skin consists of the epidermis (the top layer) and the dermis (the lower layer). Our epidermis is made of dead skin cells. Every minute of the day we lose about 40,000 (up to 3,000,000) dead cells per hour while newly formed cells (from our dermis) rise to the surface to become the epidermis. Think of it as a cyclical, never ending process which can be referred to as the skin's rotation. Blood vessels in the dermis supply nutrients to support active growth of new cells. They contain collagen and elastin fibers essential in maintaining skin strength and flexibility.

Our epidermis is tough, so this is why applying moisturizers (e.g. lotions and anti-wrinkle creams) over and over again won't do the trick. Once skin damage is done, repair becomes difficult, but not impossible. Please allow me to tell you a little yet vital secret: *Nutrients must penetrate past the layer of dead skin cells and into your living layer of skin (dermis) in order for the anti-wrinkle creams to be effective.*

The stink on skin

Bound by protective external secretions that kill bacteria, the skin has a symbiotic relationship with bacteria and fungi. The two can only be disrupted by chemicals in antibiotics, synthetic forms of medicine, or those with the wrong pH balance. When we sweat, we release toxins we've absorbed from drink, food or smoke. People who don't release toxins from these sources have the tendency to release an awkward body odor. This is how the skin acts as a conditioner and heater to the body.

It's hot in there

Blood vessels expand to cool you off, or shrink to preserve body heat. Adjusting to temperature is required for survival. It creates a proper environment for your internal organs to function properly.

Dr. Tai asks: "Did you know?"

*Extreme sensations like feeling "cold" or "hot" qualify as environmental stressors.

Let me see you S-s-stretch!

Each of the skin's layers contain connective tissues and collagen fibers. Because they provide flexibility and strength, connective tissues such as elastin and collagen are what I like to call "rubber band" fibers.

Breaking skin

The skin has a great deal of stretch ability to express the changes muscles make. Muscle movements produce tears in the skin's outer layer. Just as body-builders break muscles to rebuild them again, people who resort to facial expression as a form of communication break their skin's muscles. Where do you think those laugh lines came from? The answer is—of course—laughing.

Smiling and frowning results in facial wrinkles. Am I suggesting monitoring the rate at which you smile and laugh as a wrinkle preventative? Absolutely not! I just want you to know that after years of producing happy, sad, frightened and fearful expressions, you should expect to see a collection of emotions etched onto your face.

In comparison to other segments of the body, facial muscles are connected to bones that have the least amount of tissue. As we age, we begin to lose fat from our faces, which makes our skin thin, loose and fragile.

Building skin: Collagen

Collagen production gives the skin texture and thickness. Collagen production starts with an amino acid called *lysene*, which is changed to hydroxylysene, then to collagen. Two important chemicals, Vitamin C and zinc, help to make collagen and push it forward to the skin's top layer (epidermis).

What the experts are saying about collagen

Dr. Boorsma, a frequent contributor to the *Investigative Dermatolgy Journal*, said in an article published in 1996 that "accumulation of dead skin gives your skin a dull look." He and his fellow researchers found an absence of collagen 4 in the epidermal-dermal junction, creating a disruption of dead cells.

(Boorsma, J., et al. "Collagen 4 in photoage skin." *The Journal of Investigative Dermatology, 1996;* 107:516.)

The same journal published a study a year prior to Dr. Boorsma's finding. Researcher N.M Craven wrote that collagen 4 anchors the skin to the basement membrane where collagen 7 is lacking. When there is an absence of collagen 7 and not enough collagen 4 to replace it, wrinkles form.

(Craven, N.M., et al. "Clinical features of photodamaged human skin are associated with a reduction in collagen VII." *British Journal of Dermatology,* 1997; 137(3): 344.)

Not new for long

Our epidermis is connected by tiny, Velcro-like protein appendages that protrude into cell membranes. These membranes are called *desmosolts*. Used cleverly, desmosolts hold all cells beside, below and above each other, becoming so connected they're inseparable.

Dead skin cells cling together; they do this by a natural mortar called the "lipid matrix," a natural construction which aids in skin building, protecting the body's delicate organs from toxins, infections and pollutants. Because they are stacked together like bricks, abrasion is the only thing that'll remove dead cells. However, with time, a person's skin changes either from environment or age, or both. Normally, the younger we are, the oilier our skin is, and conversely, the older we become the drier our skin is. For this reason, skin goes through a wear-and-tear process. At 20 we try to dry the skin, and at 40 we try to moisten the skin. Please remember that our skin is a vital organ—and as the thyroid may become dysfunctional from yo-yo dieting, our skin can be just as exhausted and deserves the right kind of break. You can start by sticking to an effective skin care routine. Consistency in skincare gets results.

Slippery skin

With age, both men and women lose *sebaceous gland activity*, which in English (ha-ha!) means that your skin isn't producing as much oil as it once did. This is when your skin becomes a menace. Oily skin is both a blessing and a burden—it's nature's free goodie. Oily skin at 40+ is the extra twenty dollar bill you found in the back pocket of the jeans you thought you lost.

I find it fascinating when people ask for ways to rid their skin of oils. Now, why would you want to go and do that?

Despite the fact that my leather story was a bit of a stretch, I'm convinced that it is a good example of what your skin is like. Instead of taking care of the leather years ago when you first purchased it, you waited 30 years later. And, how in heaven's name do you expect to resurrect your skin? By dehydrating it of its natural oils and then adding synthetic moisturizers to hydrate it?

Americans spend billions of dollars a year on cosmetics! Today, these numbers are rising at a rapid pace since more and more people are concerned with their skin. Everyone is spending money to rehabilitate their skin, as if four seasons weren't enough! (This is where I throw my hands up in the air.) Try to be as gentle as possible with your skin. If you're going to wash, massage. If you're going to wipe, sponge. If you're going to buy, don't waste; stay close to the natural products.

Treat your skin with great food
Vitamins, antioxidants and herbs

Marketing groups, advertising agencies and PR firms know what people want for their skin. People want natural, wholesome ingredients and smart professionals play up all of those things in the campaigns they produce. Your skin needs vitamins and nutrients so with a huge commercial banner they present "VITAMIN C" and "GRAPE SEED EXTRACT." On packaging, these very same ingredients are printed in boldface, italicized and underlined, yet they can't even get through the outer dead layer of the skin to do any good.

Testimonial

"When my 5-year-old granddaughter said, 'Grandma, your skin is falling,' I wanted to pull her tiny ears off!

"For years, before my granddaughter made such a comment, I thought I was better looking than most women my age. For nearly fifteen years, I've worked in a leading upper-class store as the gentlemen's department manager, receiving a great deal of attention from avid shoppers who stopped by the men's section just to exchange smiles. I was convinced that people found me attractive.

"Suddenly, what became an issue was my skin. Children are usually very honest, and my granddaughter's frankness slapped me across the face. Her comment, 'Your skin is falling,' was an observation that received my attention for weeks. It is falling, and I am obligated to 'pick it up.' I tried everything my colleagues from different departments suggested I use to no avail.

"Opting to stay away from joining the masses, I do not consider cosmetic surgery as an option. Having examined dermal delivery systems closely, I've found that without liposomes, creams are washed away. I've used everything and can tell you that antioxidant liposomes have made a difference in my complexion. I'm not sure why everyone doesn't use them. I wish I had a way of telling all the customers in our store to save their money and spend it where it's well deserved—liposome creams. It's only been a few months, and with consistent use, I can see a difference. I give it one year before I voluntarily become a liposome spokesperson. "

—Russlana, 53

Antioxidants

The body is a battlefield where hormones are constantly over-producing or under-producing chemicals, functions, reactions, etc. When hormones are out of balance, various damaging chemicals counteract each other and pose the threat of destroying body parts. This process can be stopped by antioxidants, which I like to refer to as the body's watchdog. Antioxidants are natural compounds that prevent and reverse the production of free radicals (out-of-control reactive compounds i.e., terrorists) that destroy essential cell organs, e.g., DNA.

Skin suffers

Due to the damage that has occurred to your skin (e.g. hormonal loss, hormonal imbalance, excessive sun exposure, chemical preservatives, i.e., paraben and methylparaben, etc.), skin's tender fibers have *oxydized* (rusted). This is where antioxidants come in—they're known for preventing and repairing areas which have been oxidized.

As skin guardians, antioxidants allow for the skin to produce collagen synthesis that manufactures and repairs many of the tissues that have been damaged. Once the skin is repaired, it produces skin metabolites that give the skin its thickness. Just as we metabolize food, antioxidants repair skin so that collagen synthesis or metabolism can occur. By cell production, skin becomes thicker, firmer and healthier. For a complete skin rejuvenation routine, you need really powerful antioxidants like: Superoxide Dismutase (SOD), Catalase and Glutathione. These are the most elite potent antioxidants known to men, period ! The next time you decide to go shopping, make sure that antioxidants like liposome creams are the first items on your list. They incorporate potent reactions that will address dermal degradation, repair and prevent radical damage.

Studying Antioxidants

In his study "Topical absorbic acid and photo-aged skin," Dr. PG Humbert (et al.) found through topographical evaluation that by using 5 percent of vitamin C, the study's participant's skin had made drastic improvements. Thus, topical Vitamin C was deemed effective.

Dr. Humbert said, "Topical application of 5 percent of vitamin C cream was a well-tolerated treatment amongst patients and led to a clinically apparent improvement of the skin."

The participants in the double-blind study reported a reduction in wrinkle depth. Although wrinkles were still apparent, they were of a much lesser extent. Participants also said that they felt their skin increase in density.

Antioxidants Dr. Tai recommends:

- **Beta carotene**
- **Superoxide dismutase (SOD)**
- **Vitamin C (L-ascorbic acid)**
- **Glutathione liposome**
- **Catalase**
- **Vitamin E**
- **White tea extract**
- **Vitamin A**
- **Lycopene (found in tomatoes—this is great stuff!)**
- **Grape seed extract, fermented**
- **Green tea extract**
- **Blueberry and/or blackberry extract**
- **Algae**
- **Pomegranate extract**
- **Alpha-lipoic acid**
- **Clove oil**
- **Thyme oil**
- **Wolfberry Nanoextract (a favorite)**
- **Mangosteen Nanoextract (a favorite)**

Dr. Tai asks, "Did you know?"

Contrary to popular belief, **grapeseed extract** found in most cosmetics isn't as potent as most people think. Why? Cosmetic companies use unfermented grape seed extract instead of fermented grape seed and skin extract—the better, rare, and more expensive kind.

Vitamin A

If you've paid attention to market trends in recent years, you'd notice the emergence of Retin-A treatments on store shelves. Everything has Retin-A. Everyone wants Retin-A. Why? Because topical Retin-A (vitamin A) treatments work by normalizing the keratinization process (skin cell and tissue renewal).

Mainly, vitamin A is used to treat dry skin, age spots, acne and sun damage. You'll find that highly concentrated Retin-A formulas work well as pore minimizer.

Beta carotene can be converted to retinal A in the human skin. Consuming foods rich in beta carotene is like applying Retin-A treatment on your face. Dr. Antille, a professor at the University of Geneva Dermatology Department, conducted a study which showed that beta carotene consumption had the same effects as applying beta carotene. Submerging yourself in a bathtub filled with Retin-A would have a similar effect as taking a bite out of a carrot (Antille, Christopher et al. "Topical beta carotene is converted to retinyl esters in human skin *ex vivo* and mouse skin *in vivo." Experimental Dermatology,* 2004; 13(9)558.)

Alpha-lipoic acid

Alpha-lipoic acid has, by far, the most unique ability to deal with free radicals. I say unique because it's an ambidextrous antioxidant—it fights radicals while revitalizing other antioxidants.

Like a war nurse, alpha-lipoic acid fights the opposing side while caring for wounded soldiers. It prevents inflammation-induced free radical damage in the skin. It also stimulates enzymatic collagen repair and reduces collagen damage. It's both water and oil-soluble, giving it versatility in its usage, making it a potent free radical scavenger. Alpha-lipoic acid recycles and renews vitamins C and E while assisting in cellular metabolism.

Studying Alpha Lipoic Acid:

In 2003, after a 12-week *double-blind study using 5 perfect alpha lipoic acid, Sweden's Dr. Beitner (et al.) concluded that "Alpha lipoic acid is a potent scavenger with anti- inflammatory properties."

Dr. Beitner showed through his study that the roughness of his patient's skin was reduced by more than 50 percent, and the amount of wrinkles had reduced distinctively. (Beitner, H. et al. "Randomized placebo controlled double-blind on the clinical efficacy of cream containing 5 percent of alpha lipoic acid aelated to photoaging facial skin." *British Journal of Dermatology,* 2003; 149:(4)841-9.)

Vocabulary you should know:

***double-blind:** a study in which neither the study's participants nor researchers know which treatment or intervention any particular participant is receiving during the study.

Alpha-lipoic acid...

1. is an extremely powerful antioxidant that's both water and fat soluble.
2. is an anti-inflammatory agent.
3. stops aging by diminishing cross linking between proteins and other large molecules, which break down skin.
4. is essential for cell metabolism and cell energy production.
5. is an extraordinarily powerful neutralizer of free radicals, as well as a powerful free radical detoxifier.
6. possesses the potential of removing toxins caused by stress, pollutants, synthetic medications and lingering free radicals.

Natural Phytohormones
The Hit List

Isoflavones
Puereria Mirifica (great stuff!)
Genistein
Daidzen

The natural ingredients listed above have natural hormones. Phytohormones are the kind of hormones your skin can tolerate. Synthetic topical estrogens most often contain hormones altered to mimic your hormones. But they don't do a good job because if they did, side effects would be few.

With a dramatic increase in life expectancy, a woman can expect to be in menopause for more than one-third of her life. This means that the drop in estrogen will have an all-encompassing impact on a woman's skin. Bearing this in mind, women should put forth extra effort to eat foods that slow the pace of hormone depletion and use products that strengthen the few existing hormones that are present within their bodies. This is where bioidentical hormonal replacement comes in. Through advanced liposome technology, you can have nutrients sent directly through your skin.

Bioidentical hormone replacement is the most exciting medical area for me. Throughout the years, I've seen individual evolutions take place. I've seen the weak and tired turn into the strong and mighty. I've seen the pale and fragile turn into the vibrant and energetic. I am myself one of them.

With bioidentical hormones, I've seen the dull and wrinkled turn into intensely dazzling individuals. Though most people who ask for skin care advice are mostly women, more and more men have taken greater interest in their appearance. Taking bioidentical hormones

Studying phytoestrogens:

In a 2001 study published in *Environmental Health Perspective*, Dr. Patricia Whitten found through careful examinations that phytoestrogens are effective because they are "powerfully active," in a way which "your skin can tolerate," by "posing no disturbance to it." (Whitten, P. L., et al. "Cross species and inter assay comparisons of phytoestrogen actions. *Environmental Health Perspective*, 2001; 109(suppl.1):5-20.)

has not only taken an effect on my own skin, but it affects the way I currently view life; I've become much more outgoing, energetic and more eager to experience life!

Phytohormone equivalent: DHEA, testosterone and melatonin

DHEA and melatonin are the most powerful antioxidant-like hormones the body produces. They're considered to be such because they're hormones that prevent the formation of free radicals by disarming NADPH before it can generate free radicals (oxygen molecules that destroy cell receptors and destroy DNA).

Free radicals attack cholesterol. Many times they attack a "bad" cholesterol known as *LDL*. The cells go to where they are needed, kind of like saying, "Lean on me, and I'll lean on you." When a cell is in trouble, others race to the rescue. When the cells reach the attacked LDL cells, they too get eaten up by free radicals. It is a trick—the nice cells are eaten up. DHEA saves the day and stops innocent cells from being gobbled up, stopping the process by obstructing the radicals from reproducing and multiplying in numbers.

DHEA

DHEA is eventually converted into testosterone, and testosterone is one of the natural hormones that maintains thick skin on the body, specifically the face. It's an abundant hormone in men, so this is probably the reason why it's been said that men are like wine—"they get better with age." This isn't entirely true, but the saying holds *some* truth, most men don't wrinkle as badly as women, for the mere fact that their bodies hold more testosterone.

Testosterone

When testosterone levels begin to deplete in men, they're still left with more of the hormone than most women. Tests can be run to prove this, but it usually shows in facial furrows. High cortisol levels contribute to wrinkling and sagging

Studying sex hormones and how they affect the skin:

Dr. P. G. Sator (et al.) published an article on "Skin aging and sex hormones in women in the *The Journal of Experimental Dermatology* [2004; 13:(4)36-40.]

The physician at Vienna's Principal Hospital said, "The skin is the target organ for various hormones, and sex steroids have a profound influence in the aging process. A decrease in sex steroids does induce the reductions of those skin functions that are under hormonal control."

FYI: Under hormonal influence are keratinocytes, melanocytes, sebaceous, collagen content and hyaluronic acid.

Dr. Sator concluded that topical applications of phytoestrogens "have a positive effect on skin aging perimeters." He further extended this thought by stating that phytoestrogens have a profound influence on skin care by slowing down the skin's aging process. Major clinical studies like Sator's conclude that phytoestrogens leave the skin dewier and smoother.

on both the skin and neck. By replenishing testosterone using microencapsulations of liposomes, the skin absorbs the nutrients that restore lost levels of a particular hormone, or hormones.

Melatonin

Besides being antioxidants, DHEA, testosterone and melatonin are intense moisturizers. DHEA and melatonin do a nice job of clearing up eczema, excessive dryness, age spots and other skin discolorations caused by aging. It takes time to accomplish this, and generally does a better job preventing dark age spots.

Studying phytohormones

In a 1999 study found in the *Journal of Pathology*, Dr. GS Ashcroft collected 18 female participants and 18 male participants in a double-blind study testing the effects of topical estrogens. The women in his group were 74.4 years old (about 74 years old), and the men in his group were 70.7 years old (about 70 years old).

Dr. Ashcroft split the group into two, giving nine male and nine female participants topical estrogens. He gave the other male and female group topical placebos. Compared to the placebo group, the group that used the topical estrogen noticed their wounds healed at a much faster pace than what they were used to.

Dr. Ashcroft's results were as follows: In one week, collagen and fibronectin production increased. Wounds began to heal 80 percent faster than what was considered normal for participants. His study proved that topical estrogen accelerates wound healing, hence the name of his study, *"Topical Estrogen Accelerates Cutaneous Wound Healing in Aged Humans Associated with an Altered Inflammatory Response."*

Dr. Ashcroft is a member of the National Institute of Health in Bethesda, Maryland. The institute emphasizes the healing power of topical estrogens in men and women (1999; 155(4):1137-46.)

Researcher J.B. Schmidt examined the treatment of aging skin with topical estrogens on 59 women ranging in age from 41 to 67. He gave the participants instructions to use topical estradiol and estriol on a daily basis for 11 weeks. He monitored the appearance and health of their skin by using skin profilometry, cornealmetry, an immuno-chemical clinical investigation of collagen type and skin biopsies.

Dr. Schmidt's results were as follows...

Week 7: Vascularization improved by 100 percent, while skin elasticity and moisture levels improved 96-100 percent.
Week 8 & 9: Wrinkle depth decreased 87-90 percent; pore size decreased from 61-73 percent.

Schmidt said, "Both estrogen compounds were found to be highly effective in preventing and then treating skin aging in perimenipausal women."

He added, "Lack of systemic and promising effects after external use, suggests that estriol will gain importance in the technology for dermatology in the future."

In both groups that used topical phytoestrogens, there was a striking increase in collagen type 3 fibers. Clinical observations proved that there was an increase in firmness and a significantly lesser amount of wrinkling.

During the treatments, the production of acid mucol, polysaccharides and hyaluronic acid generated an increase in the amount of water in the participant's dermis. Subsequently, this elevated their skin's moisture levels. (J.B. et al., "Research treatment of skin aging with topical estrogen." *International Journal of Dermatology*, 1996; 35: 669-674.)

Besides wrinkles, there's bruising

The skin doesn't repair itself as quickly as it does when we are young. As a matter of fact, wound healing may slow down from 400-600 percent. The lifecycle of a skin cell is 28 days, as we age, this may turn out to be a lot longer.

With age, skin not only droops and sags but also becomes thinner. When I was 15, I used to get into mock fights with my brother. He would punch me on the arm and kick my leg. He'd push me and beat me to a pulp. I'd always get up, brush my shoulders off and walk away without a single bruise. Many, many years later when I turned over 50, if someone tapped me on the shoulder a bruise developed. With age, people bruise and break down at accelerated rates. By using topical treatments of phytohormones (DHEA, estriol and testosterone especially), one can prevent bruising, skin break down, and scarring from occurring so quickly.

Swedish researcher G. Roupe found delayed immune responsiveness in skin after reduced numbers of fibroblasts and mast cells in the aging dermis. Collagen bundles become fragmented, less elastic and more brittle. Roupe added that skin tumors and other dramatic changes to the skin are also age related, this could be the reason why as we age, we bruise easier. (Roupe, G., et al. "Skin of the aging human being. Lakartidingen, 2001; 7; 98(10):1091-5.)

Phytoestrogen equivalent: Estrogen

Estrogen (turn to estrogen chapter to learn about estrone, estradiol and estriol) are produced in the reproductive organs, adrenal glands and fat tissues. As testosterone is predominantly found in men, estrogen is found in women. During puberty, and pregnancy, a significant amount is produced. After menopause, a significant amount is lost. Estrone becomes the major estrogen and the adrenal glands play a much more important role then the ovaries do.

&Dr. Tai's Anti-Aging Health Secret&

You owe a lot to your skin—it protects and markets you. It's the most faithful of organs because it'll stick by your side forever. This is why I emphasize taking care of it with proper nutrients and avoiding negative habits like smoking and consuming alcohol.

As I stated earlier in the chapter, the skin is a very complex organ. Dermatology students go to school for years and years to understand its function and to help people improve its appearance. Certain prescriptions and specific procedures such as microdermabrasions, spot removals, wart removals, chemical peels, laser peels, are conducted by dermatologists to make the skin as beautiful as it is amazing.

In the world of dermatology, the sun is a controversial topic. I've heard many dermatologists tell their patients that basking in the sun is completely out of the question as it tears the skin and produces wrinkles. Every day, you can protect your skin from the harmful effects of the sun's rays and help control the damage caused by free radicals, glycation and other factors of aging. The key is daily exfoliating and then using a light penetrating moisturizer with ingredients that deliver stimulating antioxidants to protect the cells that rise to the surface. If the right SPF is used (SPF 40), sun damage can be mimized. Avoid chemical preservatives in creams and lotions such as paraben and methylparaben and use a pH-balanced formulation.

Chapter 16

Building your skin with natural ingredients

When you had the most of every hormone, it showed on your skin. Do you remember your adolescent years? Remember puberty? Remember when you were in your twenties? These were all periods when your hormones were hustling and bustling. Take a photo of yourself today and compare it to a photo of yourself fifteen years ago. When you put the two pictures beside each other you'll see it's like comparing a verdant rainforest to a lonely wasteland. The chances of your enjoying the sight between photos one and two are slim to none. If you're a part of the slim-to-none ratio, we need to roll up our sleeves and get started on a highly confidential mission entitled "Project: YOU."

Allow me to reintroduce myself as beauty drill sergeant—Dr. Tai. I'm here to help YOU save YOUR hormones and your LIFE. If you follow my instructions, you'll notice a difference in your skin, libido, energy and attitude. All I ask is that you get some discipline into you, do away with negative thoughts and self-damaging habits, and whatever you do, don't quit on yourself.

Treat hormone loss, bad food and laziness as your enemies, like they're walking towards you with a pointed stick. You will defend yourself, but in this very specific instance you won't join 'em, you'll beat 'em.

Steal from the rich, give to the poor
Plants have hormones too, lots of 'em

Estrogen, the reproductive female hormone, has receptors all throughout a woman's body, including her skin. Countless studies have shown that estrogen hormones play a vital role in skin thickening, capillary blood

---

Dr. Tai explains...

* **Collagen:**
  * Acts as a scaffolding for our bodies, giving it shape and thickness.
  * Controls cell shape and differentiation.

* Elastin:
  * Like a rubber band, elastin allows many tissues in the body to resume their shape after stretching and contracting.
  * Helps skin to return to its original position after smiling and frowning.

flow, and *collagen and *elastin replacement. After age 25, we begin to lose our hormones at a gradual and consistent pace, which results in skin thinning and deep wrinkling.

Hormones play a vital role in how our skin appears. Therefore, by using hormones through plant extracts known as phytoestrogens, we can decelerate the aging process. Use naturally low levels of phytoestrogens like the one found in Pueraria Mirifica to produce levels of *collagen and *elastin at a pace where results are clearly visible.

Bioidentical estrogen is FDA approved and long-term benefits have been acknowledged. Unlike synthetic hormones (metabolites from horse urine), bioidentical estrogen is extracted from plants like Puereria Mirifica, soy and yams. Since these substances are completely natural, a bioidentical hormone plan can be tailored for both men and women. Dosages are flexible and vary with symptoms. In contrast to the unlimited freedom one has using bioidentical hormones, people taking synthetic hormones have a limited amount of freedom. Since synthetic hormones pose the risk of side effects, one must follow doctor's orders specifically as they're given. With bioidentical hormones, you can customize to your needs.

Puereria …. Mi, mi, ri, fi—what?

For centuries, the women of Thailand have been using Pueraria Mirifica as a restoring and invigorating folk medicine. Uncommon in the U.S., the bulb-like plant is considered sacred by women throughout Asia. For this reason, it's been passed down through generations to improve complexion, remove wrinkles, and fortify and enhance the skin's overall condition. It's one of few plants that contains the chemical structures soya and alfalfa, two compounds which make Pueraria Mirifica a phytoestrogen. As with other phytoestrogens, Pueraria Mirifica is crushed into a powder and purified.

In 2004, a Thai researcher, Dr. F. Lamlertkittikul (et al.) showed that Pueraria Mirifica, his homeland's plant, did more than tighten skin—it also helped with the night sweats perimenopausal women are accustomed to experiencing. Dr. Lamlertkittikul found that perimenopausal and postmenopausal women who were experiencing hot flashes and night sweats used Pueraria Mirifica in capsule form. His study's results concluded that the herb relatively alleviated symptoms in perimenopausal women. (Lamlertkittikul, F. et al. "Efficacy and safety of pueraria mirifica for the treatment of vassal motor symptoms in perimenopausal women." *Journal of the American Medical Association, Thailand*, 2004; 87(1):33-40.)

In 2005, researcher Dr. G.C. Jeon (et al.) published an article for the Experimental Molecular Medicine Journal entirely based on the anti-tumor activity of the plant that's not just saving their skin and sleep, but also their lives. Jeon found that Puereria mirifica had an estrogen like effect by "activating estrogen receptor sites." (Jeon, G.C. et al. "Anti-tumor activity of spinasterol isolated from puereria roots." *Experimental Molecular Medicine, 2005;* 30 (37): 211-20.)

Ginseng... cha-ching!
Hitting the jackpot

You probably haven't heard of Puereria Mirifica, the first plant I mentioned, but I'm sure you've heard of ginseng. It's everywhere, because it's good stuff. That's not to say that Puereria mirifica isn't, it's just that ginseng is simpler to pronounce and it's reaped the rewards of a much more sophisticated marketing strategy. Athletes use ginseng for strength and endurance; this is why almost every energy drink stashed away in rows in giant convenience store coolers contains ginseng. Increasingly, I find ginseng tea being served both cold and hot in health-conscious restaurants and cafes, and I find it in a variety of healthful products as one of many energy-boosting ingredients. Internationally, ginseng is known as being good for you, but why, and how? How educated are you about a plant that'll help your body in more than a few ways?

The small perennial herb with funny, coarse-toothed stems has been used to remedy chronic fatigue, various types of depressions, infections (related to immune weakness), hormonal imbalance and damaged skin.

Ginseng and the sun

Because of daily or regular sun exposure, tanners are notorious for having pleated wrinkles, which can be attributed to the unremitting ultraviolet radiation attack tanners undergo for their desire to darken their skin color.

Dr. S. Kang of the University of Michigan's Department of Dermatology found that ultraviolet radiation damage generates a *reactive oxygen species* (ROS) which damages not only the epidermis (top layer of skin) but the skin's cells and its metabolic pathways.

Dr. Kang and his fellow researchers found a rapid and significant increase in hydrogen peroxide levels in vivo (inside) human skin when exposed to the sun. (The release of hydrogen peroxide causes instantaneous aging.) Both genistein and N-acetylcysteine prevented ultraviolet radiation damage to skin proteins. These two active compounds, cysteine and acetylcysteine (amino acids derived from soy), are very important because they can be converted inside of the cell and transformed into glutathione, a very powerful antioxidant that slows the process of photo aging on skin. (Kang, S. et al. "Topical ginesteine prevent ultra-violet light induced signaling in human aged skin in vivo." *Journal of Investigative Dermatology,* 2003; 120(5):835-41.)

Thousands of miles away, Dr. S. Choi, a professor at the Seoul National University, claims that Ginsenocide Rb2 a rare purified extract of ginseng stimulates fibronectin, keratin and collagen, which results in epidermal formation. (Choi, S. et al. "Epidermis proliferative effects of panax ginseng Rb #2." *The Journal Archive of Pharmacy Research,* 2002; 25(1): 71-6.)

Coenzyme Q10
Boosting cell energy

For centuries, the sun has been worshiped and used to represent power, royalty, burning passion and patriotism. In other cultures, the sun has been used as a prophetic symbol for prosperous futures and brighter days. To dream of the sun is to hope, to think of the sun is to smile, and to feel the sun is to feel warmth, but feeling an excess of the sun's rays is damaging.

With an increasingly depleted ozone layer, rays of sunshine aren't as innocent as they appear to be. In fact, I'm convinced that the sun is a hypocrite. How can something that feels this good be so bad? With a tan you look healthier, you feel younger, your eyes appear brighter and your smile is definitely whiter, but citizens of the Sunshine State will be the first to tell you that there are more skin cancer treatment centers in Florida than there are coffee shops.

Because of excessive exposure to UVA and UVB rays, which penetrate deep into the lower layers of the epidermis, skin cancer and melanoma have become two of America's most-treated illnesses. Yet there are more tanning salons in the U.S. than anywhere else in the world.

I know I'm going to feel like the mom who hands her kid a condom after the "sex talk" by telling you this, but if you're going to do it, protect yourself. Wear sunscreen SPF-45 and, if you can, increase your intake of coenzyme Q10 to protect your skin against aging and most importantly against life-threatening skin diseases.

With time, skin cells such as keratinocytes lose most of their resistance to UV radiation. CoQ10 is involved in cellular energy production. As a powerful antioxidant, it protects cells from oxidative stress to avert further damaging.

CoQ10 does an excellent job of preserving the skin by increasing its oxidative resistance. Yet, surprisingly, it wasn't until the 1980s when researchers began to pay attention to CoQ10, partially because it's a compound that's found naturally in the body. Similar to CoQ10, idebenone is another coenzyme that works in organelles like the mitochondria (the source of your body's energy) to improve electron energy production within the body. These two enzymes facilitate electron transportation, which make them useful in the photoaging process.

Similar to vitamins C, E and K, CoQ10 is a powerful antioxidant that will help replenish skin that's been damaged by the sun. You don't need a microscope to tell if your skin's been damaged by the sun—all it takes is a mirror. Deep lines, freckles, spots and facial spider veins are all excellent signifiers that the sun has disrespected your face. Combining CoQ10 with natural antioxidants found in rice, gamma oryzanol works well in conjunction with essential fatty acids linoleic or linoid acid.

Try to eat foods that are chock-a-block full, jam-packed with essential fatty acids, and although I'm not one for carbs, good carbs like the kind found in wild rice will also aid in antioxidant skin protection. For added antioxidant protection, try to use a topical liposome treatment made from CoQ10, SOD, glutathione, and catalase antioxidants will guarantee more rapid results.

Testimony
Smoking under the sun: Puff, puff, pass…

"Using bioidentical hormones was my last resort, I'd tried everything to look younger. I'm 37 years old and I used to look much older. My boyfriend who is seven years younger than me disagreed as an approach to make me feel better about myself. However, I have mirrors and I know what I look like.

"Since I was 20 I've smoked. I started out as being a social smoker and then it worsened; I started chain smoking. My skin was once supple—I was known for the most squeezable cheeks, the kind you want to pinch and kiss, but there came a point where I was surprised anyone wanted to shake my hand. My habits were to blame. I was obsessed with the sun and I couldn't keep away from smoking.

"I'm originally from New York, and in the summertime I would frequent Jones Beach or Long Island beach with friends. For hours I would sit under a scorching sun drenched in coconut-scented tanning oil without an SPF. For recreation, my friends and I would sing songs, joke and smoke until we nearly suffocated ourselves. At 26, I could see my face change dramatically. By then, I started to realize that I

had to start taking care of myself or else I was going to develop a cancer of some sort. But I couldn't stop—smoking and tanning had become a part of the life I led—it was my lifestyle. I don't remember myself without a tan or without a cigarette in my mouth.

"I've tried every beauty trick in the book. I've had my face scrubbed, rubbed, peeled, lifted, steamed—the list goes on and on. As I started to approach 40, I realized with my habits, there was no saving. I saw a doctor and asked him if there was a medical approach I could take, and he told me that with increased hormone production there was a way to mend damages. Again, bioidentical hormone therapy was my last resort and in less than one month, I could see a difference. I wish it would have been my first choice. I cut down on smoking—from one pack a day I'm down to five cigarettes per day. And if I'm feeling pale I'll rub a self-tanner and use bronzing powder as a sunshine alternative. I'm on testosterone liposome cream, a thyroid supplement and IGF-1 liposome sublingual spray. My eyelids are less puffy, my lines aren't as deep, my body feels firmer, I have less cellulite, and, surprisingly, an increased sexual appetite. I regret a lot of things I've done to myself and I still have ways to go, but I think, mentally, I've got a good strategy: I need to quit smoking and continue using the bioidentical hormones."

—Lizzy, 36

Argania and Anti Aging

Recently, dermatological institutes have adopted a technique Moroccans have used for centuries—instead of concentrating on herbal extractions, the institutes have focused, like most Moroccans, on collecting active fruit enzyme extractions to satisfy the skin's appetite.

The skin eats, and though much of the world's population hasn't realized this, most Moroccans have. For centuries, Moroccans have routinely used Argania spinosa fruits, found on a tree that resembles an olive tree, in that fruit leaves are narrow and project a light green color. Oil from the fruit tree may be an exotic topical luxury for most Americans, but for North Africans the plant is common. Found in the back yards of most Moroccans, they often make use of it, Argania spinosa is a plant that is revered in some parts of the world and taken for granted in other parts. The oil from the fruit tree provides a tight network of molecules which grabs the skin's surface while producing a close-fitting transparent weave that penetrates easily into the skin, neutralizing collagenaze-- skin bullies that break down collagen.

Perky Peptides

Letting your skin **inhale** *peptides* will only make it want to **exhale** *brilliance*.

Peptides are molecules that make up chains of amino acids and form building blocks of proteins. I find that peptide extractions are more effective when derived from fruits instead of herbs. Though both fruits and herbs are plants, I find that fruits have a higher concentration of peptide activity.

Dr. Jean Reduz, of Mondor Hospital in Paris and president of the World Congress of Dermatology, used a penta-peptide treatment on 49 women with photoaged skin (skin that's been damaged by the sun). After weeks of using the penta-peptide, all 49 women showed a substantial improvement in the depth of their wrinkles.

> **Vocabulary you should know**
>
> ***Snare:** An electrical type of protein connection between a nerve and a muscle that makes contractions.

Peptide molecules are really just small collagen "lites" composed of amino acids glycene, thrionine and serene, which are attached to an organic acid. When applied in a liposome form, peptides like the one found in the Argania spinosa fruit penetrate through the skin's top-layer.

In 2002, at the 20th World Congress of Dermatology in Paris, Dr. Carl Linter and his colleagues conducted a double blind study to show efficacy in peptide usage. Over a four-month period, Dr. Linter found a 9-percent increase in skin thickness among his study's participants, further concluding that penta-peptides work 150 percent faster than retinal cream.

Multiple personalities: Penta-, hecta- and septa-peptides

Not all peptides are alike: Penta-peptide aids in collagen production, and hecta and septa peptides bind to the *snare complexes of neuromuscular junctions. No need to squint your eyes or reread—all of this just means that larger (larger in molecule—hecta and septa) peptides act like Botulinum Toxin-A (Botox), a venom used for skin injection as a form of facial muscle paralysis.

> **No worries, Dr. Draelos:**
>
> "Critically active compounds" can be deposited into the skin by way of using transdermal topical solutions like liposomes. There are peptide liposome treatments that are made available for use—look and you shall find.

These complex peptides (penta, hecta and septa) don't exactly bind the snare complex. Instead, they inhibit acetylecholine binding, which increases communication between nerves, thereby slowing down muscle contractions. To sum it up: Peptides minimize the effects of wrinkles.

In February 2005, The Dermatology Times quoted Dr. Zoe Diana Draelos on some of her peptide thoughts. Dr. Draelos said, "Peptides have the biggest problem in the penetration of the dermis. In order to actually work in the neuromuscular junction, critically active compounds need to be finally deposited when applied to the skin in order to provide the benefits the complex peptides are capable of bestowing."

L-caffeine, L-carnitine, Caffeine & Paullinia Cupana
4Cs and Cellulite

While on the beach, I, like many others, will notice cellulite before I notice a "Baywatch" body. That's quite possibly because it's been the subject of a massive part of the research I've conducted since developing an interest in skin. Perhaps it's because, besides wrinkles, cellulite requires the most amount of skin care. The legs and thighs are the longest muscles on the body, and they're also the most problematic areas for women, influencing women to keep their bodies covered even during the most sweltering summer days.

Contrary to European women who sunbathe and swim half-naked, do you ever wonder why so many American women go swimming wearing a long T-shirt and a pair of shorts? What, you think they're cold? Then why go in the water? You think it's the ozone layer? Sweetheart, that's what SPFs and umbrellas are for. Though I could be wrong, in most instances I haven't been—on beaches, if a woman is fully clothed, she doesn't want to attract attention to the parts of her body that have captured much of hers.

Cellulite is small extrusions of fatty tissues in between compartments of fibers under the skin. These tissue fibers form alladus, an excess amount of fat that causes the skin to dimple. Ironically, cellulite hasn't been tagged in medical journals as a skin condition. Nope. The first time I've ever seen anything medically related to cellulite was in an article that skin-care specialist Dr. William Colemen wrote on cosmetic surgeries. Dr. Colemen accurately described cellulite as (ahem), "A term best applied to the egg carton appearance of the skin [of the buttocks and thighs]."

excess fat = cellulite

A significant driver in the formation of obesity is excess estrogen. Because estrogen leads to fluid retention and edema, blood vessels break. When they break, they push parts of the skin out. This turns into a microcirculation of subcutaneous tissue. Though a woman's estrogen depletes as she ages, this means nothing when it comes down to cellulite. Once it's there, it's there. It would be appropriate to think that when women age, they have less cellulite, since there are fewer fat-producing hormones in her body. But you see, with cellulite, once you have it, you're stuck with it, unless you find a product that directly targets external fat projections.

I used to think that once cellulite happened to a woman it was difficult to reverse its presence without surgery. That is, until I was confronted by a French dermatologist during my stay in Paris for an anti-aging conference. She said that for years, French women have been successful in their attempts to avoid cellulite by walking instead of driving, keeping slim, and utilizing caffeine outside of an espresso cup.

L-caffeine, L-carnitine, cysteic and paullinia cupana seed extractions are all excellent energy stimulants, and they're even better when they're combined or mixed into a liposome topical treatment. A group of female volunteers varying in ages rubbed a liposome energy stimulant solution with L-caffeine, L-carnitine, cysteic, paullinia cupana seed extraction on their butts and thighs. Using ultra-sound imaging, researchers found that the appearance of cellulite on the group of female volunteers was reduced by 0.6 mm (millimeters). From their study, researchers concluded that liposome microencapsulations of energy stimulants reduce the appearance of fat and improve skin textures.

Chapter 17

Look younger in 30 days

Every square inch of your home contains traces of "you," from the wall paint you chose to the dust on your coffee table. Although you can't see it, your skin sheds approximately 3 million dead cells each hour. Like certain reptiles known for skin shedding, people's skin is constantly changing, from firm and moist to saggy and dry. If you'd prefer a correlation, skin goes through a process much like reincarnation—it dies and then it's born again. Old skin cells slough off and new skin cells rise to the top. It's a process that's constantly repeating until a certain age. The older people become, the more difficult it becomes for the epidermis to release skin cells. Therefore, no matter how many times 80-year-old people decide to scrub their faces, they aren't releasing nearly as many dead skin cells as their 20-year-old grandchildren would.

Dr. Tai asks, "Did you know?"

If skin was stripped off the body, it would be approximately 10 feet long and two feet wide.

Measurements may vary slightly depending on height and weight of an individual.

Skin after a certain age

Skin on older people is obstinate and stubborn. If older people's skin is so tough, then why does it sag and wrinkle? Because, as we age, dead epidermal skin cells build up, and it becomes increasingly harder for nutrients to get through without an active delivery system. As you age, the dead layer of your skin becomes thicker, while the dermis (living layer) becomes thinner. If you're a diabetic or an aged person (who has not balanced hormones or has lived a lifestyle of sun exposure, smoking, and excessive alcohol consumption, etc.), cuts and wounds won't heal as they once healed. As you'll find in this chapter, as we grow older, even exfoliating dead skin becomes more sluggish because dead skin cells gather and develop a tighter bond than when we were much younger.

In this chapter we'll examine how to resurrect old skin, so you don't have to mask it with makeup or go to radical extremes like cosmetic surgery. This brings me to another point: Why do people choose cosmetic surgery?

The reasons why people chose cosmetic surgery:

- They don't have a skincare regimen.
- They won't stick to a daily skincare regimen.
- They don't have the patience to wait for topical solutions to affect their skin.
- They're skeptical as to how effective creams are.
- They want immediate results.

The dirt on cosmetic surgeries and cosmetic companies

I don't entirely blame people who have had cosmetic surgery, because it's the only effective way of getting rid of something they don't like, either semi-permanently (with things like Botox and collagen, both of which wither away with time) to permanently (reconstructive surgeries, implants, etc.). With cosmetics, every company makes the same claims and promises the same things, yet they all have different campaigns. Every cream typically has the same ingredients but there are two differences: the packaging and the various names and faces that represent them—names that are paid royalties to back these companies.

What gets me is when I see an 18-year-old model represent an anti-wrinkle cream. Wow, do I laugh! What kind of wrinkles can an 18-year-old possibly possess? And are these companies so confident that their products will deliver skin that looks like their spokesperson's skin? Getting a much younger model to represent a product meant for an older group of consumers is one thing, but what about an older model? You don't think those belles are wearing makeup? You don't think their images have been photoshopped, airbrushed or tweaked? If you think for a minute that there are people in the world that look like that without some sort of help, you're wrong! Wrong, wrong, wrong! Everyone needs help—we're human, not demigods and goddesses. Some people inherit freakishly awesome genes, but even they have some form of default.

I can't help you with the color of your eyes or the shape of your nose, but I can help you with the texture of your skin, hair and nails (since the two are part of the skin), the way you sleep at night, how you feel during the day and the energy you feel. The energy, mental acuity, and awesome self-confidence is all in the hormones that must be consumed and applied.

Active delivery: Pleoliposomes

Most of the synthetic forms of medicine need to be approved by FDA before they can be publicly available, and this process generally takes up to 20 years and one billion dollars. When you see an advertisement for a new drug, it isn't necessarily new, it's just new to you, the public. Before John Doe and Suzy Chapstick are on familiar terms with drugs, medical communities know what's hip and happening in laboratories. This was also the case with pleoliposomes, created 20-some years ago. They have just recently been made a big deal since they've just recently been made available.

*Dr. Tai clarifying...

Through careful scrutiny, I've evaluated various studies on phosphatidylcholine extract of soy and have found that when sweeping statements are made about the plant, it's solely because most studies' supplementations are dose, time, age, and gender-dependent. Ultimately, phosphatidylcholine and soy is a plant that your body can recognize easily since it's made from a lipid matrix similar to our own cell membrane.

Friends, countrymen, lend me your eyes and minds
Liposomes something to think about

I did not portray liposomes as such a topic of importance in previous chapters, only because I wanted to give you choices. As far as delivery systems are concerned liposomes are the most effective way to get nutrients into areas (epidermis and dermis) that need most of their help (besides injections). If the admiration for liposomes were a religion, I would be a follower, along with all of the many others whose lives have affected. I love liposomes like dentists love teeth, like hairdressers love hair, like bakers love croissants. Liposomes are, by far, the most effective way to deliver nutrients into a person's body.

Made from a natural cholesterol lipid matrix, the cells in your body are made from phosphatidylcholine (fosfet-d'l-ko-leen'). Like extractions from the ever-popular soy bean,* phosphatidylcholine is a major constituent of all cell membranes. Because our skin is made from phosphatidylcholine, it recognizes everything else that is, and this is how liposome formations are allowed to proceed past the dermis and into the dermis. Liposomes are microscopic bubbles that technology has skillfully crafted for your body to recognize. They are directly transported through your skin and into your blood, minus the side effects and delayed results. Liposomes transform phospholipids into aromatic pearls of power-packed skin essentials by using microencapsulation, a technique used to help the various extracts in products maintain potency and freshness.

Nutrients

Nutrients + Liposome-> epidermis-> dermis—a stunningly beautiful complexion

What the experts are saying about liposomes

In 2002, the Dermatology Department at the University of Ljubljana concluded liposomes "improved skin's oxygenation by stimulating the healing process of damaged skin."

Kristl, J; Abramović, Z; Šentjurc M. et al.; Pharmacy faculty, University of Ljubljana, Slovenia. "Skin oxygenation after topical application of liposome benzyl nicotinate as measured by EPR oximetry in vivo: influence of composition and size." *American Association of Pharmaceutical Scientists,* 2003; 5(1): 2.

The University of Dublin's Pharmacology Department reported 95 percent of liposome formulations target and diffuse skin cells.

Prancoise Audibert, Ph.D. "Liposomes in the therapy of infectious diseases and cancer." *Journal of Cellular Biochemistry, 2002;* 38 (S12B):244-62.

According to leading natural medicine authority Dr. Michael Murray, "Liposomes increase the absorption of herbal extracts" and "deliver more water-soluble substances into the skin with more efficacies."

Murray, Michael. "Phytosomes herbal support increase the absorption of herbal extracts." *Dr. Murray's Natural Living.* 20 Aug. 2006.

It's all inside

While cosmetic makers focus on your exterior, you should focus on your interior. It's your dermis that matters, but it receives the least amount of attention and care only because it's difficult to get to. With liposomes, products will multi-task effectively to reverse the effects of skin aging by filling facial furrows and soothing your skin's driest and most neglected areas.

They are by far the most effective way to deliver nutrients into a person's body. Instead of receiving 365 insulin injections a year, diabetics will soon be placed on transdermal liposome insulin. Liposomes have the same effect on body as injections do but without shots and without pain. You can use liposomes on the skin, but they work just as well when sprayed under your tongue or into your nose.

Getting through past tight parts

Our skin includes numerous sebaceous glands. Within the glands there are tiny hair follicles that have a small opening. Only liposomes can pass through these tiny openings. Because they are tiny enough to be absorbed by your body, they can pass through sweat glands and skin cells without interruption.

The smaller the molecular weight (500-1,000 daltons), the easier it is for an import to cross through the skin's barrier. The outer encapsulation of phosphatydlcholine has an ability to wiggle its way through the skin since it measures 200-500 nanometers. Being so small, liposomes possess the amazing capacity to reach beneath the skin's deepest layers.

Fat and water soluble

Dr. Tai's fun fact:

Physics line of transdermal diffusion:

The equation laboratory technicians use to determine how a liposome is made

J=K D/h (c0-c1)

J: amount of material passing through the skin.

K: stratumcorneum (the skin)

D: diffusion coefficient of the corneum

h: underneath stratum corneum thickness

C0: concentration of the active substance

C1: molecule size

Unlike many delivery systems, liposomes can be both fat- and water-soluble, depending on the nutrients they're transporting. To be fat- or lipid-soluble means that nutrients are absorbed by fat stored in the body and retained, whereas with water-soluble systems, nutrients are retained only briefly and then released via sweat and/or urine.

Doses of water-soluble delivery systems are therefore usually higher than fat-soluble doses. A prime example of a water-soluble oral supplement is Vitamin C, which can be consumed in large amounts (1,000 mg+) on a daily basis. If you've ever wondered why your urine changes from a pale yellow to lime green during nutrient supplementation, it's generally because the water soluble nutrients you've added to your diet are slowly being released as the day progresses. Liposome encapsulations of bioidentical hormones (what a mouthful!) are typically lipid-soluble, which means natural hormones are released into the skin and body slowly and consistently.

Expiration dates?

Another advantage that liposomes have over other forms of topical delivery systems is the length of their shelf life. (Before liposomes were used as vehicles for delivery, they were used to keep ingredients from spoiling.) Their prolonged bioactivity allows for long-lasting skin supplementation that continues to work for you long after you've stopped thinking about it. The active ingredients used to be mixed with all of the dozen other ingredients. After sitting on the drug store shelf for six or more months, the active ingredients are not so "active" anymore and have lost their freshness. On the other hand, microencapsulation of liposome keeps the active ingredient "fresh" until the moment you use it.

Loyalty looking lovely

"Promising ingredients can only do so much. The delivery system is what counts. Cosmetic companies can be as enthusiastic as they like. Eventually, the public will find out what's the real deal and what's not."

—*Marcia, 46*

Marcia said these words to her dermatologist after she was on a liposome treatment for 30 days. She said that when she took her second saliva test, her doctor saw a significant transformation in her total hormone count and Marcia noticed a major difference in her skin, unlike with cosmetics. Today she promotes bioidentical hormonal therapy and liposome delivery systems by showing off her gorgeous face and body.

How it happened for Marcia

Marcia was a prime example of a skeptical patient. She'd tried so many different kinds of anti-aging products and had spent her grocery money on wrinkle creams instead of food and supplements that were packed with anti-aging nutrients. Being a smarter consumer would have been more beneficial to her both financially and visibly, but, again, she was one of those "I didn't know any better" end users. Now Marcia knows, and she's now trying to convince her husband. She's a first generation Italian-American, and her husband Celestino migrated to U.S. at the age of 13 (he's now 49). Celestino used to poke fun at his wife's attempts to maintain her youthful sex appeal, because she claims both their families are too accepting of the ravages of age. Wrinkles, sagging skin and weight gain are all common amongst both Celestino's and Marcia's family members, but for Marcia it was important that she not join the majority.

Since I introduced Marcia to bioidentical hormones and liposome delivery, she's changed a great deal and has expressed her content to me through phone calls, letters, emails and periodic drop-bys, which are usually accompanied by a basket of sugar-free candies and fruits or vegetables from her backyard garden.

Marcia keeps in touch and tells me that her husband has become a believer in her anti-aging strategies. Though we once thought he would not accept Marcia's routines as valid, Celestino tells her that she's growing more vibrant by the day.

During a mid-afternoon phone conversation I had with her some time ago, she said, "He's convinced that what I'm doing has been working. He wants to try, but he's too macho. He says he'll leave that to the ladies. I swear I know he wants to try, but he doesn't know how to ask me, and I don't know where to start with him. I know he needs a saliva test before he tries the liposomes but I don't know how [to get him to do one].. He loves the sun and has such a large appetite. I need to find a way to calm his appetite and get some of those wrinkles off his forehead."

P.S. Celestino is now taking Weight & Inches Specialist to control his enormous appetite and cravings and Max-Thyroid Specialist to boost his metabolism. So far so good.

The truth hurts

Men have been more willing of late to try and use skin care products because they've finally realized how important appearance is. I will make no attempt to be philosophical with you—I'll leave it to your spiritual leader to tell you, "No, it's the inside that counts." Although, I believe in this—the world will judge you based on what they see.

As jobs become scarce, prices soar and the economy falters, first impressions have become increasingly crucial. In a fast-paced world, rarely does anyone want to give you a second chance. As an architect, Celestino professed to his ever-so-caring wife that he'd have

Dr. Tai's "Did you know?"
Forehead wrinkles

Wrinkles are folds in the skin concentrating on areas where there is frequent and constant bending. The skin loses collagen and elastin fibers by continuous bending of all three layers. The dermal and epidermal junction has defects and thinning, and these areas thin because of lack of collagen.

Loss made worse by the elastic tissue being over-stretched and torn into bits and pieces increases the visibility and magnitude of wrinkles.

(Braverman, I.M., et al. "Studies in cutaneous aging the elastic fiber network." *Journal of Investigative Dermatology*, 78; 434-43, 1982.)

more clients when he was a certain weight and a certain age. I'll tell you why this is: A youthful look denotes energy and bright ideas. Obese people have been burdened with the stereotype of being lazy—sad but true. Aged persons with a multitude of wrinkles have been thought of being not with it, tired, stressed, incompetent and over-worked—again, sad but true.

Now, imagine you were hiring and two people had a similar portfolio. Would you give the job to the overweight, wrinkled person or would you be more prone to hand the offer to the bright-faced individual? If you were to choose "Bright Eyes" over "Oompa-Loompa," then you've answered much like the rest of the world's population.

Mama Mia! Marcia's old man

Celestino's deep forehead wrinkles etched an insecure and worried expression on his face. He appeared unsure of himself, which made him come off as a rookie instead of a veteran in his field. His clients were surprised that he'd been an architect for 26 years, his expression made him come off as a worried college grad looking for a job. The look of desperation pushed people to pity Celestino, and that didn't do much to help him pay his bills. I suggested to Marcia that she ease up on the pushiness and to leave some of her products behind and continue to go about her business. Sure enough, with all that was going on in their lives, he would have adapted some of her ways.

In six months, Marcia looked five years younger, and Celestino reached his last straw when one day, at the supermarket, a stock boy asked what such a beautiful woman was doing with an old guy like Celestino.

Of course, the stock boy was joking, but, Celestino got the point. Marcia laughed while telling me the story, but Celestino didn't find as funny. The two Italian lovebirds had become partners in regaining their beauty, health and success.

Dr. Tai's daily skin care plan

Cleansing
Toning
Moisturizing
Eye serum
SPF-45

Dr. Tai's evening skin care plan

Exfoliating
Toning
Night Caviar
Triple Antioxidants
Eye serum

(See Dr. NanoDerma Products)

Ready, set, go!

They got around it spectacularly. Celestino cut out the carbs notorious in Italian cooking, omitting pasta, lasagna, bread sticks and tiramisu from his meals. Instead, he eats blueberries, salmon, spinach greens and a gallon of water a day, and is taking supplements to control overeating like Max-Digestion Specialist and Weight & Inches 30 minutes before every meal. In addition, he exercised and used natural hormone replacements (DHEA, progesterone, melatonin and cortisol support). Along with controlling his diet and using bioidentical hormones, he adopted a consistent skin care plan. He and Marcia used Diamond exfoliator daily and used liposome creams for their faces and everything else below the neck.

Celestino turned negative ideas of himself into productive steps for a positive outcome. In 28 days Marcia's husband lost two inches around his waist and had more energy than when she first met him. Celestino appeared younger, happier, fresher and "more alive."

Ciao Bello! Ciao Bella!

Celestino and his wife Marcia are just as excited about liposomes as I am. Both are frequent users who've implemented sublingual and topical (liposome application) of bioidentical hormones into their daily routines. Together, they both walk daily and eat foods rich in color, excluding sugars and white flour from their diets. Marcia exfoliates daily to strip off dead skin layers and applies moisturizers twice daily, in the morning and evening. For the time being, her husband exfoliates thrice a week, but he's slowly shifting gears to daily. He doesn't like to spend a lot of time washing his face over a sink, so he cleanses and exfoliates in the shower.

It took both Marcia and her husband less than 30 days to turn a life-changing plan into a habit. The happy couple have become nothing short of an inspiration for me!

Purifying the impure

If Marcia and Celestino, two fans of tanning and carbs, can do it, so can you! Marcia was developing crow's feet near her eyes and Celestino had nasty forehead wrinkles. Both had developed dark spots on the sides of their faces, which was explained by the fact that both Celestino's and Marcia's family members were avid smokers. Marcia claims she's never touched a cigarette, but because both of her parents still smoke, she often reeked of cigarette smoke. Secondhand smoke is just as bad as firsthand smoke, and Marcia had been around it for such a long time that she smelled of smoke. Cigarette smoke had clogged her pores and she'd released a heavy odor when she sweated, which meant that her skin was in trouble.

Both Marcia's and Celestino's skin had been tormented by smoke, excessive tanning, sugar and dehydration. They hadn't been consuming enough water, so the first step to good skin was raising the bar on H_2O consumption, and the second step was ridding both their skin of the nasty gunk that'd been clogging their pores.

Dr. Tai's "Did you know?"
What comes in must come out

Diet and environment effect scent.

If you have a diet which consists of fried and greasy foods, you'll smell worse when you sweat than people who don't. Because skin detoxifies the body through sweat glands, if you smoke, your sweat will have a much sharper scent.

Soap sucks!

When Marcia was asked what she'd been using to clean her skin, she said, "Soap." Soap! The worst thing to wash your face with is soap! It leaves a residue that just clogs more pores. Think of washing your car. What happens when soap bubbles are left to dry on your car window? Spots are left behind, and your car has just become dirtier than ever. Cleansing is the key step to enhance the appearance of your skin. Any dermatologist will tell you that cleansers are not supposed to leave filmy residues behind. If your skin feels tight and blotchy after you pat it dry, you didn't wash it properly! Marcia heard it from me, and I had advised she steer clear from highly fragrant cleansers that stripped her skin's natural moisture. Most importantly, she needed to stay away from the bars—the soap bars, that is.

pH

Everything has a pH, a measure of hydrogen ions in a solution and its acidity and alkalinity. The pH value is a number without units, usually between zero and 14. pH indicates whether a solution is acidic,

Dr. Tai's fun fact:

Measuring pH levels

Acidic: below pH of 6.5
Neutral: pH of 7.0
Alkaline: above pH 7.0

Examples of acidic substances:
Orange juice, cola

Examples of alkaline substances:
Bleach, ammonia

neutral (pH 7) or alkaline. Soap has an alkaline pH, which is opposite of your skin. (This is why many people experience allergic reactions and severe skin drying from soap.)

The skin's pH

Soap strips all of the natural oils and fatty acids from the face. The skin has a special pH which varies from 5.5 to 6.0. The microenvironment of the skin understands exactly how to protect itself from bacteria and infections, and it knows exactly how to replenish missing fatty acids, natural acids and oils. It's natural to do a perfect job in moisturizing and facilitating the exfoliation of the outer dead skin layers into a mild exfoliant, breaking away of the dead cells, and stimulating the new to the surface. It also has the natural protection and anti-inflammatory properties required to keep your skin looking healthy.

Harsh cleansers, soaps and glycolic acid pads

Somehow a marketing machine in the cosmetic industry has created the need for people to strip oils from their skin. People are beginning to use more and more glycolic acid cotton pads and harsh cleansers. Again, all of these things are unnecessary. Believe it or not, the oils of your skin are Mother Nature's way of delaying wrinkle formation. They're also Mother Nature's way of protecting your skin from harsh pollutants and chemicals. Think of fly paper, the sticky paper used to catch pesky flies that have entered your home on a hot summer day. Well, that's exactly the function oily skin fulfills—it catches pollutants and retains them until you decide to give it a light wash followed by an invigorating scrub.

Anti-Bubble:
The more lather, the worse:

Throughout the years I've seen people play up the misconception that bubbles are what cleans the skin. You know you've seen commercials where tiny little bubbles

Dr. Tai's lighthouse: "just looking out"

Many cleansing products often contain detergents that can irritate the skin. Some examples: sodium lauryl sulfate (SLS) and sodium laureth sulfate (SLES). Look out for chemical preservatives, i.e., paraben and methylparaben. Published research reveals they may cause skin cancer.

Before you buy, read the label and make sure cleansers don't contain SLS, SLES, paraben, or methylparaben.

are working hard at cleaning toilet bowels, sinks and faces. These powerful little suds are going through an uphill struggle getting dirt and grime off of surfaces so things sparkle brilliantly. These are lies! Don't believe the bubble commercials, because bubbles don't do anything except leave a residue behind. Foam or no foam, if a cleanser doesn't have the right ingredients, it won't help clean your skin and, if anything, bubbles will hinder the process.

Uh-oh! Did I burst your bubble?

A good cleanser is light, gentle and non-abrasive. Even if your skin isn't sensitive, it's better to choose a solution meant for sensitive skin types. The lighter the better, since cleansing is preparation for the next more important and more intense stage of the cleaning process: exfoliating.

Exfoliating

It used to be that exfoliating treatment was advised once a week, then it was bumped to thrice a week. I'm telling you to exfoliate your skin every day! If you want your night serum to work properly for you, you must slough away dead skin cells in order for a new cellular turnover to occur. Once pollution, smoke, excess oil, dried-up sweat and various forms of bacteria have been cleaned off your face, you must scrub in order to ensure cleanliness. Exfoliating is like giving your face a massage.

I've witnessed people scrub their faces so aggressively I've been almost positive they'd strip a layer of skin off. I'm exaggerating, but it isn't necessary to go overboard with the exfoliating process. Stick to gentle strokes in circular motions focusing on the cheeks, forehead, chin and nose (the area where blackheads mostly congregate). People make the common mistake of not exfoliating their necks. What makes you think your neck is any less important than your face? Scrub your neck gently—you need to slough off skin cells to prepare for moisturizing, and moisturizing the neck is the way to steer clear of sagging skin and turkey necks.

> **Dr. Tai's quick tip!**
>
> Take care of your neck as if it were part of your face! Age shows up most on the neck and the back of your hands. It's a dead give-away!
>
> **Wash, exfoliate** and **moisturize!**

Different kinds of exfoliants

Battery-operated gadgets that promise to give you an invigorating skin stimulating massage are offering something you can achieve for yourself. All you need to exfoliate is a jar of natural enzymes and 0.5 micron diamonds that are hypoallergenic, non-irritating and great skin exfoliants.

I've heard many complaints about the various ingredients found in exfoliants. Everything from synthetic beads to sand exfoliates can leave the skin irritated. I thought about how I could solve this problem by creating my own exfoliant. My favorite by far is Diamond Exfoliant. As a formulator, I've created an exfoliant made up of micronized monocrystal diamonds! You better believe it! The story behind the idea was that I realized it's never been done and it's the world's highest-powered super-mineral, super tough as a gem but super gentle as a micronized exfoliant.

Diamonds for your face

Diamonds are millions of years old (about 70 to 150 million) and are formed 150 kilometers below the earth's surface. Extreme heat and pressure or volcanic eruptions transform carbon atoms into diamonds by bringing ore to the surface. When volcanic activity stops and cooling takes place, diamonds remain in the magma and are collected. Diamonds are a mineral form of carbon and are the hardest known substance.

I suggest using the "Diamond Micro-dermabrasion," which was created to leave your skin feeling as dazzling as the gem itself. It's natural, non-allergenic, non-irritating and pulverized to half of a micron to exfoliate skin. Diamond Microdermabrasion has the extraordinary capability of lifting dead skin cells that have accumulated over time and have caused your skin to dull. It's natural and non-irritating, a high-powered super-mineral which ensures clarity and will offer you a dazzling complexion. For a soft buffed glow, I recommend natural moisturized liposomes to reduce inflammation and aid in the process of healing damaged skin.

Dr. Tai's lighthouse: "just looking out"

Steer clear from exfoliators with walnut pieces and aluminum beads. These agents will leave miscroscopic abrasions on your skin.

Aluminum toxicity has been associated with Alzheimer's and Dementia.

> **"If you want to appear a bit healthier, over-the-counter skin peel and microdermabrasions can help."**
>
> —*Dr. Pamela Phillips*
> *Mayo Clinic*

Exfoliating isn't supposed to hurt

Forget the magnifying mirror—if you were take it a step further and examine your skin with a microscope, what you'd see would be scary. Over time, skin cells accumulate, and this why your skin needs to be prepared by cleansing (remove excess oils) before you can exfoliate (sloughing cells). A good exfoliant contains non-allergenic micronized particles that won't irritate or scratch the surface of your skin. All you need is a lift—no cuts, or scratches. Use micronized diamond exfoliant that doesn't have jagged-edged ingredients like seeds or nutshells or toxic ingredients like aluminum.

Natural Enzymes at Work

Exfoliating treatments using natural cleansing food enzymes increase the rate at which the dead cells in the stratum cornium are peeled off, consequently speeding outer cell layer renewal. It's within these layers that the strong support of collagen gives the skin wonderful texture and thickness.

> **Ashes to ashes**
> **Dust to dust**
> **I relinquish my dead skin cells**
> **Because I must.**

Exfoliating pleases a lot of people. The result of daily usage is a fresher, vibrant, and more lively face. Your skin will appear one hundred times healthier than it once looked. Exfoliating weakens dead skin cell links by breaking the lipid matrix they've created for themselves, a sticky bond made from the oils your face has produced.

Moisturizing

Moisturizers are created to block excess water from leaving the ambient air and entering the surface of the skin. They've been created to fill the tiny crevices between the surface skin cells, lubricating the skin and making it more soft and smooth. Moisturizers for the face shouldn't be heavy! Heavy moisturizers only clog pores. The two heaviest creams you should use are the one you apply before bed and the cream applied around the eyes. Eye cream should be used before bedtime as the high water content within the moisturizer works on the thinnest part of your face while your body rests.

The skin needs water in order to keep moist and supple. Heavy oily moisturizers hold a light blanket over the skin. While non-oil, light lotions are made from water. Due to the water-based composition, your skin stays moist until your next wash.

Cream explained:
Moisturizers are made in two ways. They can contain tiny droplets of oil-in-water moisturizer, which generally has a lighter feel (lotion-like) to it than its counterpart, the water-in-oil moisturizer, which is heavier and much more cream-like.

I recommend that those with only the driest of skin take on water-in-oil type moisturizers, although these are generally used as night creams. Those with severely dry skin should use a minimum amount of night cream during the day. Using an excessive amount of night cream during the day will give the skin an oily, unkempt appearance. You want to hydrate the skin, not make it look as if you could fry an egg on it.

SPF and makeup

I realize that women don't leave the house wearing just their moisturizers. Although a lasting anti-aging skin care plan requires cleansing, exfoliating and *moisturizing, SPF and makeup should also be considered.*

Consider this…

- Hygiene is extremely important in the anti-aging process. Before beautiful skin, concentrate on clean skin.
- The skin needs water in order to keep moist and supple. Oily moisturizers hold a light blanket over the skin. Non-greasy, light liposome lotions are made with water sodium PCA, which holds 500 percent of its own weight in water. Due to the water-based composition, your skin stays moisturized until your next wash.

- Find a light liposome moisturizer with an SPF of 45 to prevent UVA and UVB rays from damaging your skin.
- Don't buy combinations of moisturizers and sunblock. They may be too heavy for your skin and pose the risk of clogging pores that'll eventually cause skin suffocation, creating blackheads, whiteheads and pimples no matter your age.
- If foundation and/or concealer are used, make sure the formula is light-weight and non-greasy.
- If you're a woman whose skin is excessively dry, steer clear of powders and switch to liquid, or, better yet, a mousse formula. Although mousse formula foundations aren't as readily available as concealer in stick and liquid form, they are lightweight and don't clog pores. Next time you go to the store, I suggest you ask for mousse.

Ꮧ Dr. Tai's Anti-Aging Health Secret Ꮧ

Skin and hair have been referred to as the "windows of age." For thousands of years, many have tried to reverse the effects of aging in order to appear as youthful as possible for as long as possible. Our skin is a multi-layered, meticulously complex organ—it covers every inch. It's what protects us from an environment that has increasingly become more and more unpredictable. With pollution taking a more prevalent role in our lives, it's difficult to preserve our skin's condition, which serves as visible evidence for our age and health. Every 10 years after the age of 20, our body's hormone levels drop consistently at a rate of 15 percent. Predictably, by the age of 45, both men and women experience a dramatic decrease of essential hormones. As a result, their bodies are permanently damaged by gradual weight gain, overwhelming fatigue, a lack of energy, decreased libido, hair and skin thinning and deep wrinkles.

Liposomes transform essential phospholipids into aromatic pearls of power-packed skin essentials by using microencapsulation, a technique used to help preserve the various extracts in our products and maintain their potency and freshness. The very best technology is at your fingertips with liposome's multi-tasking skin system that effectively refreshes dull skin, smoothes facial wrinkles and revives epidermal conditions. The active delivery system leaves your skin looking and feeling noticeably softer and clearer, achieving the youthful glow you never thought you would be able to obtain.

Age discriminates, and it seems to concentrate on our faces. The largest segment of our population is the Baby Boomers. The free-spirited hippies and dance club divas have turned into frantic forlorn workaholics who waste their pay in hopes of discovering youth in a jar or perhaps in a needle. Americans are facing more than a 30-percent increase in the general population over the age of 60. And with a rising life expectancy, the economics of lifestyle must change in order for us to FEEL STRONGER, LOOK YOUNGER, AND LIVE LONGER.

SECRET VIII

"It ain't over 'til it's over."
—Yogi Berra

Chapter 18

Dr. Tai's Asian Diet

Over 67% percent of Americans are overweight and 32% percent are obese. You may not yet be a part of this growing epidemic, but a recent poll taken by Yale University researchers shows that more than half of the Ivy League University's students would rather have a year taken away from their life than be diagnosed or appear to be obese.

Obviously, appearance plays a major issue here, but health effects are most important. People who are obese are playing with a time bomb waiting to explode. Obesity causes an explosion of health ailments and precipitous hormone downfall.

We are "*Super Sizing*" America. For 50 cents more you can get double or triple size of what ever you are eating. And for bonus, a 64-oz. sweet syrup drink to go! At the same time, more Americans today are going into stores to buy appetite suppressant drugs, spawning a jet-fast growing billion dollar industry. Fancy weight loss centers with sexy names are now appearing in every mall--there is someone there to offer you an easy way out, telling you how the "Hollywood stars" do it.

Is this what you want? If the answer is YES, then STOP reading right NOW! This chapter is not for you!

However, if you want a simpler and more satisfying lifestyle, you should make a pledge right now that for the rest of your life, you will adhere to a healthier lifestyle. This weight loss chapter will be an enlightenment for you. Read and re-read.

This chapter will teach you how to...

- **Rev-up your metabolism**
- **Balance your personal hormones**
- **Stop cravings and allergic responses to food**
- **Undertake a new and improved healthy lifestyle of eating**
- **Adopt a personal philosophy and mental attitude towards food**

My own story... Dr. Tai, the "Fatso"

I am now confronted with a mirror. I see a change in the way my jeans fit and bulging jowls underneath my chin. What are those bags of fat sagging under my armpits? Oh my goodness! Are these *really* my thighs?

This is the way I felt one morning. All of a sudden, I was 190 pounds and bulging!

Our society has many deadly diseases but the one that consumes us most is Obesity. Over 60 percent of Americans today are overweight and over 30 percent are obese. Just imagine the giant medical epidemic problem this creates! It affects you and me, our friends, our family members, and our neighbors, but it also affects our sons and daughters. This is going to lead to an epidemic of older and harder diabetes, hypertension, stroke, heart disease, cancer... shall I go on?

It is much harder for your body to lose weight today than it was 15 or 30 years ago. When we reach and pass age 40, fat grips us like a crazy monkey on our backs--we can't shake it off no matter how much we struggle. It affected me a great deal--I lost confidence in myself and my entire outlook on life was different. It had taken a toll on my health. With heart disease prevalent in my family, I was literally playing with a time bomb. So how did I solve this problem? How did I get rid of this truck tire around my waist?

New diets emerge on a daily basis: Atkins, Cabbage, Grapefruit, South beach, Mediterranean, Healthy Fat, Cortisol. Here's another one to add to the extensive list: *"Dr. Tai's Asian Diet."* I don't want to be another doctor that dispenses ineffective advice. We've heard "eat less, exercise more" used in a hundred different ways. It's not that difficult, *really*. You really don't have to kill yourself or starve yourself to lose weight. In fact, the more people tell themselves they "have to lose weight" the more I've see them gain it instead.

Metabolism gone haywire!

I told you in previous chapters that you lose hormones with every passing year. By the age of 50, you will have lost 50-70 percent of those protective hormones that keep your metabolism at a high rate.

Having a higher metabolism means you burn more calories, even on idle, and lose weight much easier. While you sit in front of your desk or sleep, you still burn more calories, so blood sugar gets used up instead of turning into fat cells.

3500 calories = 1 pound of weight

Where has all the muscle gone?

As you get older, you lose muscle mass—1 to 1.5% of muscle every single year. At that rate, in 10 years, you will lose 10-15% of all your muscle.

Lower muscle mass equals lower metabolism because muscle burns more calories than fat, even when it is at rest. Fat does not require or consume a large number of calories; mostly, it just sits there passively. So what happens to these extra calories? They turn into FAT!

This is a vicious cycle spiraling towards less muscle and more fat every single year. Do the math. If you gain only 2-3 pounds a year, in 10 years, you'll gain 30 pounds. In 20 years…60 pounds. I know because that was the story of *my* life two years ago.

Dr. Tai's Summary

You are eating the same foods in the same quantity, and practicing the same habits as you did when you were 20-30 years old. Now that you've lost 40% of your metabolism, if you haven't adjusted the way you eat, the resulting extra calories have probably turned into fat deposited around your waist. Now you know why!

So what to do?
Maintain a high thyroid function

Special supplements of iodine and iodide and a diet rich in sea kelp and fucoidans help to maintain a higher thyroid function. The average American diet does not have a natural high source of balanced iodine and iodide like the average Asian diet of more seafood and seaweeds. You may review the thyroid chapter for information on special supplements for thyroid health. (See Max Thyroid and Thyroid Specialist from Health Secrets USA.)

Easy does it!

Simple exercise. I'm not talking about sweating like a pig. I'm talking about simple walking, small incremental amounts of exercise, a healthy shift in lifestyle--small changes like choosing to walk the stairs, walking outside to enjoy a beautiful day, taking your dog (or your husband or friend) for a brisk 20-minute walk. Fresh air and exercise will improve your mood and get you breathing heavy. But most importantly, it will enhance and turbocharge your metabolism.

Once your metabolism kicks in, it is like an engine that continues to run so you will naturally burn more calories. Exercise is a daily investment with great return to your good health. One walk in the morning for 20 minutes, one walk in the afternoon, and 30 minutes of chores throughout the day--like housework or work in your garden--can lift your spirits and help to speed up your metabolism. This small addition of everyday activity will burn an extra 500 calories a day, which when multiplied by seven days equals 3500 calories. Again do the math. 3500 calories equal one pound...times four weeks per month...equals four pounds. Multiply this times 12 months per year and that equals 48 pounds a year, give or take 3 pounds. Net? 45 pounds a year. Not bad for a little "easy does it." (OK, so even if you only lose only 2 pounds per month, we're talking about 24 pounds a year!) This simple change in lifestyle will pay BIG dividends.

Measure once and measure again

Don't weigh yourself daily! Watching the scale too closely will only frustrate you. It's easy to become discouraged by small swings in weight. Weigh yourself no more than once a week--better yet, weigh once a month, on the first day of each month. And remember that weight does not tell the whole story about your body. Losing fat and gaining muscle may not change your total weight, but looking leaner and muscular will give you a wonderful body and a beautiful shape, which is far more important than weight alone. ***Emphasize shape, not weight.***

You don't have a number "tattooed" on your forehead. People don't know how *much* you weigh, but they sure know you are BIG, your waist is HUGE, and your butt is BULGING. The shape of your body matters! Measure your chest, your neck, your buttocks, waist and thighs, and keep those measurements in your drawer to remind yourself where you started and where you are going. Re-measure monthly and keep a record.

"It's the lifestyle, stupid!"

Whatever you decide to do, ***do it daily***.

You may want to find someone to go with you on this journey to a new healthy lifestyle. It could be a spouse or significant other, but your next-door neighbor will do fine too. This will help you keep going on the days that you don't feel well.

Having company helps you stick to the plan better. So get going…find someone to join you or find a group and join them… if all else fails, call *me*.

Killing you softly

It's the toxins in your gut, stomach, intestines, colon, liver, in fact, all over your body—they're clogging your system, and perhaps even "killing you softly." We need to wash away toxins by drinking at least eight 10-oz. glasses of water with lemon a day, or eight glasses of unsweetened tea. (Better yet, use MaxDigestion Specialist [see Resources] to help clean and detoxify your GI tract.) This is an internal cleansing program which elder Chinese people have practiced for a thousand years. In China, Japan, or other Asian countries, you rarely find fat people. They're slim and trim and their lifestyle fits perfectly in our modern society.

Green tea is the drink of choice. You can brew the tea ahead of time and keep it fresh in the refrigerator if you like. The Asians *never* use sugar in their tea yet drink 8 to 10 cups a day. They start with 2 cups of hot tea before breakfast, drink 4 cups of tea in the afternoon, add 2 cups of tea with dinner, and then end the day with 1 or 2 cups before bedtime. Some people find green tea difficult to drink at night, so you can substitute chamomile tea at night. Its powerful antioxidants clean and remove toxins from the bowel while calming before sleep. My own preference is jasmine tea. And oh, yeah…this doesn't mean adding cream and sugar…Plain tea only. As you lose and melt away your body fat, the acid by-products need to be washed away by this simple, elegant Asian cleansing program–tea.

Food Addictions

Do you have a craving for certain foods? Are you a lover of sweets? Chips? Bread? Cola?

My friend Jean, a beautiful young lady with a major pre-occupation, ate chocolate on a daily basis--sometimes the whole box when she was feeling down. She couldn't help it. It was an addiction. She had to eat her chocolate several times a day, and sometimes all day long. Her favorite pastime was watching TV with a bag of chocolate. For each program she watched, she finished a whole bag. Just guess how many programs she watches each day!

Is there food that you depend on daily? Do you crave potato chips, candy bars, cookies, sweets, soft drinks? Most people who crave for food, sweets and soft drinks have a special stash they hide away in a very secure place where no one can discover or take it from them. God forbid they should run out during one of their craving attacks. They hide their precious cravings in their car, their purse, the bottom drawer of their desk, so it will always be available whenever the craving attacks.

When is a food craving an addiction? When you look at it or someone offers it and you can't resist it. You have just finished a sumptuous meal, and moments later, you reach for the bag of potato chips. That's addiction! Works the same for candy, ice cream, colas…Yes, even wine, liquor…or cigarettes…and cocaine! Get it? It's **Addiction**.

Joseph, the owner of a bowling alley, was horrified one day when unbeknownst to him, he got up in the middle of the night and sat on the living room couch eating his beloved potato chips. The next morning, his wife woke him up, caught with his hand still tuck away in the potato chips bag*! **Now that's addiction**!!!

Now come the really hard part for us to accept. Craving of any food is a quintessential sign **of food allergy**. Most people who are allergic to a food, candies, sugar, chocolates—they have a craving for it. Don't get me wrong--we are not talking about itching throat, running nose, red eyes, skin hives. We are talking about a low grade, chronic, nearly imperceptible immune abnormality, filled with inflammation that slowly destroys the organs and your body. We are talking about feeling anxious, moody, fatigued, sleepy or experiencing a light headache, a "foggy" brain, impatience and short temperedness when you don't have your FIX! This is a highly addictive cycle of allergy to the food you crave. The more you eat, the more you want. The fatter you become, the more overwhelmed by the inflammation which leads you to more craving. (see chapter on Food Allergy – Food Intolerance.)

For example, a kid and his first cigarette. To be cool, he takes his first drag of cigarette in the back alley with his friends. In less than 5 minutes, after a few puffs, he coughs and chokes himself near death. His skin turns a few shades of green and he wants to throw up! His friends call him a sissy, and to prove otherwise, he continues to smoke, overcoming the resistance of his lungs and body in general.

Originally, the cigarette's completely obnoxious and foreign substance made him very very ill, but only one month later, his body has adjusted and worse yet, now the body craves that irritating cigarette smoke. He cannot go without puffing it. He craves it! He's hooked!

This same exact mechasim of addiction goes for food your parents encouraged you to eat. Remember the famous words, *"Clean your plate. Remember the starving kids in China?"* Feeling guilty, you finished your dinner though you were already satisfied, full, and not hungry. As a reward for having done what your parents told you to do, you were given more apple pie, ice cream, or cookies as reward for eating more despite the fact you did not want it anymore.

Today, sitting alone in your beautiful kitchen or living room, devouring a full box of chocolate, *you are addicted*. Who would have thought that you and the junkie on the corner with cocaine and syringe in hand are suffering from the same disease. That street corner addict started innocently on the path of cocaine maybe as a joke, a dare, or a recreation but now would be willing to sell his mother for a fix. Of course, in your case, it's bread, chocolate, chips, and cola. On the surface, it is innocent enough, but the excess sugar converts into excess weight and slowly piles on until you're obese—killing you softly, killing you slowly.

Dr. Tai's Asian Diet

Asians always start (and finish) meals with a large bowl of clear soup/broth, around 12-14 oz., made of chicken, beef, pork or seafood boullion garnished with a medley of chopped seasonal vegetables. For the main course, they have a variety of lightly cooked, steamed, or sauteed vegetables. The average person eats no more than 3 fingers of very thinly sliced meat or seafood (which makes it appear like a lot) accompanied by a small portion of rice, and of course, we finish with one more bowl of clear soup.

Today, you may modify this meal by choosing soup with a large salad mixed with a variety of vegetables of different colors, texture, and flavors. You may jazz up your salad with eggs, thinly sliced meats, or seafoods. Sprinkle with nuts, tomatoes, and onions if you like. Be mindful of salad dressings; keep them simple and light. The best ones are made with extra virgin olive oil, lemon juice with a little zest, or rice or wine vinegar, all of which play an important role in enhancing the digestive enzyme in your stomach, the acid responsible for efficient digestion. This is a very important part of the diet; as we get older, our stomachs do not make as much acid as is needed for digestion.

Lastly, a typical dessert is, in small portion, a medley of different fresh fruits cut in cubes. Do not follow the typical American habit of buying a single fruit like watermelon and eating it completely in a sitting. Small amounts of different fruits make a fresh fruit salad with more variety, more color, and more taste—with heavy emphasis on blueberries, raspberries, and strawberries. Your meal will be delightfully complete, clean, and light. Eating this way, you can easily lose 2 pounds a month. That's 24 pounds a year!

This is my secret. I did it in two years and lost 40 pounds in weight. I am today 155 pounds and have a 31 inch waist. With a 5 foot 11 inch frame, that's a reasonable weight I can live with and maintain.

If, in a weak moment, you break away from this diet for one day, you can make up the next day by eating more vegetables to correct the infraction early and quickly. This way, you will not have much to deal with when it becomes unmanageable. Remember, this is a lifestyle change.

Forbidden foods

You must remove high glycemic foods, drinks, and fruits from your diet. These are the sweet, sugar-laden foods and drinks that easily convert to glucose in your bloodstream, causing an hyper-insulin reaction. Refined sugars, candy bars, chocolate, mints, soda and cola, bread, chips, pastas, pizza, cookies, cakes, pies-- you get the idea. I always laugh when I see the ingredients of these "Good for you" granola bars laden with sugar, corn surup, and processed honey, even if they claim to be "low fat." They still convert excess sugar into fat when eaten.

Try to stay with fruits in the berry family--strawberries, blueberries, raspberries, etc. Stay away from sugary fruits such as oranges, apples, bananas, and pineapples, and their juices.

Americans are notorious for having sweet tooths. This seems to be getting a lot worse. Thirty years ago, the average American ate 70 pounds of refined sugar per year. Today, the average American eats 150 pounds of refined sugar! Think about it. That's like eating your own body weight in refined sugar. Someone like myself who eats fewer than 10 pounds of sugar a year have a surrogate American somewhere eating more than his share plus my share to boot. No wonder we are an increasingly obese society. Even Europeans, the inventors of chocolate and pastries eat less than half of the sugar intake per year of the average American.

Line up the suspects
Common Food Allergens

Eggs, chocolate, coffee, corn, wheat, potatoes, refined sugar, milk, cheeses, ice cream, cookies.

Common Allergy Symptoms/ Food Intolerance

Feelings of weakness, cravings, irritability, shakiness, shortness of breath, moodiness, depression, headaches, anger, impatience, lack of energy, fatigue, sleepiness, mental fogginess, lack of concentration, arthritis, constipation, hyperactivity, skin blemishes, aches and pains, etc.

Authors on food allergies

Dr. William Philpott M.D. says in his book *Brain Allergies* that addictive food triggers a rise in the brain *opioid* and *enkephalin*, two natural narcotics produced by the body. Opioid and enkephalin produce at unprecedented rates and form addiction (Keats, 1980).

Dr. Marshall Mandell M.D. in his book *Dr Mandell's 5-day Allergy Relief System* (Pocket Books, 1979) conducted a five-day study on schizophrenic patients. Dr. Mandell said in his book "It was hard to treat patients. Neurotics were found to be 88 percent hypersensitive to wheat and 50 percent of them were hypersensitive to milk. Of all the patients he tested for hypersensitivity 92.2 percent showed hyper-sensitivity to food.

In 1995, Dr. Rudy Rivera, author of *Your Hidden Food Allergies Are Making You Fat* (Prima Lifestyles, 2002) conducted a study at the HCA Medical College, Center for Sports Medicine in Houston, Texas. He gathered one hundred overweight patients and surveyed their eating habits for 4 weeks. Dr. Rivera excluded foods he saw most of his patients were addicted to. After seeing the study to completion Dr. Rivera found that half of his participants lost an average of three pounds of fat and gained one pound of lean muscle.

After the study, Dr. Rivera said "Food intolerance and hypersensitivity causes the body to react abnormally to common foods. One abnormal malfunction triggers and impacts the next like a series of dominoes resulting in excessive mucus production, chronic inflammation and contractions of the lungs and other biochemical processes."

Portion Control

The latest restaurant marketing craze towards profitability comes in four words: "ALL YOU CAN EAT," a home run into the mental and emotional needs of the American people.

Over and over again, $15 get you into the biggest "feeding frenzy," reminiscent of hungry piranas gorging on the banks of the Amazon River.

People insist on eating at least $50 worth of food so they can walk away smiling and believing that they got the best deal yet, bragging to their friends and anyone that will listen how they "broke the house." You ate until you couldn't eat anymore! All those King Crab legs, roast beef, pasta, cookies, ice cream, to the point where you promised and swore that you will never eat like this again for the rest of your life. Liar! You'll be back again next week, only two pounds heavier.

Now, I ask you, who got the worst deal? The restaurant owner is still in business, making money and laughing all the way to the bank. He is so profitable he's investing in bigger and wider chairs so that you won't feel how fat you have become. You, however, walk away feeling stuffed to the point of feeling ill. You will gain two pounds and one inch around the waist to show you won.

And…you paid $15 for the food! But that is the least of it. You will probably spend 10 times more sweating in the gym, working off the extra weight you have added to your aging body and you will spend an additional $100 on supplements and diet aids. Think about it and ask yourself what created this problem? Is it really worth it? We are penny wise and pound foolish.

Portion control is an extraordinary secret to a powerful weight-loss lifestyle. Asians use small bowls and eat with unmanageable chopsticks. That's portion control! In a modern adaptation, I suggest using smaller plates, chewing your food slowly, and savoring every minute of the meal. It is the "Zen of Eating." In other words, be in the moment and enjoy the tasty fragrance of *now*. Spend at least 20-30 minutes savoring your favorite morsel of food while in conversation with a friend or loved one. It takes at least 20-30 minutes for your stomach to tell your brain that you are satisfied and full. Otherwise, you are bound to overeat. If you eat out, take two-thirds of the food for carry out and drop it off at a friend's house as a gift and share. Better he or she be fat than you…Ha! Kindness does pay off. I promise YOU WON'T GO HUNGRY!

Don't eat and run. Enjoy your food. Put your fork down between bites. You can eat again whenever you like. You don't have to stuff your face to the point of no return. Ask yourself…when was the last time there was no food for you? When was the last time you went hungry? When was the last time you went a whole day without eating? (Except maybe when dieting…) Perhaps some people in "third world" countries will go several days without food to eat, but not the average American.

It is far better to eat three to five small meals a day with small snacks in between and not having to ever go hungry. In fact, it is far better that you start to eat *before* you are hungry. This way, you will eat a small amount just to satisfy, not to gorge. The purpose here is *not* to eat until you cannot eat anymore. The purpose is just to eat so you can enjoy food, be satisfied…and stop eating. Get it?

You live in a world of "abundance," yet you eat until you can't eat anymore as if you come from a world of "scarcity." When you open your refrigerator, is it empty? How about your freezer, is it empty also? How about your cupboards? I bet not. I don't think so. If you act as if you are homeless and have nothing to eat, you will overeat!

Neanderthal Man:
The genes are still kicking, same behavior...different time.

I will wager that you have too much food in your house, more than you can possibly eat in three months. Make an inventory of your food. And don't forget about all those stashes of food in your garage...Oh! the basement also! Got it? I assure you there is no food shortage, and you are not starving. Get it through your head that you are surrounded by food. You can have all you want and no one will stop you. I promise!!! And, by the way, you can forget forever about that starving Chinese kid your mother talked about...he's here in America and had to *lose* 40 lbs. No kidding—that starving kid is me!

Cheers!

Alcohol encompasses unnecessary calories you could gain from healthy foods. Weekend trips to the bar will add extra pounds; most alcoholic beverages range in the hundreds of calories; three drinks can equal the total calories of a packed meal. Besides the extra calories, alcohol aromatizes or converts your good hormones into excess estrogen and then into fat. Fermented potatoes (in vodka), grapes (in wine), and yeast (in beer) all have high levels of sugar especially when combined with syrups or fruit juices. Waves of high sugar cause the pancreas to overproduce insulin, which will in time cause glucose receptor sites not to respond and become insensitive, potentially leading to secondary diabetes. Impaired and abnormal insulin will lead to greater fat deposits due to sugar excess. Increased insulin production will cause you to crave for more sugar.

Now you know where the term "Beer Belly" came from. Fat deposits most often gather in a person's mid-section, the hips, stomach and back, creating bulges of "love-handles."

Max Digestion

When the right proportion of Vitamin C meets L-Glutamine, a peptide, the combination produces fantastic benefits for your body. The two work together to heal the stomach's inner lining. *Max Digestion Specialist* is a formula I created, which consists of calcium, magnesium, vitamin C, and L-Glutamine with 80 other essential micro-minerals.

Directions:

• One teaspoon of Max Digestion in a 12 oz. glass of water.
• Drink one half-hour before eating, or take five to ten minutes before eating foods that you crave.
• Be consistent and in a few months, your cravings will diminish. Watery stool will detoxify your G.I. tract and cleanse your entire gut. It is not abnormal to have watery stool during this process; when the G.I. tract is repaired, the stool will return to a soft solid.

In 2005, I received a United States certified patent for Max Digestion Specialist and its ability to help achieve satiety (food satisfaction) and rid a person of food cravings.

Research on Calcium and Weight Loss

Researcher P.N. Hopkins (et al.) found that a diet consisting of high calcium results in an average weight loss of 24.6 pounds in 16 weeks. (Hopkins, P.N. et al. "Risk of valvular heart disease associated with use of fenfluramine." *International Journal of Obesity & Related Metabolic Disorders*, 2003; 11:3(1):5)

M.B. Zemel (et al.) found through his study that people lost 10.56 pounds in one year after simply adding a cup of plain yogurt to their daily diets. ("Regulation of Adiposity by dietary calcium." *The Federation of American Societies for Experimental Biology*, 2000; (9):1132-8).

1000 mg of additional daily calcium intake resulted in a 17.6 pound difference in body weight for Dr. Davies' patients. (Davies, K.M. et al. "Calcium intake and body weight," *Journal of Clinical Endocrinology and Metabolism*, 2000; ae5(12):4635-8).

Researcher Dr. R.P. Heany studied the effects of calcium on both children and adults. He saw that 300 mg of calcium resulted in a kilo (approximately 2.2 pounds) loss in children and three kilo (6.6 pounds) loss in adults.

(Heany R.P. et al. "Calcium and weight: clinical studies." *Journal of the American College of Nutrition*, 2002 Apr; 21(2):152S-155S).

Here's how Hunger works:

The "Satiety Center" is located near the hypothalamus, the center of the brain. When we consume a formula made with essential minerals the body needs in order to feel properly fed, the brain tells us that we should stop eating. People with "Dysfunctional Satiety Center Syndrome" continue to eat because their brains fail to signal when enough is enough.

Pairing "dysfunctional" and "syndrome" to any word gives us the impression that there is a rare and scary condition when, in fact, the condition is very common. People who crave certain foods have developed an allergic reaction to those foods and as a result, have desensitized their satiety center and suffer symptoms like constipation, diarrhea, weight gain, headaches and moodiness. Max Digestion cleans the stomach's inner lining and repairs whatever has been damaged by inflammation caused by food intolerance. In a sense, **Max Digestion** "resurfaces" the intestines by mending them. Once the intestines are cleared, the body receives a fresh start. Once the cravings have left, the satiety center gains a break from constantly being triggered and regenerates itself.

Chapter 19

Delayed Food Allergy/Food Intolerance

"Food intolerance and allergy have become an increasingly serious problem in recent decades. Food allergy might be the cause or aggravation of almost any disorder, and, often enough, it is the cause."
—*James C. Breneman, M.D. author of Basics of Food Allergy*

Just imagine, millions of poor souls in America suffering "nightmarish" symptoms of major medical conditions that puzzle established medical doctors coast to coast, leaving them dumbfounded and scratching their heads, wondering what is causing this massive epidemic of chronic migraines, painful irritable bowel syndrome, unmanageable obesity, exhausting hyperactivity syndrome, life draining chronic fatigue syndrome, painful arthritis, skin problems, lack of energy, insomnia, asthma, anxiety…

WOW! That list can go on and on. How many people have told you they have been suffering from these persistent symptoms for decades and these patients often report that countless unproductive visits to doctors and specialist, only to be told that nothing else can be done for them, that they just have to "live with the problem."

All the above frustrating experiences and conditions I have described can in actuality be caused by ONE dangerous culprit…*Delayed Food Allergy or Food Intolerance.*

"An estimated between 30%-90% of American population suffer some kind of food intolerance with a variety of diseases ranging from obesity to cravings and lack of energy to diabetes and asthma."
—*Rivera, Rudy. M.D. Your Hidden Food Allergies Are Making You Fat*
Three River Press, NY 2002.

What is Delayed Food Allergy & Food Intolerance?

It is developed when your body rejects individual ingredients of food in your diet by "turning on" your own body's immune system, antibodies, and chemical mediators.

Severe food allergies are life-threatening and rare (incidence less than 5%) in our population. In severe allergies, the reaction of antibody IgE is immediate and violent, e.g., wheezing, hives, diarrhea, swelling, and shock.

A far more common *delayed* food allergy is known as *food intolerance*. Some authors claim that food intolerance affects potentially 30-90% of Americans. Food Intolerance or Delayed Food Allergy is a chronic severe immune response of Antibody IgG that rejects the specific food ingredient acting as a food allergen. This may be caused by an enzyme deficiency or chemical sensitivity.

This negative delayed food allergy response from your body may last from several hours (migraine headaches occur 48 hours after allergic foods are eaten) or several days; these destructive food allergens bound to antibodies circulate in our blood stream. Called Immune Complex, over time, they become deposited in nervous systems, blood vessels, joints, organs, and other vital tissues.

Food Intolerance and Delayed Food Allergy can occur from any vital organ or essential body tissues in our body, resulting in over 100 allergic symptoms. These are the root causes of over 150 significant specific medical diseases. A conservative estimate is that over 80 million Americans suffer from the signs and symptoms of clinically ravaging food allergies, which, to my amazement, they are totally unaware.

"It's a great disappointment that doctors don't bother to consider food intolerance because removing certain foods from certain people's diets can be helpful with so many problems." *John W. Gerrard, M.D. Professor of Pediatrics. University of Saskatchewan, Canada.*

"Failure to recognize and control food allergy throughout life accounts for much unnecessary morbidity, invalidism, and even mortality." *Albert H. Rowe, M.D. author of "Food Allergy: It's Manifestation and Control."*

"No drug, no medical therapy, and no diet alone can improve your health or help you lose weight if you continue to bombard your body with your own personal poison (food allergy)." *Rudy Rivera, M.D. author of "Your Hidden Food Allergies Are Making You Fat" Three Rivers Press, NY.*

> "Fatigue is very often reported as a symptom of food intolerance, specially in connection with migraines, morning tiredness, and irritable bowel syndrome." *Professor Dr. Jonathan Brostoff. "The Complete Guide to Food Allergy & Intolerance." 1992.*

Common Signs & Symptoms of Delayed Food Allergy/Food Intolerance

Uncontrolled weight gain
Respiratory diseases. ie. Asthma, bronchitis, etc.
Chronic fatigue, feeling tired and lacking energy
Degerative arthritis. e.g., Rheumatoid
Skin diseases. e.g., Psoriasis, eczema, etc.
G.I. tract disorder. e.g., colitis, stomach pain, etc.
Hyperactivity in adults and children
Anxiety & Tensions
Chronic diarrhea
Nausea
Depression
Bloating & cramps
Rashes & itches

Chronic muscle pain
Allergies and sinusitis
Infertility
Diabetes type II
Migraine and headaches
Frequent panic attacks
Frequent colds and infections
Poor appetite
Frequent ear infections
Dizziness
Wheezing & Sneezing
Fluid retention

Obesity: A National Epidemic

Institute of Medicine – Declare war on epidemic of obesity.

Harris Polls Report – In individuals over age 25, the percentage of Americans who considered themselves overweight in:

1983 – 58%
1990 – 64%
1995 – 71%
2002 – 80%

JAMA (Journal of American Medical Assoication) – December 2001 study reports an alarming statistic—a more than 50% increase in children obesity over the past 12 years.

National Center for Health Statistics – One in five children age 4-12 is overweight.

In March 1994, Harvard Medical school's Harvard Heart Letter said, "Medical researchers and weight loss experts no longer regard being overweight as a simple failure of willpower. Instead, obesity is considered a chronic disease, like depression or diabetes."

Over 50 million Americans are dieting and statistically 95% will fail.

Weight Loss Made Easy

"A very high percentage (80%) of obese patients have serious food allergy/addiction. They will never be able to adequately conquer the problems of obesity...until their allergic–addictive foods have been identified and eliminated from their diets."

—*Dr. F. Fuller Royal. Clinical ecologist, Food Sensitivity and Environmental Medicine*

In 1995, a landmark research conducted at Columbia/HCA Medical Center in participation with Baylor Medical School, performed a control study of 100 overweight participants with additional health problems. i.e. Lack of energy, insomnia, chronic fatigue. Divided into 2 groups: 50 subjects were control group and 50 subjects had eliminated food allergies identified by a simple finger prick blood test over a 4 week period.

The 50 subjects that eliminated food allergens from their diet lost an average of 3 pounds of fat and gained nearly 1 pound of lean muscle. In contrast, the 50 control subjects following their own diet plans lost 1 pound of fat and gained 1 pound of muscle.

The difference between these two groups in "lean-to-fat ratio" showed a 6 pound difference at the end of the 4-week study. Dramatically superior, the 50 "Allergy-Eliminated" group improved significantly and dramatically in 20 of 24 disease symptoms when compared to the control group.

"We found that you can change people's health dramatically when you remove their intolerant foods from their diets. [Removing] food intolerance is extremely helpful in improving health and losing weight. It is much more effective than traditional dieting."

—*Dr. Gilbert Kaats, Ph.D. Director, Health and Medical Res. Foundation, San Antonio, Tx.*

How does Food Detective work?

The Food Detective uses the principles of enzyme immunoassay (ELISA). This highly sensitive technique is normally carried out in a biochemistry laboratory. However, scientists have simplified the procedure, allowing it to be carried out by medical and alternative practitioners. The test detects IgG antibodies to fifty-nine commonly eaten foods. Each numbered well on the Food Dectective reaction tray is coated with a different food extract and is identified by reference via a table provided in the instruction manual.

Food Detective at Home or Your Doctor's Office

All materials required are provided. Access to a sink is necessary for disposal of the used chemicals. The chemicals used in this test procedure are non-hazardous.

1. A pin prick blood sample is collected, using the lancet and capillary tube provided.
2. The sample is dropped into diluting fluid which is then poured into the Food Detective reaction tray and left for 20 minutes.
3. The tray is washed and Detector Solution is added.
4. After 10 minutes the tray is washed.
5. Chromogen solution is added and left for two minutes.
6. Blue spots (slight) appear where food antibodies are present.
7. Aftet two minutes the tray is washed and dried, and the results can be read by the naked eye.
8. A positive and negative control is provided to monitor test performance.
9. A report is then completed for each individual.

Which foods are tested?

OAT	WHEAT	RICE	CORN	RYE	DURUM WHEAT
GLUTEN	ALMOND	BRAZIL NUT	CASHEW	COLA NUT	WALNUT
COW'S MILK	EGG	CHICKEN	LAMB	BEEF	PORK
WHITE FISH*	FRESHWATER FISH*	TUNA	SHELLFISH*	BROCCOLI	CABBAGE
CARROT	LEEK	POTATO	CELERY	CUCUMBER	PEPPERS*
LEGUMES*	GRAPEFRUIT	MELON*	PEANUT	SOY BEAN	COCOA
APPLE	BLACK CURRANT	OLIVE	ORANGE & LEMON	STRAWBERRY	TOMATO
GINGER	GARLIC	MUSHROOMS	YEAST	NEGATIVE control	POSITIVE control

* White fish – Haddock, Cod, and Plaice
* Freshwater fish – Salmon and Trout
* Shellfish – Shrimp, Prawn, Crab, Lobster and Mussel
* Peppers – Red, Green, and Yellow
* Legumes – Pea, Lentil, and Haricot
* Melon – Cantaloupe and Watermelon

This Food Detective Test can be ordered from Health Secrets USA (See resources)

"**Delayed Food Allergies / Food Intolerances are commonly reversible. If you strictly eliminate the allergic foods for 6 months, you can bring most of them back into your diet and remain symptom-free. (Run a Food Detective follow-up test).**"

—Dr. James Braly, M.D. Delayed Food Allergy Testing.

Frequently Asked Questions

Q. Do I have to collect the blood sample at any particular time of day?
A. No, samples can be collected at any time of the day.

Q. Could I be reacting to the chemicals in food rather than to the food itself?
A. Addictives are small molecules, which usually do not cause an immune response. However, some chemicals can produce intolerance symptoms without involving the immune system. They are best avoided if you suspect them but are difficult to test for.

Q. I have avoided eating a specific food for sometime. Will this food show up in my test?
A. If you haven't eaten a certain food for more than 6 months, it may not be positive in the food IgG test.

Q. Is Candida infection affected by baker's yeast?
A. No, they are quire different and unrelated organisms. Antibodies to baker's yeast, however, are associated with Crohn's Disease, a form of inflammatory bowel disease. If you suffer from bowel pain and have a strong reaction to baker's yeast, then you should seek advice from your health professional.

Q. Is gluten intolerance the same as wheat intolerance?
A. No, gluten is a protein, which is present in wheat, rye and barley. For some people it causes changes in the intestinal villi resulting in Coeliac Disease, which can be very harmful. Non-coeliac wheat intolerant patients may be reacting to other wheat proteins, separate from gluten.

Q. If I react to cow's milk, what should I do about other dairy products?
A. Antibodies to cow's milk are found in about 40% of patients. If you are positive for cow milk, avoid all milk products, i.e., yogurt, cheese, cream, etc.

Chapter 20

Extreme Anti Aging Technology

Xeno Stem Cell / Live Cell Technology

What do all these famous people have in common?

Frank Sinatra, Charlie Chaplin, Sophia Loren, Liz Taylor, Bob Hope, Alfred Hitchcock, Hirohito of Japan, Gustav VI King of Sweden, King Saud of Saudi Arabia, Sultan of Brunei, Winston Churchill, Dwight D. Wisenhower, Joseph Kennedy, James S. Rockfeller, Pope Pius XII, Jackie Onasis, Pablo Picasso

They have all enjoyed the treatment of cell therapy.

> *Sources:*   *Prof. Dr. James G. Defares M.D., Cell Therapy, page 16-20.*
> *E. Michael Molnar, M.D., Forever Young, page 79-91.*

The basic theory behind cell therapy was stated best by Paracelsus, a 16[th]century physician who wrote: "Heart heals the heart, lung heals lung, spleen heals spleen; like cures like." Paracelsus and many other early physicians believed that the best way to treat illness was to use living tissue to rebuild and revitalize ailing or aging tissue. Modern orthodox medicine lost sight of this method, so it may use chemicals to interrupt or override living processes. While chemicals and drugs work only until they are broken down by the body's metabolic processes, cell therapy has a long term effect, because it stimulates the body's own healing and revitalizing powers.

Father of Modern Cell Therapy

Dr. Paul Niehans M.D., a Swiss surgeon, is considered the "Father of Cell Therapy." Cell Therapy has been available in Europe for decades (70 years) and has been used by millions of people.

Definition

Cell therapy is a treatment intended to regenerate or rejuvenate the body's tissues and vital organs by the injection [or ingestion via oral supplement] of healthy live or freeze-dried cells derived from animal organs or embryos. It is sometimes called fresh or live cell therapy (or Xeno Stem Cell Therapy).

What is Cell Therapy?

Cell Therapy is a non-toxic, holistic, and supplemental natural repair of the tissues and organs on the cellular level. Injecting or taking orally lamb embryonic cell tissues that are sterile, harvested at proper critical stages, and freeze dried (lyophilized) in vacumm low temperature, properly treated (nanotechnology) and stored with inspection and certification by New Zealand government's Seal of Approval from the Minitry of Agriculture and Food Department. (MAF)

This refurbishing and regeneration of cells in the areas targeted, stimulates the immune system. Live cell therapy (Xeno Stem Cell Therapy) is not intended for replacing tissues but rather for stimulating the repair, growth and function of your existing "fatigued" tissues. Live Cell Therapy repairs the DNA/RNA of old and dormant cells within the individual, creates new electrical systems called synapses, and re-invigorates connective tissues.

Dr. Niehans wrote, "Cellular Therapy is a method of treating the whole organism on a biological basis, capable of revitalizing the human organism with its trillions of cells by bringing to it those embryonic or young cells or parts (organelles) which it needs. Cells from all organs are at our disposal. The doctor's art is to choose the right cells. Selective cellular therapy offers new life to the ailing or diseased organism."

—*Source: Cornell Lumiere, Feeling Younger Longer, 1973*

Freeze Drying

Cell Therapy was developed in 1930 by Dr. Paul Neihans, quite by accident, while desperately trying to save a dying patient using cells from an animal's gland. The patient recovered miraculously and went on to live to the ripe old age of 90. Dr. Neihans discovered another breakthrough while working with scientists to successfully develop a method of "freeze drying" cells to insure the sterility of the preparation. The freeze-dried cells currently used in the live cell therapy undergo a process of change to remove the cell surface coating and minimizes the risk of an allergic reaction.

The Nobel Prize in Medicine and Physiology was awarded to Dr.'s Peter Medawar and Macfarlane Burnett in 1960, for their work in transplantation immunity. They showed that lyophilized tissue will not provoke an immune reaction. They also showed that fetal cells are less antigenic than any other types of cells. These studies were performed transferring allogenic spleen cell suspensions and leukocytes, which in the fresh state are highly immunogenic, from A-mice to CBA-mice.

When lyophilized cells are implanted (injected), they are broken down by macrophages (tissue histiocytes). According to Dr. Trotsky of Israel, in 1985, he injected lyophilisied cells into a research group of 300 adults and children, with the incidence of only 10% of the subjects experiencing (CTLHR) cell therapy local histamine reaction at the injection site. This clinical study, 5% of the subjects had lethargy or flu-like symptoms lasting 2-3 days, 5% experienced a slight rise in temperature lasting a few hours to days, 30% experienced some symptoms of malaise lasting 10-15 days, 50% without any side effects.

How does Cell Therapy work?

Dr. Franz Schmidt, M.D. believed that there are no untreatable diseases, only diseases for which doctors have not yet found therapeutic solutions. He advocated that physicians should think "holistically" and utilize treatment methods that support the complex interactions of the biologic systems. He felt that it was a pitfall of "linear thinking" to only focus on identification of a single cause for a disease.

Embryonic cells from specific tissues (Lamb) are freeze dried. The tissues are tested thoroughly for sterility before given to the patient. The live cells are absorbed by the patient's body and act as a small stimulant to "wake up" the individual's own corresponding cells. The frozen cell material is engulfed by the special white cells called "macrophages" and are taken to the corresponding human organ, for example, liver to liver, kidney to kidney, etc. where it is re-invigorated. The healthy lamb cell material attaches to the fatigued human cells and helps to correct, revitalize, and repair. With the help of radioactive traceable lamb cells, research has shown that the material injected into humans is quickly dissolved and taken by the white cells within hours to the corresponding organs and tissues. Live cell therapy may not have appearant healthy benefit to some for a few weeks after treatment as each individual responds differently.

Studies conducted in German universities found that injected cells tagged with radioisotopes migrate to the organ in the human body corresponding to the organ from which they were taken. The reasons for the effectiveness of cell therapy, however, are not yet understood. It is thought that live cells may revitalize an "old" organ by "reprogramming" its genetic material. Another theory holds that the fresh cells stimulate secretions that restore the proper functioning of the targeted organ. Rebecca J. Frey, Cell Therapy, Gale Ency Med, 1999

The purposes of cell therapy include:

- Stimulation of the immune system
- Slowing the effects of aging, including memory loss, and sexual dysfunction as well as external appearance. [Skin, hair, and nail]
- Revitalization of specific body organs.
- Treating specific diseases and disorders, including arthritis, lupus, cancer, HIV infection, cardiovascular and neurological disorders, and Parkinson's disease.

Dr. Schmidt argued in his books and published articles that once doctors begin to think about multicausal interactions that it made sense to address diseases by supporting primary cellular structures and cellular processes (Schmidt 1960, 1973, 2000, 2001). He thought that cell therapy was effective because it could specifically repair undeveloped, diseased and age degenerated organs and tissues by supporting and revitalizing the cells of these organs. He also understood that cell therapy can facilitate cell growth, cell proliferation, and normalization of cellular functions in underdeveloped organs and repair and replace damaged cells in diseased and aging degenerated organs and tissues. (Schmidt 1973, 2000, 2001)

Why Embryonic cells?

The preference for fetal cells over the cells of fetal or newborn animals is because they are more compatible with the target host due to the lesser likelihood of allergenic, anti-immune responses. If the injected material is embryonic and is given in reasonable amounts, it is practically free of side effects and is accepted and handled as its "own" by the human body.

How do animal cells correspond to human cells?

Animal cells work in human organisms because in specific organs there are no essential differences between the enzymatic and functional capacities of human and animal cells. On a cellular level, the tissues function essentially the same.

Mechanism of Action
Two major mechanisms of action for revitalization of fatigued and diseased tissues and organs.

8 Powerful Secrets to Anti-Aging

1. The theory described genetic information contained in DNA and RNA of the "old" cells is defective because of either overused, age, or disease. The old cells' genetic codes have been corrupted, creating gaps, or incorrect information which can lead to major problems causing the cellular genetic misinformation and the cells to reproduce inefficiently. The organ or tissue cells do not look or function as well as they should. The new fresh and young cells from the embryonic lamb bring fresh genetic information contained in their still new DNA and RNA. This theory represents that new cells carry potentially the correct genetic message to the old aging cells. The new cells also are able to replace the misinformation with the correct original genetic code. Therefore, these old cells with their genetic mistakes are revitalized and corrected. Once this new DNA information is in place, the gland, organ and tissues begin to function correctly once again as if they were as young as the donor embryonic cells.

2. The cells age the same way as we do as human beings. As the cells age they gradually lose their ability to function precisely as they were originally intended. The effects of fresh embryonic cells are to stimulate secretion and natural compounds that activate the aging or diseased cells to return to their proper functions. The injection of embryonic cells provides the recipient organism with a greater number of bio-chemical substrates and enzymes that are found in very high concentration and unique composition in the fetal and embryonic cells, tissues, and glands.

Screening and Treatment

Individuals who wish to use Cell Therapy should seek the help and supervision of a doctor or health professional for a complete medical history and physical examination. A detailed evaluation should be conducted with focus on identifying the conditions and the organs involved.

Each individual receiving the cell therapy is given a succession of weekly shots for a series of individual tissues or organs targeted for repair and rejuvenation. Depending on the individual condition, a selection of multiple combinations of tissues and organs will be customized specifically to facilitate cellular repair of aging organs or tissues involved.

Overall internal cleansing and detox for 2 weeks is recommended before cell therapy for maximum health benefit and clinical outcome. A blended diet of vegetable, fruits and fish is recommended, with minimal or complete avoidance of red and processed meats; processed or refined sugar and high glycemic carbohydrates, breads, and fruits; and complete prohibition of alcohol, tobacco, and caffeine.

Individuals may use Max Digestion Specialist, one teaspoon into 10 oz. of water three times daily for a total GI tract cleansing and repair. Using a double dose of Cordyceps Sinensis from Max Performance Specialist with meals will support liver and kidneys. Proper hydration with eight glasses of lemon water daily, sipping slowly. A complete support of essential vitamins, minerals, and micro-nutritients (Daily Energy and Daily Wellness) and also liposome encapsulated glutathione should be taken daily for antioxidant repair.

Adequate sleep of a minimum of 8 hours or more daily is a must, as well as consideration for optional oral chelation of heavy metals like mercury and lead should be considered. (See LipoDetox, made of micro-encapsulated liposome of EDTA).

Very Rare Risk(s)

After millions of cell therapy treatments, there have been virtually no allergic reactions. Freeze dried cell therapy is generally well tolerated and virtually never triggers life threatening allergic reaction. Nevertheless, similar precautions generally used in all injectable or oral supplements must be taken. Supervised tests to screen for potential side effects and severe allergies should be performed. (Have available EpiPen.)

Precautions

Proceed with caution in treatment of individuals with severe end stage renal failure, acute fulminating viral liver disease, end-stage liver cirrhosis, acute severe upper respiratory infection, active asthmatic attack, or a history of severe and multiple allergic reaction. Always approach with care dealing with individuals with uncontrollable advanced diabetes, uncontrolled hypertension, and severe active infections with clinical symptoms. Cell therapy is *not recommended* and never used for pregnant or breast feeding mothers.

If individuals have experienced a small area of redness about an inch in diameter at the injection site for cell therapy, this can be expected to last for 2-4 days with no adverse consequence. These are fairly normal and routine local reactions that resolve on their own with no consequence or treatment needed. Ten days of complete rest are recommended for individuals receiving Cell Therapy.

Oral Cell Therapy

Cell Therapy can be given orally in "nano-cell" particles encapsulated and specially prepared and formulated for site specific absorption in the small intestines. The multiple phase encapsulation is designed for specific enzymatic breakdown not in the stomach but in the small intestine where the whole cell peptides are transported through "Active Junction Cells" directly into the mesenteric arteries and blood circulation.

Oral Organ Extracts

- In support of Hippocrates theory and Niehans therapy, Dr. W. Boecker directed a double-blind clinical trial on 1436 patients with cirrhosis of the liver. Half were given a placebo, and half took a liver extract. Sixty-seven percent (67%) of those taking the liver extract had significant improvement in liver function (more than placebo).
- A double-blind study of 600 patients suffering from hepatitis, Dr. Kiyoshi Fujisawa at the Jikei University School of Medicine in Tokyo, showed that, in only 12 weeks, 35% of the patients taking a liver extract showed substantial improvement (better than placebo).
- Dr. Pietro Cazzola conducted a study of 130 patients with malfunctions of the immune system and reported that treating those patients with thymic gland extracts improved their conditions.
- Dr. D.M. Kouttab of the Roger Williams Hospital and Brown University, reported health efficacy for extracts of the adrenal cortex.
- Dr. Franco Pandolfi of the medical school at the University of Rome directed a double-blind clinical trial on elderly hospitalized patients. Half of the patients were given a thymic extract and half took a placebo. Those taking the extract had fewer infections over a six-month period than those receiving the placebo.
- Dr. V. Vangemi followed 25 patients taking thymic extracts after cancer surgery and found that none of them got infections. Tests showed that their immune systems were substantially bolstered by the thymic extracts compared to controls.
- Dr. Massimo Fedrico guided a double-blind trial of 134 people undergoing chemotherapy. Half of the patients were given thymic extracts, and the other half received placebos. In only three months, but not during the winter cold season, those taking the thymic extracts had 30% fewer infections thatn the placebo group.
- Dr. G. Laurora and researchers form the Cardiovascular Institute conducted double-blind trials on patients with each stage of arteriosclerosis (clogged arteries). Half of the patients received mesoglycan, (animal aorta) and half took a placebo. A small section of one artery was scanned with high resolution ultrasound before and after treatment. At the end of 18 months, the occlusion of the arteries of the patients taking the placebo increased seven times more than those taking mesoglycan. Several clinical trials have shown that mesoglycan also deters blood clots and reduces the risk of strokes, even for people who have severely clogged arteries.

- Dr. F. Vecchio found that patients given mesoglycan (aorta tissues) for only 15 days experienced a 20% drop in "bad" cholesterol and 44% increase in "good" cholesterol.
- Autistic children could theoretically use brain cells or gut cells to achieve maximum efficacy and revitalize their organs.

Injectable Cell Therapy

Injection is available to physican and health practitioners for a highly effective and fast delivery. Total sterile technique should be followed with alcohol or iodide prep to the skin.

Freeze dried cell tissues come in sterile vials, reconstituted using 5cc of saline or sterile water injected into the vial. Shake the vial vigorously for two minutes until completely dissolved and use for injection within five minutes. Discard unused portion. You may choose to use a single syringe injection with an 18-gauge needle for deep subcutaneous (abdominal) or intra-muscular injection. Others may choose instead to use a divided dosage of two 3cc syringes given separately. 2 x 3cc each = 6cc.

Aftercare

After injection, a light and gentle massage of the area is helpful for 5-10 minutes. Light walking also helps to disperse fluid throughout the tissues. It is not advisable to sunbathe, or engage in strenuous exercise, hot baths, saunas, or excessive perspiration. Rest and proper hydration, including refraining from long trips or flying within 7-10 days of treatment is advised.

What are Normal Results?

- The initial phase is characterized by marked improvement in skin and general level of well-being.
- The reaction phase which lasts for approximately two weeks, is marked by tiredness and return of some earlier symptoms.
- The healing phase, which takes six to nine months after treatment to attain, is defined by long term improvements in stamina, skin tone, and general health. Improvements continue over several years, but treatment may be repeated as frequently as on quarterly or yearly intervals.

—*Source: Rebecca J, Frey, Cell Therapy; Gal Encycl. of Medic., Gale Res. 1999.*

Conditions Appropriate for Cell Therapy

Cardiovascular diseases
Neurological diseases
Loss of vitality due to aging
Aging with organ degeneration
Hormone inbalances
Mental exhaustion and memory loss
Pre and Post operative healing

Sexual dysfunction
Skin, wrinkle, facial rejuvenation
Systemic lupus erythematosis
Cancer
Weakness of immune system
Physical exhaustion and lack of energy
Rejuvenation due to chronic illness

Physicians Published Uses of Cell Therapy

- Old age and loss of vitality (Schmidt 1983, Guberman 2000, Kment 2000)
- Down's syndrome (Schmidt 1983, Feldmann 2001)
- Asthma and allergies (Mueller 2001)
- Alopecia Areata (Schmidt 1983)
- Burns and keloids (Leyh 2000, Shuck 2000)
- Orthopedic, osteoporosis, and arthritis (Eickschein 1999, Herbert 2000, Schuck 2000)
- Menopause and Andropause (Schmidt 1983 & 2000)
- Migraine (Babillotte 1999, Sulman 1999)
- Senile Dementia (Wolf 1999)
- Infertility (Mueller 2001)

From a May 1986 published report by Dr. Robert Bradford, Dr. Henry W. Allen, Dr. Michael L. Culbert—

Cell therapy may be beneficial in:

Neuromuscular disorders, epilepsy, multiple sclerosis, amyotrophic lateral sclerosis (ALS), Parkinson's disease, stroke paralysis, muscular dystrophy, sexual disorder, impotence, menopause, andropause, obesity, hypothyroidism, dermatologic disease, psoriasis, eczema, arthritis, pancreatitis, arteriosclerosis, liver cirrhosis, allergies, hip malformation, congenital dysplasia, spiral problems, cleft lip, lung disease, kidney disease, auto immune disease, antiaging rejuvenation.

—Source: "The Biomedical basis of Live Cell Therapy."
The Robert Bradford Foundation, Chula Vista, CA.

Summary

Doctors who practice cell therapy believe that cell therapy acts like an organ transplant and actually makes the old cells to "act younger." This biological "lesson" is not quickly forgotten by the cells.

In Europe, the effectiveness of cell therapy is widely accepted. In West Germany, for example, more than 5,000 physicians regularly administer cell therapy injections. A great proportion of those injections are funded by the West German social security system. Several million patients (up to 20 million) around the world have received cell therapy injections since the mid-1950's. Source: Dr. E. Michael Molnar, M.D., Forever Young, 1985, page 79-91.

Cellular Therapy is supported by more than 3,000 scientific publications, a number which grows day by day. These works can be found in the library of the International Center of Cell Investigation in Heidelberg, Germany, and some of them contain definitive conclusions regarding the mechanisms of action based on studies with radioisotopes and histochemical studies.

Freeze dried embryonic lamb tissues and gland are available: Male/Female Placenta, Hepatic (Liver), Immune system, Renal (Kidney), Skin, Male/Female specific Gland, Spine/Lumbar system, Pulmonary/Lung, Olfactory, Muscle, Bone, Marrow, Bone system, Cardiovascular, Cartilage, Central nervous system, Ear Nose & Throat, Gastrointestinal, Joint & tendons. (See Resources: Health Secrets USA)

Chapter 21

Is there Life after 50?
By Katherine M. Lee

Yes!!! Life after 50 can be your best years yet!

Please allow me to share my story with you. Many, many moons ago, when I was in my teenage years, people who were in their 50's looked very old to me. Their hair turned all grey and railroad tracks surfaced all over their face and neck (we used to tease the old folks saying their wrinkles looked like railroad tracks). They looked tired all the time and didn't feel like going out or even taking a short walk around the house. Their conversations were always about their illnesses, aches and pains. Their health was literally "Over the hill and down under!" I thought that life was over after one turned 50 and I dreaded the thoughts of being there someday.

My family owned an import/export herbal medicine company in Hong Kong. Every weekend, my mother would choose different kinds of herbs from the warehouse and take them home, adding thoroughly cleansed animal organs or meat (depending on which organs of our bodies she thought needed nourishment). She put all the herbs, organs or meat in an earthen crock-pot of water and simmered them for eight hours or longer until they reduced to about one-fourth of the original amount of liquid. She then insisted everyone in the family drink his or her individual portion because "it was good for our eyes" or "good for our livers." She made a new soup every week to benefit different parts of our bodies.

An obedient child, I drank all the soup my mother allotted for me. Sometimes I even drank the portion for my elder sister to protect her from being punished by my mother. My sister refused to drink the soups, complaining about the bad taste and awful smell of the herbs. Well, guess what? The real punishment came much later. My sister has had more health problems in one year than I have had in my whole lifetime! I credit my good health to my mother's good herbal soups. I hardly get sick other than an occasional cold or flu.

Time passed and I found myself running several businesses and raising two beautiful sons. Life was wonderful. But as I approached the big "FIVE-O," I couldn't help but pay more attention to friends and relatives who were about my age who complained about their aging health problems: hot flashes coming on just about any time of the day (they were often awakened in the middle of the night in a pool of their own sweat, soaking the entire bed). They would sometimes cry for no apparent reason at all, just watching a simple TV commercial! They were losing self-confidence, and had no courage to take on new projects while old tasks piled up and were not getting done. They felt very negatively about people, weather, food, just about everything they looked at, including themselves. "I feel ugly and I look ugly!" my friend said angrily. She had no desire for sex, sometimes feeling disgusted when her husband even tried to sit a little closer to her. A number of friends sadly became victims of breast cancer, spending every day combating the disease. I am very sad to say that at this writing, a dear friend who thought she was recovering from breast cancer just passed away at home from a sudden recurrence. May she rest in peace. She will be sorely missed.

Weight gain was the most common problem among my friends over 50; they also started to forget names, phone numbers, the names of their favorite foods, and sometimes even their own children's ages. The horror stories went on and on.

I began to wonder. If the statistic was right that the average life span for women is 80 years old, would I go through the next thirty or so years of my life in misery??? *Oh, my God,* I began to think, *this fearful feeling is one of the symptoms of menopause! I'm doomed now.*

The day I had feared since my teenage years had arrived. I was over 50 years old! One good thing was that my two sons were both grown, graduated from University of Michigan, and were working and living in New York. I had all the free time and extra money to do whatever I wanted for my own enjoyment. I wanted to truly live it up in the second half of my life, but this beautiful picture would be ruined if I was to spend the rest of my life going to the doctors, staying at the hospital, or making constant trips to the drug stores.

Whether I liked it or not, I began to feel the symptoms of aging. Like every woman who has entered "The Land of Menopause," I started to lose control of my weight. (I felt that I could gain weight just by breathing air!) So I restricted my intake of food and stayed good for a while, but then I felt deprived of life when I could not eat a favorite dessert or portions that would satisfy my appetite.

So I cheated. I ate everything in sight till I was happy again. Well, the reality check came when I couldn't zip up my pants. I became angry with myself and got depressed with life. I didn't seem to be able to get out of this vicious cycle!

At night, I had a phobia of my bed; as soon as I looked at it, I started having cold sweats. I tossed and turned almost every night, unable to fall asleep! And just when I would finally fall asleep, the alarm would go off!!! I had little energy for work. I caught myself falling asleep during meetings. It was tough trying to pretend I was awake and alert with the rest of the people in the meeting room!

I had fear of talking with people; even if there were only two people in the room, I found myself forgetting what I was saying even as I was saying it!!! How could this happen to me!!! "Someone help me, please!" I cried.

Fortunately, all those years of listening to my mother's preaching on the value of different herbs began to pay off. I started using different herbs to treat my aging symptoms. But there were problems—the good old herbal soups failed to work fast enough to help with my sudden onset of hot flashes! I needed something that worked right there and then! Another problem was that I didn't have time to sit home all day to simmer those herbal soups! I had to find another way of doing this more efficiently.

Thanks goodness for Dr. Tai! He was a Godsend.

First of all, his well researched knowledge in herbal medicine is so vast and far beyond my mother's words of wisdom. Secondly, he has incorporated advanced technologies in his products to speed the delivery of all the good herbs to the blood stream, so I can feel the benefits right away. So now, at age 55, since Dr. Tai balanced my hormones, my life is better than ever!!!

According to my Saliva Hormone test results, my biological age is now in my 30's! Not just because the report says so—I can feel it physically and mentally! I can feel that my energy level is as good as it was in my 30's. Another bonus that I didn't expect was that now I have the kind of self-confidence and courage that I have never experienced before! I feel the world is in my hands, and there is nothing that I cannot do. All problems have become happy challenges to me. I can work long hours every day without any breaks.

A few pumps of Dr. Tai's AndroWomen in the morning are all I need to feel that I am on top of the world. At night, a couple pumps of Progesterone Specialist help me feel so calm and peaceful that I sleep like a baby. No more phobias of my bed! DHEA & Pregnenolone Specialist keeps me in good mood all day long. Besides running my businesses, I am also deeply involved in the community as a volunteer. I am a board member of the Brownfield Re-Development Authority in the city in which I am living; a trustee at St. John Oakland Hospital in Michigan, the president of the City of Troy Heritage Foundation and the president of the Council of Asian Pacific Americans in Michigan. I'm not trying to show off my credentials—I merely want to share with you the amount of extra work I took on *after the age of 50* when most people seem to lose their zest in life. These are all passions I chose for the second half of my life!

I am now able to give speeches in front of thousands of people without any fear, whereas in the past, I would rather die than speak in front of two people in the room. I have fun in everything I do so the outcome always comes out well. Sometimes I have new ideas come to me in the middle of the night that I can't wait to get up in the morning and act on. It is a fun thing to see if I can beat my alarm clock every morning, and I can!

I travel at least twice a month all over the world without feeling much jet-lag. I look in the mirror and can honestly say I like what I see. Using Dr. Tai's latest formulation of skincare products have made big improvement with my skin. The fine lines on my face are disappearing; I have baby soft skin now instead of the rough, dry skin I had a few months ago.

I hope you, too, will experience the excitement I have for life at the age of 55. I wish you joy and happiness in the "Land of Menopause"!

Don't accept the old advice to "age gracefully." You don't have to compromise with life.

You are in the driver's seat. So drive!

Chapter 22

Conditions and Supplements

ACNE

Acne can take the form of blackheads, whiteheads, pimples, and even deeper lumps (cysts or nodules) that occur on the face, neck, chest, back, shoulders and even the upper arms. Acne is a disease that is not restricted to any age group; adults in their 20s—even into their 40s—can get acne. While not a life-threatening condition, acne can be upsetting and disfiguring. When severe, acne can lead to serious and permanent scarring. Even less severe cases can lead to scarring. Hormones affect acne and its severity. The hormones that cause physical maturation also cause the sebaceous (oil) glands of the skin to produce more oil. The hormones with the greatest effect on sebaceous glands are androgens (male hormones), which are present in females as well as males, but in higher amounts in males.

Caused by infectious bacteria (Propriobacterium Acnes) that live in pores and sebaceous glands, acne can be controlled and resolved in a number of ways. There are many treatment options available for a person to utilize. Natural ingredients can help a person avoid acne breakout. Some products may be too harsh for the skin as they dry the skin of its natural pH. People who are prone to developing acne should use non-drying/ non-peeling treatments which show the results they promise.

1. R. Coptidis, A. Dahurica, A. Lappa (Burdock)—used for most skin disorders, arictium lappa, or burdock, is used to remedy various sorts of skin diseases and infections. It cools and dries open sores on the skin.

2. Citrus extracts—as an anti-bacterial, extracts from citrus fruits are used against a broad range of bacteria. External uses of citrus extracts have prevented bacteria from causing infections.

3. Lichochalcone (Licorice extract)—an anti-inflammatory and anti-bacterial agent licorice reduces redness and has been used for centuries as a skin disease preventative.

4. Saliyclic acid—Saliyclic acid has been used to treat acne, warts, dandruff, psoriasis and similar conditions. In acne treatment, salicylic acid slows skin cell

shedding in hair follicles so they do not clog the pores and cause pimples. It also has a keratolytic effect, causing dead cells to slough off. The top layer of skin is removed, and pores are unclogged.

5. Usnea extract—A liquid extract of dried tree lichen extracted with hot alcohol, usnea is like licorice and citrus extracts, an anti-bacterial.

*Note: The listed natural ingredients are essential to your internal skin care program. You can find the following ingredients in Dr. Tai's proprietary formulas: **AcneDerm Cleanser, AcneDerm Gel, AcneDerm Urgent Care.**

ADRENAL FATIGUE

Adrenal fatigue is a condition that has the ability to baffle both patients and doctors alike. Patients experiencing adrenal fatigue aren't responsive to most treatments; they wake tired and they go to bed tired. Unable to cope with minor forms of stress, adrenally fatigued persons have difficulty running errands or going to work. Beyond the scope of severe symptoms, laboratory diagnoses of clinical adrenal exhaustion can be confirmed by taking a five panel salivary test. If you're suffering from adrenal fatigue, your morning cortisol level will be just as low as your evening level. There are no simple treatments available for rapid recovery. However, there are natural supplements to remedy your inability to cope with stress. Patients who are adrenally fatigued report experiencing insomnia, digestive problems and bone/joint problems. More serious than most people would like to think it is, adrenal exhaustion can further deteriorate the immune system, causing inflammations and frequent colds, headaches and sore throats.

Formulas with adrenalinum, astragalus, eleutherococcus, glycerrhyza acid and panax ginseng can increase NK cell activity (cells that build muscle), increase cell proliferation/ATP synthesis, promote and enhance recovery, improve libido, increase sperm count and sperm survival, reduce muscle soreness, promote oxygen efficiency and improve blood cell viability and function.

1. Adrenalinum, Astragalus (Huang Qi) and Eleutherococcus—The active principle of the medulla of the suprarenal gland is employed as a chemical messenger in the regulation of the activities of the body. Adrenalinum strengthens heartbeats, increases glandular activity, alleviates depression of respiratory center, contractions of muscular tissue of the eye, uterus and vagina, and relaxes muscular tissue of the stomach, intestines and bladder.

• Astragalus (Huang Qi) tones spleen deficiency problems such as poor appetite, fatigue and diarrhea. Astragalus was used by practitioners of traditional Chinese medicine to strengthen the body's overall vitality, improve digestion and support the spleen.

• Russian athletes use Eleutherococcus to increase endurance and resistance to stress, and researchers have referred to the plant as an adaptogen, a substance that promotes adaptation to environmental stress of all kinds.

2. Glycerrhyza Acid—Glycerrhyza acid helps to retain the cortisol hormone in the body and its activities for greater periods of time, therefore diminishing the loss of cortisol through excretion, leaving you able to keep net cortisol levels at a much higher level. Also known as Chinese licorice, it's known for its abilities to loosen and help expel congestion in the upper respiratory tract and stimulate mucous secretions of the trachea. Glycerrhyza produces new cells in the stomach's lining.

3. Panax Ginseng—Panax ginseng has been known to have a relaxing effect on the muscles in the lungs. The resulting airway relaxation may help calm asthma symptoms and other airway-constricting lung conditions. Most importantly, panax ginseng helps fight fatigue, increase stamina and enhance libido.

*Note: The listed natural ingredients can be found in Dr. Tai's proprietary formulas: **Max-Performance Specialist, DHEA and Pregnenolone liposome, Human Growth Matrix and Max Adrenal.**

ALZHEIMER'S

MEMORY LOSS

LEARNING DIFFICULTIES

Research reports that over 50 percent of individuals aged 75 to 80 have some form of Alzheimer's. With age comes a loss of natural compounds that are part of functioning brain physiology. Much of these natural compounds help with neural transmission of cell-to-nerve communication, more commonly referred as synapses or "nerve talk." Natural compounds such as Huperzine-A and GABA contribute to the efficiency of improving memory, logic, and reasoning by way of boosting cell synapses.

In 2004, researcher M. L. Fiovaranti (et al.) found that another natural compound Cytidine diphosphocholine (phoshpotidylcholine type lipid) had shown excellent results in improving short- and medium-term memory function. Memory lapses or rapid recall were proven to have improved with Cytidine diphosphocoline, and even better results showed when combined with natural memory enhancers like huperzine A and GABA.

1. Cytidine diphosphocholine, Huperzine A and GABA—aids in brain anti-aging and memory sharpness. Used as a preventive against Parkinson's disease. Improves neuro-receptors, and enhances short- and long-term word recall. Increases nerve to nerve electrical conductivity.

2. Vitamin A and E—Vitamin A is required for night vision and healthy skin. It assists the immune system, and because of its antioxidant properties, it is great for protecting against pollution and cancer formation and other diseases. It also assists the sense of taste as well as helps the digestive and urinary tract, and many believe that it helps slow aging. Vitamin E is a powerful antioxidant that works to protect cells in the body from damage caused by free radicals. Free radicals are highly reactive substances that result from normal metabolism as well as from exposure to factors in the environment like cigarette smoke and ultraviolet light. Vitamin E is especially important in protecting blood cells, the nervous system, skeletal muscle and the retinas in the eyes from free radical damage.

*Note: The listed ingredients can be found in Dr. Tai's proprietary formulas: **Sharp Memory, Brain Power Specialist, Max-Performance Specialist and bioidentical DHEA and pregnenolone.**

ANDROPAUSE

Andropause is a result of low testosterone throughout a man's body. Testosterone peaks in both men and women in their early 20s, and afterward testosterone quickly and drastically declines. By the time people near age 50, they've lost almost 75 percent of testosterone, leaving them weak, flabby and forgetful. A testosterone loss can be the potential cause of osteoporosis and heart disease. Through natural supplementation, problems that form as a result of a testosterone deficiency can be avoided.

Research proves that testosterone improves self-perception, raises confidence, enhances sexual desire and firms body tones as it reduces fat. Aggressiveness, bossiness and unwanted hair growth are side effects of a testosterone excess. When taking bioidentical testosterone make sure not to overdo it.

1. Cordyceps Sinensis—Traditional Chinese doctors use the Cordyceps mushroom to energize, improve health, and treat so many ailments that it was classified as a "life extender." Cordyceps was designated as the first anti-aging supplement in history to be enjoyed in royal courts by the kings and queens of ancient Chinese dynasties.

2. Cistanche—Like cordyceps cistanche is an effective mushroom known to help male impotency.

3. Evodia—influences the metabolism of supplements, raises body temperature, and influences the secretion of catecholamines from the adrenal glands.

4. Tribulus—A beneficial herb for sexual activity and improving muscular strength; tribulus supports erection and helps with arousal.

*Note: The listed natural ingredients can be found in Dr. Tai's proprietary formulas: **Max-Performance Specialist, Man Power Specialist, Human Growth Matrix, DHEA and pregnenolone, Andro Man and Max Men.**

ARTHRITIS

FIBROMYALGIA

MUSCLE AND JOINT PAIN (back, neck, shoulders etc.)

There are over 100 types of arthritis and rheumatic diseases including osteoarthritis, rheumatoid arthritis and fibromyalgia. The illness can cause pain, stiffness and swelling in the joints and muscles. Though arthritis can affect anyone, people over the age of 45 have a higher likelihood of developing arthritis. After years of extensive laboratory research pain relief and anti-inflammation was found in eight herbs from a blend of 4,605 plant extracts. A combination of the right herbal extracts can be more effective than synthetic pain relievers, which can cause a chain of negative side effects. Through "medicinal teapot extraction," herbs have the potential to perform their best anti-inflammatory abilities, remedying the most paralyzing joint/muscle pains. When you stop inflammation, you will STOP PAIN at its root.

1. Boswellia Serrata—an Ayuverdic herb of frankincense has been used as anti-inflammatory for a thousand years. Boswellia acid the active ingredient, has been found to block the destructive leukotrienes enzymes, which trigger inflammation that can be painful.

2. Curcumine—has a unique ability to inhibit and neutralize destructive enzyme 5-LO from leukotrienes, as well as COX-2— culprits of inflammation and pain (Journal of Ethropharamacology, 1993).

3. Ginger—Often overlooked and forgotten, ginger is one of the oldest anti-inflammatories and pain relievers known to mankind. Ginger extract (gingerol—the active ingredient) is proven effective at relieving arthritis pain.

• The Journal of Osteoarthritis Cartilage reports a study at Tel Aviv University of 29 patients suffering from knee osteoarthritis. Half received ginger extract, the other half a placebo. At the end of 12 weeks, the ginger group showed knee pain was reduced significantly while joint mobility increased significantly.

• Another study at University of Miami enrolled 247 subjects with severe osteoarthritis of the knee. Subjects were divided into two groups, a "ginger" group, and a "placebo" group, for six weeks. 63 percent of the ginger group's participants reported significant improvement, while the placebo group showed no improvement (Journal of Arthritis and Rheumatism, 2001).

• In a 2004 Chicago Daily Herald article, Dr. Patrick Nassey was reported to have found that ginger reduces the pain associated with knee arthritis (Chicago Daily Herald, 2004).

• At a university study in Denmark, Dr. Srivastava reported 56 patients comprised of rheumatoid arthritis, osteoarthritis and muscle spasm pain who used ginger, experienced pain relief and saw that their swelling had decreased. All of the patients with muscular pain experienced relief and most importantly, no side effects were reported after several months to several years of consumption (Medical Hypothesis, 1992).

4. Glucosamine sulfate—A natural component of our joint cartilage, tendons, bone, ligament, nails, hair, etc. There have been many published studies on glucosamine sulfate proving its value in reducing rheumatic symptoms and rebuilding damaged cartilage of joints. Our own body's cartilage cells use for repair of joint as well as inhibits enzymes that destroy cartilage. By blocking the destructive mechanism of cartilage degeneration, glucosamine can halt and even reverse the disease process and relieve rheumatoid symptoms. However, beware of the many glucosamine forms available.

5. Grape skin—Magazines and catalogs try to sell lower quality grape seed for its content of active ingredient "resveratrol," but scientific evidence disputes this kind of salesmanship. Research performed on quantitative analysis by Xingjian Medical School in China shows that contents of resveratrol are much higher in wine than in fresh grapes (Journal of Agricultural and Food Chemistry, August 2003).

6. Methylsulfonylmethane (MSM)—A critical sulfur required for proper repair of injured cartilage, ligaments and tendons. Although naturally present in our food (found in vegetables, fruits, fish and meats), it is not available at sufficient quantities for our joint needs (Qie (et al.) 1998). Reports show that a strategic use of MSM increases therapeutic efficiency of glucosamine because of its sulfur presence.

• Dr. Lawrence from UCLA's Medical School found that arthritis symptoms improved in 80 percent of his patients.

7. Quercetin—This very rare ingredient has been considered the ultimate weapon against inflammation. Dr. Morikawa of Sagami Women's University in Japan reports that quercetin is the "champion of anti-inflammation" because it suppresses inflammatory response in animals (Life Science, 2003).

• Dr. Woo from Chubu University says quercetin is able to suppress bone loss which may stop cartilage degeneration (Biology and Pharmacy Bulletin, 2004).

8. White Willow—Centuries old, this natural remedy provided pain relief for all conditions. It's the grand father of all analgesics; with a number of strong clinically proven efficacies, white willow is an essential for pain management (WeinMed Wochenschr, Germany, 2002).

*Note: The listed natural ingredients can be found in Dr. Tai's proprietary formulas: Max-Performance Specialist, Max-Pain Specialist, Antioxidant Specialist, Biogenic PH, Human Growth Matrix, Max-Arthro Specialist.

Gluthione
1. detoxifies the liver.
2. improves lung function.
3. improves heart function.
4. increases energy, endurance, and stamina.
5. protects the skin from UV rays.
6. strengthens immune function.
7. helps alleviate some AIDS-related symptoms.
8. alleviates multiple sclerosis, lupus, and ALS symptoms.
9. alleviates ADHD and autism symptoms.
10. lessen cancer and chemotherapy side effects.
11. improves diabetes and sugar metabolism.
12. decreases the chances of developing cardiovascular disease and athrosclerosis.
13. nulls adrenal fatigue fibromyalgia development.

CELL DIVISION

You are as old as your cells are. Cells have a limited number of cell divisions in a human lifetime. Studies show that by age 20, most cells that make up your body have used up half of the divisions available in their cell lifespan.

By the time a person is 40, there may be only 30 percent of possible cell divisions left. When cells use their naturally allotted divisions, the end result is death. Recent research has given new hope to the task of rejuvenating and extending the lifespan of cells. While this seemed impossible only a few years ago, astonishing scientific research has made possible longer cellular life spans. This has been achieved using special antioxidants that can actually keep cells looking and acting younger by

900 percent! Antioxidants prevent memory loss, cancer, senility and heart disease. Glutathione an antioxidant our body produces is not absorbed into the body when taken by mouth. One way to get around that is to take it by injection. Another way is to take amino acids precursors—that is, the molecules the body needs to make glutathione—but there is no solid proof this works and most doctors doubt its validity. **A new innovative way is to microencapsulate in natural essential phospholipids to make a liposome, where it keeps the Glutathione fresh and delivers it effectively into the blood stream.**

Glutathione is a super antioxidant that is important for good health because it neutralizes free radicals that can cause permanent cell damage. Because glutathione exists within the cells, it is in a prime position to neutralize free radicals. It also has potentially widespread health benefits because it can be found in all types of cells, including the cells that make up the immune system.

Jerry Appleton, MD (Chairman of the Department of Nutrition at the National College of Naturopathic Medicine) says glutathione removes foreign chemicals such drugs and pollutants from the liver. "If you look in a hospital situation at people who have cancer, AIDS, or other very serious disease, almost invariably they are depleted of glutathione."

He added, "The reasons for this are not completely understood, but we do know that glutathione is extremely important for maintaining intracellular health."

Appleton said glutathione and other antioxidants are far from interfering with chemotherapy and appear to reduce side effects without decreasing efficacy and may, in fact, improve the efficacy of the chemotherapy in fighting cancer.

Glutathione is also used to prevent oxidative stress in most cells and helps to trap and neutralize free radicals that can damage DNA and RNA. There is a direct correlation between the speed of aging and the reduction of glutathione concentrations in intracellular fluids. As individuals grow older, glutathione levels drop, and the ability to detoxify free radicals decreases.

Preliminary evidence suggests that glutathione may eventually prove to be useful in the management of some forms of cancers, atherosclerosis, diabetes, lung disorders, noise-induced hearing loss and male infertility. It also helps prevent various heavy metal and chemical toxicities.

Glutathione also has been researched for AIDS-associated cachexia, cystic fibrosis, Parkinson's, ADHD, autism, multiple sclerosis, cancer, mercury poisoning, lupus, ALS and various other liver diseases.

*Note: The listed natural ingredients can be found in Dr. Tai's proprietary formulas: **Glutathione Liposome.**

DIABETES II

SYNDROME X

The American Diabetes Association reports that diabetes is one of the fastest growing diseases in the world. Currently, diabetes affects 16 million people in the United States. An additional 14 million people have potential diabetes or have high risk of developing diabetes that has yet to be diagnosed. Worldwide, this epidemic claims more than 100 million lives annually. In the United States, diabetes is the seventh-leading cause of death. Diabetes is also one of the leading causes of adult blindness, kidney failure, atherosclerosis, cardiovascular diseases, premature aging, obesity and syndrome X (The American Diabetes Association, 2005).

Type II diabetes is a non- insulin-dependent diabetes that develops in later life, often called adult-onset diabetes. Most people with Type II diabetes don't show signs of any symptoms until it is too late. To cope with this problem with natural alternative complementary medicine, attention has been given to research of natural medicinal plants from all over the world, including India and China, for the control and modulation of high blood sugar.

1. Corosolic Acid—From the Banabas plant. Dr. Yamazaki, a professor of pharmacology at Hiroshima University's School of Medicine, said that corosolic acid is able to activate and transport glucose across the cell membrane resulting in lower blood sugar levels just as insulin does. When corosolic acid is taken orally, it can produce a drop in blood sugar. Insulin can be distributed solely through injection. Benefits of corosolic acid have been documented in a variety of animal studies. Rabbits taking oral doses of corosolic acid had lower blood sugar. Corosolic acid also improved blood glucose transport into cells to fuel energy in rabbits studied. Corosolic acid has the ability to lower blood sugar even after the treatment has stopped.

Dr. William Judy from the Southwestern Institute of Biomedical Research in Bradenton, Florida confirmed the use of corosolic acid in a randomized double blind crossover trial using 12 subjects of six women and six men with Type II diabetes. Dr. Judy tested their ability to tolerate sugar. Over the course of 22 weeks, the participants aged 46 and older took 48 mg daily. The participants who took corosolic acid were had a 31.9 percent drop in blood sugar.

2. MHCP (Methyl Hydroxy Chalcone Polymer)—The USDA Agriculture Research team was able to extract an active compound from cinnamon called MHCP. The USDA Agriculture Research team found that cinnamon makes human cells more sensitive to insulin through multiple test tube studies.

• MHCP is an active compound that assists in the transport of glucose and increases the sensitivity of the receptor sites in order to process the hormone insulin as reported by Dr. J. Karalee from the Department of Biochemistry at Iowa State University (American Journal of Nutrition).

• Dr. Richard Anderson and Dr. Marylyn Polanski from the USDA's Agriculture Research Department discovered that MHCP can stimulate glucose uptake by working synergistically with insulin to mobilize sugar into the cells.

*Note: The listed natural ingredients can be found in Dr. Tai's proprietary formulas: **Max-Performance Specialist, Max-Glucose Specialist.**

EDEMA

Water retention

Many people believe that the kidneys don't play a vital role in our lives because it's possible to live off of one of the two. Contrary to popular misconception, the kidneys are just as important as any other organ in the body. As filters, kidneys process hundreds of quarts of blood a day to sift through waste and the extra water which eventually becomes urine. Edema is a visible illness, meaning that it's possible to see the illness take effect. A person with edema will look as bloated as they undoubtedly feel even if they haven't eaten anything. Edema forms in patients with kidney problems because urine releases protein. If the body releases too much protein, it releases albumin, which is needed to maintain blood flow.

1. Lobelia—an extremely powerful muscle relaxant to improve respiration and circulation to relieve vascular tension and balance high blood pressure.
2. Magnesium—Alleviates premenstrual symptoms of fluid retention.
• Dr. A.F. Walker conducted a study using magnesium on female patients who frequently experienced water retention. Dr. Walker concluded that all of his patients were relieved from the water retention they were accustomed to experiencing (Women's Health Journal, 1998).
3. Poria—an ancient edible fungus found on the roots of aging pine trees. Poria has an uncanny ability to ease bodily tensions around the kidney area. Poria improves circulation and immune system function as well as expels excess mucus.

*Note: The listed natural ingredients can be found in Dr. Tai's proprietary formulas: **Water Specialist, Pregnenolone Liposome and Max Performance Specialist.**

FIBROCYSTIC BREASTS

OVARIAN FIBROIDS

UTERINE FIBROIDS

The human body produces its own estrogen part of this process is called aromatization. After the age of 50 years old, this process is more accelerated and becomes even more prominent, setting up potential major problems for woman with familial history of breast cancer, uterine and ovarian cancer. For men, aromatization exacerbates prostate hypertrophy and increase risk of cancer due to increased levels of estrogen this is why a man at the age of 55 has as much, or even more estrogen than a woman at 55. In an article published by researcher C.K. Osborne (et al.) entitled "Estrogen self proliferation and implication for treatment of breast cancer" (Cancer Treatment Research, 1988) Osbourne reported an increase of estrogen lead to cervical, ovarian, breast cancer as well as endometriosis. To relieve the body of forming excess estrogen extensive research confirmed that vegetables from the "brassica" family have active indol-3-carbinols (13C) that act as estrogen hormone modulators. When 13C is ingested in the stomach and mixed with the stomach acid, another very active and more powerful ingredient Diindolylmethane (DIM) is produced, which is a vital natural compound known to have potent anticancer and antitumor properties. Both 13C and the converted DIM have proven to lower the circulating estrogen, estrodial (E2) by quickly neutralizing excretions from the liver (Benabadji, S.H. et al., "Anti-estrogenic and antioxidant diindolylmethane." Octa Pharmacology, 2004).

In order to receive a sufficient amount of I3C and DIM a person must eat: large quantities of broccoli, 103 pieces of Brussels sprouts and one fourth head of a raw cabbage. Many people find these dietary requirements impossible to meet on a daily basis, therefore, the National Cancer Institute and the National Cancer Prevention Center has shown interest in the natural cancer prevention agents for breast, cervical, endometrial, colorectal cancers as well as prostate cancers, I3C and DIM (Balk, J.L. et al., "Indol-3-Carbinol for cancer prevention." Alternative Medicine Review, 2000).

Chrysin, evodia and resveratrol work synergistically through different pathways and mechanisms as "anti-excess estrogens" to formulate a balanced blend that isn't available anywhere else in the world.

1. Chrysin—A naturally occurring bioflavonoid extracted from the plant Passiflora-coerulea. Researchers have found Chrysin to have the ability to inhibit the conversion of testosterone into estrogens.

2. Evodia—Influences the metabolism of supplements, raises body temperature and influences the secretion of catecholamines from the adrenal glands. **A powerful anti-inflammatory.**

3. Resveratrol—Highly concentrated in grape skin (abundant in red wine), resveratrol has been reported to reduce the risk for cardiovascular disease. Researchers have attributed the cardioprotective quality of resveratrol to have similar effects of estradiol, a major protective estrogen. **Must be fermented to have the intended beneficial effects.**

*Note: The listed natural ingredients can be found in Dr. Tai's proprietary formulas: **Estrogen Defense, Progesterone specialist, Max Pain Specialist.**

HEART DISEASE

CHOLESTEROL

ARRHYTHMIA

Certain herbs possess the capacity to repair, protect and restore the heart to its healthiest and strongest condition by controlling blockage of coronary arteries that deprives the heart muscle of blood and oxygen. The same herbal formulations can decrease the chances of Arrhythmia from developing, a disorder of regular rhythmic heart beats. Millions of Americans are living with atrial fibrillation, which can occur in a healthy heart. Though, atrial fibrillation may also indicate a serious problem and lead to stroke, heart disease and/or sudden cardiac death.

Powerful natural herb extracts lower total cholesterol and LDL yet simultaneously increase HDL. Proprietary forumations neutralize the toxic amino acid Homocysteine so damaging to the cardiovascular system.

1. Inositol hexanicotinate—Vitamin B3 niacin is well accepted by mainstream medical community to lower cholesterol but unfortunately niacin when taken in quantities to lower cholesterol can cause severe flushing, headaches and occasional liver inflammation. A more powerful alternative, inositol hexanicotinate has been extensively studied as a safer alternative to niacin without side effects.

• Dr. A.L. Welsh said "inositol is improved, powerful, and more effective than niacin." (International Medical Records, 1961).

2. Octacosanol—A natural compound made from sugarcane that lowers low density lipoprotein (LDL) a bad cholesterol that clogs arteries.

• Dr. Gourini-Berticold said that poli- (many)cosanol reduces low density lipoprotein (LDL) up to 29 percent, and raises high density lipoprotein (HDL) by up to 15 percent (American Heart Journal, 2002).

- Dr. G. Castano said that policosanol in postmenopausal women lowered LDL by 25 percent and rose HDL (good) by 27 percent (Gynecology and Endocrinology, 2000).
- After testing policosanol on 28,000 patients Dr. J.C. Fernandez J.C. concluded that policosanol is "effective, safe, and well tolerated" (Current Therapy Research, 1998. Journal of Gerontology, 2000).

3. Pleurotus—A complex species of mushroom that shows activity against cancer, high cholesterol, antitumor, immune response, anti-inflammatory, antiviral and antibiotic.
- Dr. Solomon Wasser reports pleurotus ostreatus lowers statin, a hypolipidic agent (International Journal of Medicine, March 1999).

*Note: The following natural ingredients can be found in Dr. Tai's proprietary formulas: **Heart Specialist, Max-Performance Specialist and Glutathione.**

HIGH BLOOD PRESSURE

Uncontrolled high blood pressure can lead to stroke, heart attack, heart failure or kidney failure. This is why high blood pressure is often called the "silent killer." The destructive force of hypertension is well researched and documented, recent publications verified that hypertension contributes to cardiovascular disease(s), Parkinson's, Alzheimer's, strokes etc. Hypertension is a difficult condition to address, especially using herbal extractions; however, with the right composition it's a condition that can be controlled.

1. Hawthorne Berry—A tonic for the heart, hawthorne berry protects arterial walls and has the ability to enlarge coronary blood vessels and strengthen the heart's pumping ability.
2. Lonicera Japonica (Japanese honey suckle)—It has antibacterial and anti-inflammatory properties, japonica is used to dispel heat and remove toxins, including carbuncles, fevers, influenza, and ulcers.

*Note: The listed natural ingredients can be found in Dr. Tai's proprietary formula: **Blood Pressure Specialist.**

MENOPAUSE

Menopause affects every woman at some point in her life. Like puberty and childbirth, it's a normal process, and like puberty and childbirth, there are symptoms due to hormonal irregularities. By using the right herbs, menopause can be enjoyed instead of avoided.

Estrogen and progesterone are two of the most important hormones in a woman's body and both hormones perish in a large amount after menopause. They can be found in a variety of phytohormones, or bioidentical hormones found in plants.

1. Black Cohosh—an herb used extensively in Europe for treating hot flashes and other menopausal symptoms. The American College of Obstetricians and Gynecologists supports short-term use of black cohosh.
- Dr. Lehmann (1988) found 80 percent women using black cohosh had improvement of symptoms of menopause and PMS.
- Dr. Ducker (1991) proved that black cohosh stabilizes the luteinizing hormone and improved the symptoms in menopause.
- Dr. Lieberman (1998) showed black cohosh is effective against menopause and is safe for use.

2. Chaste Tree (Vitex agnus)—Chaste tree berry is an effective and well-tolerated treatment for the relief of PMS symptoms including depression, anxiety, cravings and water retention. Chaste tree extracts may protect women from uterine cancer, fibroids, and from ovarian cancer and cystic changes of the ovary. Chaste tree restores and balances reproductive hormones by sending messages to ovary to increase progesterone.
- Dr. Amman (1979) used chaste tree for relief of menstrual water retention. After conducting a 1500 participant study on chaste tree for five months, Dr. Amman found that 35 percent of patients had total menopause relief experiencing no symptoms. 90 percent of all his patients had improvement of symptoms from menopause.
- Dr. Veal (1998) showed that when taken orally, chaste tree berry restored hormones in menopause patients.
- Dr. Halaskun (1998) found that taking chaste tree relieved perimenopausal/menopausal patients of breast pain.

3. Dong Quai (Angelica sinensis)—Treats muscle cramps and pain associated with difficult menstrual periods. It comes from the carrot family and is known in Asia as a "female tonic." It is a muscle relaxant and helps convert all androsterones to estrogen, progesterone and testosterone in the liver.
- The research of Dr. He (1986) showed patients taking dong quai were able to regulate menstrual abnormalities and provide relief of PMS symptoms.
- Dr. Osaka (1990) showed dong quai relaxed muscles and improved blood flow by expanding blood vessels.

4. Isoflavones—concentrated active ingredients of soy. Isoflavones like daidzen helps curb sugar cravings, reduces insulin fluctuation and binge eating. Studies have showed that consumption of daidzen decreases fat storage while increasing muscle mass and may also attenuate the increase in fat deposition and prevent loss in lean tissue during menopause. Genistein, another kind of isoflavone, has estrogenic and antioxidant activities. It may also have anticarcinogenic, anti-atherogenic and anti-osteoporotic activities.
- Dr. Xu (2000) shows isoflavones decrease the risk of breast cancer, and increases bone loss protection by reducing calcium loss in researched animal studies.

• Dr. McKenna (2001) used isoflavone concentrate to treat his patients experiencing PMS symptoms as well as menopause symptoms. He used isoflavones because he said they were "safe, have low toxicity, and can be tolerated well."

6. Red Clover—Like genistein and daidzen, red clover provides 18 amino acids important in protein metabolism. Research shows red clover is good for heart disease. It decreases cholesterol and the risk of cancer in the colon and breasts.

*Note: The listed natural ingredients can be found in Dr. Tai's proprietary formulas: **Max Menopause Specialist, Estro-E, Max Estro, Progesterone Specialist.**

MIGRAINES

Headaches and migraines usually occur to women during menstruation or ovulation. From this we can conclude that headaches and their more severe forms—migraines—are usually caused by hormone fluctuations. However headaches and migraines can also be triggered in a variety of ways like by stress, improper diet, lack of magnesium, dehydration and/or constipation with toxins of the bowels.

1. Curcumin—One of the finest anti-inflammatory herbs. Known for its unique ability to inhibit and neutralize destructive enzymes 5-LO from leukotrienes, and COX-2—the main culprits for inflammation and pain (The Journal of Ethropharamacology, 1993).

• Dr. Kaug, a contributor to the Journal of Pharmacology, confirmed that curcumin "significantly inhibited" COX-2 (The Journal of Pharmacology, 2004).

• According to Dr. Goel, curcumin protects against colon cancer (Cancer Letters, 2001).

• Dr. Susan Lark reported that curcumin was able to reduce morning stiffness and swelling as comparable to synthetic phenylbutazone without side effects (American Journal of Natural Medicine).

2. Ginger—Often overlooked and forgotten ginger is one of the oldest pain relievers known to mankind. Using a special concentrated extract of gingerol (the active ingredient) is proven very effective at relieving arthritis pain.

3. Glucosamine sulfate—Fundamental and natural component of our joint cartilage, tendons, bone, ligament, nails, hair, etc. There are multiple clinical studies and published reports proving its value in reducing symptoms and rebuilding the damaged cartilage of your joints.

4. Quercetin—A bioflavonoid that's been documented to have anti-cancer activity.

• Dr. Morikawa from Japan's Sagami Women's University found that quercetin suppressed of inflammatory responses in animals tested in vitro (Life Science, 2003).

5. Vitamin bound peptide—highly effective in cleasing colon detoxing the bowel by removing food alleagens and lower inflammation. Good bye, migraine.

*Note: The listed natural ingredients can be found in Dr. Tai's proprietary formulas: **Max-Digestion Specialist.**

OBESITY

Appearance can mean a lot to a lot of people. However, when obesity is concerned, there is more at stake than just vanity. Excess weight might make a person feel and look unattractive, but it can also be a precursor to more serious health complications such as Type II Diabetes.

A diet high in sugars and carbohydrates is highly unhealthful and potentially dangerous to the system. High sugar levels create two-part problem within the body. First, when sugar levels rise, the body responds by over-stimulating the pancreas by producing too much insulin. Second, when sugar peaks, it is converted to fat. In response, the pancreas drops insulin down below the normal level and the body begins to enter hypoglycemic, or starvation, mode.

Using fermented, soybean-derived Touchi extract cortisol and sugar levels are neutralized. Touchi extract has been proven to be a naturally safe and effective way to regulate and control borderline and mild- Type II Diabetes and controls high and low insulin (American Society for Nutritional Sciences, 2001).

Appetite and craving suppression are the keys to weight loss. Over 70 percent of Americans are overweight and nearly 30 percent of Americans are obese. The phenomenon of overeating has long been believed to be due to a lack of "control" on the part of a person. However, this is far from the truth. Most often, overeating is due to a Dysfunctional Satiety Center (DSC). When a person eats, the hypothalamus (a small gland located at the base of the brain) sends a message (via hormone) to the brain that the body has received food. Unfortunately, however, an abnormal hypothalamus does not register when food has entered the stomach. There is a non-functioning circuit between the stomach and the brain. As a result of this lapse in communication between body and brain, those with an abnormal hypothalamus are prone to overeat.

Ginsenosides normalize the internal "switch" and allows the stomach to quickly respond when consuming food by regulating a dysfunctional system and virtually eliminating the possibility of overeating.

1. Deer antler extract—contains "Master Growth Factors." Master Growth Factors are: IGF-1, IGF-2, Epidermal Growth Factor, Neural Growth Factor, Vascular Growth Factor, and Transfer Energy Factors. All which increase immunity, improve well being, promote higher fat burning metabolism, and increase both energy and power.
 • Dr. C.E. Broder from Benedictine University conducted a double blind study that showed deer antler with Master Growth Factors significantly improved total maximum strength as well as had a 9.8 percent improvement in aerobic (oxygen) capacity on participants.
 • The same researchers also noted that IGF-MGF reduced LDL cholesterol by 12.2 percent and improved HDL by 8.4 percent.
2. Elutherococus (Siberian Ginseng) and Spirulina (a natural sea vegetable)-both have natural antifatigue properties.
3. Green tea extract—with polyphenols and ECGC, both power antioxidant properties stimulate and improve metabolism while neutralizing damage done by free radicals caused by instable dieting. Green tea improves the body's metabolic rate and gives the body a "jump start" when diet and exercise aren't enough.
4. Rhodiola Rosea—modulates mood swings, a commonplace occurrence among dieters.
5. Vitamin bound peptides- repair stomach lining and revitalizes micro-villi (small fingers in digestive tract) for nutrient absorption. Consistent use of vitamin bound peptides have been documented to cease or stop food allergies.
6. White bean extract (Phaseolus Vulgaris)- inhibits digestive enzymes. White bean extract prevents the body from absorbing excessive carbohydrates by diminishing amylase carbohydrates. Reduced to its essence, white bean extract promotes weight loss.

*Note: The listed natural ingredients can be found in Dr. Tai's proprietary formulas: **Weight and Inches Specialist and MaxDigestion Specialist.**

OSTEOPOROSIS

35 million Americans have osteoporosis. 1.5 million have spontaneous fractures a year and 150,000 die from them. If that doesn't scare you, it'll probably scare someone who cares about you. Americans experience more than a million fractures per year from osteoporosis, a disease that occurs when bones become so porous and weak they eventually collapse. This usually occurs mostly among women who are post-menopausal, but don't let that fool you. Men are great candidates for osteoporosis, too. As a result of demineralized bones, two milion men a year suffer from osteoporosis. The National Osteoporosis Foundation reported that 1 out of 8 men are diagnosed with osteoporosis, and from it, other illnesses may develop (Dr. Lauren Lipson, 2004).

1. Fulvic/Humate—helps aid in strontium absorption found in bone strengthening formulations.

2. Strontium—A crystallized and enhanced form of calcium. Technologically improved, it's 200 percent more powerful than calcium and is necessary, especially if osteoporosis has started to take its effect.

• Researcher P.J. Meunier conducted a few case studies on strontium and its effects on osteoporosis. Meunier and his team of researchers gathered 353 people who suffered at least one vertebrae (back and spine) fracture due to osteoporosis. Each study participant took strontium but some took a lesser dose than others. Those that took a daily dose of 680 mg daily had a much greater increase in vertebrae bone mineral density per year than those that did not take it on a daily basis (International Journal of Osteoporosis, 2002).

• In addition, a 2004 study produced by the New England Journal of Medicine showed the subjects that consumed strontium had a 14.4 percent increase in back-bone density and an 8.3 percent in thigh bone density.

*Note: The listed natural ingredients can be found in Dr. Tai's proprietary formulas: **Bone Specialist.**

PROSTATE INFLAMMATION
Benign Prostatic Hyperplasia (BPH)

Our bodies produce and process a variety of enzymes and chemicals, one of which is HETE, an enzyme that feeds inflammation.

Produced by 5-LO (lypo-oxygenase), as long as there is HETE within a body, there's a way for cancer to develop and thrive. However, there are a variety of natural ways to stun 5-LO and HETE production.

Dr. J. Gosh at the University of Virginia Cancer Center and Dr. L.A. Herzenberg said, "The inhibition of 5-Lipo-oxygenase (5-LO) triggers massive apoptosis in human cancer cells" (Proceeds from the National Academy of Science, 27 October 1998; 95(22): 13182-13187).

Studies like Gosh and Herzenberg's prove that 5-LO and HETE production induces cell death, hence hormone death. 5-LO and HETE play a critical role in prostate health and herbs like beta sitosterol, green tea, saw palmetto, Scutellaria baicalin, ginger and Panax ginseng have been used for centuries to decrease the size and weight of the prostate, but it's rare to find a blend encompassing all nine ingredients.

8 Powerful Secrets to Anti-Aging

1. Beta- Sistosterol—A standardized combination of plant phytosterols found in vegetables and herbs.
- Dr. Bernges (et al.) of the University of Bochum, Germany conducted a double-blind study including 200 men. After the one-year study had been completed, Dr. Bernges wrote, "Significant improvement and urinary flow parameters show effectiveness of beta sitosterol in BPH [benign prostatic hyperplasia]" (Lancet, 1995).
- For 30 years, 32 researchers at the Minneapolis VA Medical Center studied the effects of beta sistosterol. One of the 32 researchers said, "The greatest efficacy among phyto-therapeautic substances is beta sitosterol. It improves urological symptoms and flow measures" (Veteran Hospital).

2. Boswellia serrata—A natural 5-LO inhibitor, Boswellia serrata was used thousands of years ago as currency. Once more expensive than gold, in scripture, the Three Wise Men were said to have brought the herb to the infant Jesus on the day of his birth.

What the experts say on Boswellia serrata:
- Dr. H. Safayhi (et al.) "Boswellia acids, novel, specific, reduce inhibitors of 5-lipoxygenase" (Journal of Pharmacological Experimental Theories, 1992).
- Dr. H.P. Amman (et al.) "Boswellic acid has anti-inflammatory actions" (Journal of Ethno Pharmacology, 1993).
- Dr. M.T. Huang (et al.) "Boswella serrata has anti-tumor and anti-carcinogenic activities" (Biofactors, 2000).
- Dr. P. Jakoksson (et al.)" Boswellic acid regulates 5-LO" (Proclamations of National of the Academy of Science,1992).

3. Flower pollen- is extracted after careful fermentation and enzymatic pollen processing. Flower pollen is a natural amino acid that possesses the ability to stop tissue inflammation, primarily prostate tissue.

4. Ginger—The USDA Phytonutrient Database shows ginger to be a critical inhibitor of 5-LO.

5. Green tea—A polyphenol extract derived from a catechin compound.
Studies conducted on Green tea
- Dr. Pashce (et al.) "Induction of apoptosis in prostate cancer by green tea ECGC" (Cancer Letters, 1998).
- Dr. R.A. Hilpakka (et al.) "Structure activity relationship for inhibition of human 5- alpha- reductase by polyphenol" (Biochemistry and Pharmacology, 2002).
- Dr. S. Gupta. "Inhibitation of prostate carcinogenesis in TRAMP mice by oral infusion of green tea polyphenols" (Proceeds from the National Academy of Science USA, 2001).
- Dr. B.D. Lyn-Cook. "Chemo preventive effect of tea extract and various components on human pancreatic and prostate tumor cell" (Nutrition and Cancer, 1999).

6. Licorice—Another herb is a root used all over the world has many powerful compounds.
- The 1999 National Cancer Institute International Conference showed that licorice extract exhibits anti-tumor activity in acute leukemia, breast cancer and prostate cancer.

7. Panax Ginseng—Probably the oldest and most-used herb in the world. Used as an anti-aging and anti-fatigue tonic.

· • Research shows the ability of ginseng to work on interfering with 5- LO. It also reduces DHT production. Dr. Liu (et al.) found that ginseng has autoproliferative effects on the human prostate (Life Science, 2000).

• Dr. Fahim (et al.) showed the intake of Panax ginseng actually decreased the size and weight of the prostate while increasing the level of testosterone for libido and increased sexual functions (Archives of And., 1982).

8. Saw Palmetto (Serenoa repens)—A small palm tree native to Florida. The fruits and berries of the saw palmetto tree have been used since the 1800s by physicians to treat various kinds of urinary problems.

• A six-month double-blind clinical study conducted by Dr. L.S. Mark, the director of the Urological Sciences Research Foundation, showed that men taking saw palmetto had 32 percent less DHT—a hormone associated with BPH (Journal of Urology, 2001).

• Dr. T.J. Wilt (et al.) used saw palmetto extract for the treatment of benign prostatic hyperplasias (The Journal of the American Medical Association, 1998).

9. Scutellaria baicalin—An ancient Chinese root herb that has been used to tonify and heal a soared pancreas.

*Note: The listed natural ingredients are Dr. Tai's patented formulas: **Max-Prostate Specialist.**

SEXUAL DYSFUNCTION (female)

60 to 70 percent of American women experience difficulty reaching orgasm during intercourse. With Viagra and Cialis available in the market, men have multiple synthetic choices of achieving erections, but women don't have it at as easy. With hormone decline, the most romantic of settings or the gentlest of caresses won't turn a woman on. Even when the lights are off, excitement after a certain age can feel as if it's a thing of the past. Throughout the world, libido loss in aging women has captured researchers' attention, until Chinese researchers recently found that aleppo oak extract, derived from a small bush native to Asian highlands, is found to be effective in intimacy and lovemaking because it stimulates a specific neuro bundle of the brain which signals orgasm. Herbs like aleppo oak can increase sensitivity, while herbs like eurycoma can generate a quicker response to sensitivity.

1. Aleppo Oak—stimulates circulation in genital areas. Women's response to aleppo oak extract has been overwhelmingly positive. The bush extract has been reported to have given women who experience orgasms multiple orgasms. Women who report to sometimes or rarely achieve orgasm have said to experience them more frequently with consistent aleppo oak use.

2. Epimedium—has been used for centuries in China as a natural aphrodisiac. The plant enhances cognitive responses for the ability to achieve gratification from sexual stimulation. It has been classified as an adaptogen because of its calming effects.

3. Eurycoma—is an energy and mental stimulator. Eurycoma is effective because once the herb is consumed it works through the hypothalamic pituitary axis by stimulating the nerves, which coerces a person to exert more energy. Clinical studies have shown eurycoma modulates the luteinizing hormone that stimulates a woman's sexual response. Because of eurycoma's energy-inducing abilities, it is suggested that athletes in training take a supplement with eurycoma extract.

*Note: The listed natural ingredients can be found in Dr. Tai's proprietary formulas: **Lady Specialist, Lafemme Specialist.**

SEXUAL DYSFUNCTION (male)

Many synthetic products in the marketplace have side effects that have the potential of inducing hypertension and overstimulating the blood, increasing the likelihood of heart attacks. Special proprietary formulation of extracts taken from all over the world can stimulate adaptogenic effects similar to the kinds our body produce. With precise measurements and careful herbal selection, men can speed metabolism and enhance sexual drive without the negative side effects of synthetic drugs regardless of age.

The ingredients chosen for this proprietary formulation was very carefully researched for its antiaging properties—adaptogenic as well as natural secretagogues of our hormones. The combined qualities of these herbal extracts work specifically on the pituitary and hypothalamus (master glands), which control and regulate our personal hormone production.

1. Butea—A plant used as a sexual enhancement tonic by older men in Thailand.

2. Epidemium—A natural aphrodisiac (see female sexual dysfunction for description).

3. Eurycoma—improves energy, reduces fatigue and enhances overall physical and sensual performance.

4. Watermelon rind extract—known for centuries in ancient Asian pharmacopeia for its fabulous erectile functions.

*Note: The listed natural ingredients can be found in Dr. Tai's proprietary formulas: **Max Men.**

STRESS

Stress is pressure, strain and anxiety; it's exhausting, nerve-wracking and hectic. Natural formulas made from passion flower, valerian and Rhodiola Rosea promise to strengthen the nervous system and ease hypertension that can lead to overeating, weakened immunity function and the development of neurological disorders.

1. Passion flower—The Native American flower of passion will do what it promises. Powerful in flavanoids, it exhibits anti-anxiety effects for extra energy. Also a mild aphrodisiac, it decreases the strain in lungs to bring more oxygen into the system (Alternative Medicine Review, 2001).
2. Rhodiola Rosea—The Russian resistance builder helps provide cardio-pulmonary protection as it works as a stress-fighting hormone that balances the adrenal glands that can throw the body's nervous system off. Rhodiola Rosea is a relief from chronic fatigue syndrome (Alternative Medicine Review, 2001).
3. Valerian—Used for thousands of years in ancient Greece and China, valerian helps provide calming and sedative affects. It provides relief from tension, headaches and gastrointestinal spasms (Herbal Medicine, 2000).
• In 2002, Andrea Tini (et al.) conducted a study testing the effects of valerian extract on 48 adults and split the group in half. Three times a day, one group was given 2.5 mg Valium (a sedative pharmaceutical drug) while the other group was given 15 mg of valerian. The group that took valerian showed significant improvement in their moods; their scans showed that their anxiety sensations reduced dramatically.

*Note: The listed natural ingredients can be found in Dr. Tai's proprietary formulas: **Stress Specialist.**

WRINKLES

Nano-encapsulated liposomes were formulated to deliver powerful plant extracts deep into the skin's sub-layers. With nano-encapsulated liposomes formulators have been able to pack microscopic bundles of natural ingredients like: Prodew a nourishing skin humectant that promotes moisture retention and kukui nut oil. Scientific research has proven that a combination of oils and herbs transported by a dependable vehicle can give the skin 500 percent more moisture than lotions and creams without liposomes. However, the true source of power for an effective anti-wrinkle system are phtyohormones, and the leader of the pack is-puereria mirifica. Puereria extracts lifts damaged collagen and reconstructs elastin turning congested, dull and wrinkly skin into an image of freshness. **Epidermal Growth Factors turbocharge skin repair and produce natural collagen and elastin to rejuvenate the skin's wrinkles.**

8 Powerful Secrets to Anti-Aging

Cleanse

1. Licorice—Licorice is included in most Chinese herb combinations to balance the other herbs and to promote vitality. It is a source of magnesium, silicon and thiamine.

2. Linden—While sometimes referred to as a lime flower, linden is not related to the lime fruit helps to increase the immune system's ability to fight infections. When used as a cleansing agent Linden rids the skin of bacteria.

3. Pinus—The oil made from its seeds has a powerhouse of beneficial antioxidant vitamins and minerals.

Exfoliate: Diamond Microdermabrasion

1. Diamond microcrystals—Hypoallergenic 0.5 micron diamond crystals that remove dead skin cells from the skin's surface.

2. Papaya—An amazingly rich source of proteolytic enzymes; the papaya fruit has chemicals that enables cell metabolization.

3. Pineapple—The fruit is abundant with the trace mineral—manganese, which is needed for the body to build connective tissues.

Moisturize

1. Kukui nut oil—Kukui oil is expeller pressed from the nut of the kukui tree. The oil is an outstanding emollient that is absorbed quickly and thoroughly, and leaves no greasy after feel. Kukui nut oil has earned its historic reputation through generations of use, providing nature's relief for dry skin, and easing the symptoms of eczema and psoriasis.

2. Niacinamide—Protects photosensitive skin, which burns easier than most skin types from penetrating sunlight. Niacinamide protects skin to any and all conditions light eruptions that can cause dramatic rashes.

3. Prodew—A complex humectant derived from research on the skin's NMF. It is an NMF base and possesses excellent humectant properties due to the synergistic effect of sodium PCA and L-proline.

4. Benzyl Nicotinate—A natural powerhouse of oxygen infusion into the skin to increase energy and repair metabolism. Published research shows improved O_2 helps to heal, energize, and repair damaged skin.

Anti-wrinkle eye serum

1. Epidermal Growth Factors (EGF)—Growth factor proteins that bind to receptors on the cell surface, with the primary result of activating cellular proliferation and/or differentiation.

2. Marine Collagen—Boosts collagen production naturally, while working effectively to smooth fine lines and increase skin elasticity. Marine collagen has be used widely amongst dermatologists to firm and tone, naturally detoxify the skin and help carry oxygen to the epidermis.

3. Mugwort—Mugwort has been used to treat a host of skin conditions; the plant is known to help metabolize nutrients into the skin.

Restoring night caviar

1. Liposome Vitamin C- Vitamin C (L-ascorbic acid) is one of the relatively few topical agents whose effectiveness against wrinkles and fine lines is backed by a fair amount of reliable scientific evidence.

*Note: The listed natural ingredients are essential to your internal skin care program. You can find the following ingredients in Dr. Tai's proprietary formulas: **Nattoyant Cleansing Gel, Diamond Microdermabrasion, Essence Flash Toner, Anti-wrinkle Nano-eye Serum, Nano-Moistutizer Day Cream, Nano-Restoring Night Caviar and Triple Nano-Antioxidant Rejuvenator.**

RESOURCES

Health Secrets USA
24141 Ann Arbor Trail
Dearborn Heights, Michigan 48127
Tel: 313.561.6800
Fax: 313.561.6830
info@healthsecretsusa.com
Website: http://www.healthsecretsusa.com

Get Healthy Again
Robert Harrison
40374 Waterman Road
Homer, Alaska 99603
Tel: 907-235-5556
Website: http://www.gethealthyagain.com

Garden of Life
5500 Village Blvd.
Suite 202
West Palm Beach, Florida 33407
Tel: 561-748-2477
Wholesale orders: 800-622-8986
Wholesale information: 561-748-2478
Fax: 561-472-9298
Website: http://www.gardenoflife.com

Saliva testing – Food Allergy/Intolerance testing

Health Secrets USA
24141 Ann Arbor Trail
Dearborn Heights, Michigan 48127
Tel: 313.561.6800
Fax: 313.561.6830
Website: http://www.healthsecretsusa.com
info@healthsecretsusa.com

REFERENCES

A

Aardal, E.; Holm, A.C. "Cortisol in saliva-reference rages and relation to cortisol in serum. *European Journal of Clinical Biochemistry,* 1995; 33:927-932.

Aardal-Eriksson E.; Karlberg, B.E.; Holm, A.C. "Salivary cortisol- and alternative to serum cortisol determinations in dynamic function tests." *ClinicalChemistry and Laboratory Medicine,* 1998; 36: 215-222.

Allollio, B.; Hoffmann, J.; Linton, E.A.; Winkelmann, W.; Kusche, M.; Schulte,-H.M. "Diurnal salivary cortisol patterns during pregnancy and afterdelivery: relationship to plasma corticotrophin-releasing hormone. *Clinical Endocrinology,* 1990; 33: 279-289.

Araneo, B., et al. "DHEAS as an effective vaccine adjuvant in elderly humans." *Annals of the New York Academy of Sciences,* 1995; 774: 232-48.

Arlt, W., et al. "Dehydroepiandrosterone replacement in women with adrenal insufficiency." *New England Journal of Medicine*, September 30, 1999; 341(14): 1013-20.

Aver, S.; Dobs, A.S.; Meikle, A.W. et al. "Improvement of sexual function in testosterone deficient men treated for one year with a permeation enhanced testosterone transdermal system." *Journal of Urology*, 1996;155:1604-8.

B

Baker, Valerie L. "Alternatives to oral estrogen replacement: Transdermal patches, percutaneous gels, vaginal creams and rings, implants and other methods of delivery." *Obstetrics and Gynecological Clinics of North America*, 1994; 21 (2):271-97.

Barret- Connor E.; Khaw, K.W.; Yen S.S., et al. "A prospective study of dehy- droepiandrosterone sulfate, mortality, and cardiovascular disease." *New England Journal of Medicine,* 1986; 315: 1519-24.

Barrett-Connor E., et al. "The epidemiology of DHEAS and cardiovascular disease." *Annals of the New York Academy of Sciences*, 1995; 774: 259- 70.

Bartsch, C.; Bartsch, H., et al." Melatonin in cancer patients and in tumorbearing animals." *Advances in Experimental Medical Biology*, 1999; 467: 247-64.

Basaria, S. and Dobs, A.S. "Risks versus benefits of testosterone therapy in elderly   men." *Drugs Aging*, 1999; 15(2): 131-42.

Bates, G. et al. "Dehydroepiandrosterone treatment of midlife dysthymia." *Biological Psychiatry*. 1999; 45: 1533-41.

Baulieu, E. E. et al. " Dehydroepiandrosterone (DHEA), DHEA sulfate, and aging. contribution of the DHEAge study to a sociobiomedical issue." *Proceedings of the National Academy of Sciences USA*, 2000; 97(8):4279-84.

Bilimoria, M.M., et al. "Estrogen replacement therapy and breast cancer: analysis of age of onset and tumor characteristics." *Annals of Surgical Oncology*, 1999; 6: 200-7.

Bolaji I.I.; Tallon, D.F.; O'Dwyer, E.; Fottrell, P.F. "Assessment of bioavailability of oral micronized progesterone using a salivary progesterone enzymeimmunoassay." *Gynecological Endocrinology*, 1993; 7:101-110.

Bradlow, H.L. et al. "Indole-3-carbinol: A novel approach to breast cancer prevention." appearing in "Cancer Prevention. From the Laboratory to the Clinic: implications of Genetic, Molecular and Preventative Research," *Annals of the New York Academy of Sciences*, September 1995; 768: 180-200.

Bradlow, H.L. et al. " Multifunctional aspects of the action of indole-3-carbinol as an antitumor agent," *Annals of the New York Academy of Sciences*, 1999; 889:204-13.

Brody, Jane E. "Restoring ebbing hormones may slow aging." *New York Times*, July 18,1995; C1.

Bush, Trudy L. "Preserving cardiovascular benefits of hormone replacement therapy. *Journal of Reproductive Medicine*, September 1998; 19 (9): 1623-9.

Buster, J. E. et al." Postmenopausal steroid replacement with micronized dehydro epiandrosterone: preliminary oral bioavailability and dose proportionality studies," *American Journal of Obstetrics and Gynecology*, 1992; 166: 1163-68.

C

Campbell, B.C.; Ellison, P.T. "Menstrual variation in salivary testosterone among regularly cycling women." *Hormone Research*, 1992; 37: 132-136.

Carlson, L. E. et al. "Relationships between deydroepiandrosterone sulfate (DHEAS) and cortisol (CRT) plasma levels and everyday memory in Alzheimer's disease patients compared to healthy controls," *Hormonal Behavior*, June 1999; 35(3): 254-63.

Carter, H.B. et al. "Longitudinal evaluation of serum androgen levels in me with and without prostate cancer," *The Prostate*, 1995; 27:25-31.

Casson, P. et al. "Oral dehydroepiandrosterone in physiologic doses modulates immune function in postmenopausal women." *American Journal Obstetrics Gynecology*, 1993; 169: 1536-39.

Chakmakjian, Z. H.; Zachariah, N.Y. "Bioavailability of progesterone with different modes of administration." *Journal of Reproductive Medicine*, June 1987; 32(6):443-47.

Chang, K.J., et al. "Influences of percutaneous administration of estradiol and progesterone on human breast epithelial cell cycle in vivo." *Fertility and Sterility,* April 1995; 63(4): 785-91.

Choe, J.K.; Khan-Dawood, F.S.; Dawood, M.Y. "Progesterone and estradiol in the saliva and plasma during the menstrual cycle." *American Journal of Obstetrics and Gynecology*, 1983; 147: 557-562.

Claustrat, B., et al. "Hormone and jet lag: Confirmatory result using a simplified protocol." *Bio Psychiatry*, 1992; 32:705-11.

Colditz, G.A. et al. "Hormone replacement therapy and breast cancer risk." *American Journal of Obstetrics and Gynecology*, 1993; 168: 1473-80.

Collaborative Group on hormonal Factors in Breast Cancer. "Breast cancer and hormone replacement therapy: Collaborative reanalysis of data from 51epidemiological studies of 52, 705 women with breast cancer and 108, 411 Women without breast cancer." *Lancet*, 1997; 350: 1047-59.

Cooper, A., et al. "Systemic absorption of progesterone from Progest cream in post menopausal women." *Lancet*, April 1998; 351(9111): 1255-6.

Cowan, L. D., et al. "Breast cancer incidence in women with a history of progesterone deficiency." *American Journal of Epidemiology*, August 1981; 114(2):209-17.

Cromer, B.A. "Effects of hormonal contraceptives on bone mineral density." *Drug Safety*, March 1999; 20(3): 213-22.

D

Dabbs, J.M. "Salivary testosterone measurements: Collecting, storing and mailing saliva samples." *Physiology and Behavior*, 1990; 49(48): 83-86.

Davelaar, "Exogenious estrogen (E2) subcutaneous protective?" *Tijdschr Geneeskd*, 1991; 135 (14): 613-15.

Delfs, T.M.; Klein, S.; Fottrell, P.; Naether, O.G.; Leidenberger, F.A.; Zimmermann, R.C."24-Hour profiles of salivary progesterone." *Fertility and Sterlity*, 1994;62: 960-966.

Diamond, P. et al. "Metabolic effects of 12-month percutaneous dehydoepiandroste-rone replacement therapy n postmenopausal women." *Journal of Endocrinology*, 1996; 150:S43-S5.

E

Eden, J.A., et al." A case-controlled study of combined continuous estrogen-progestin replacement therapy amongst women with a personal history of breast cancer." *Menopause*, 1995; 2: 67-72.

Elakovich, S.O.; Hampton, J. "Analysis of Couvaestrol. A Phytoestrogen, in Alpha Tablets Sold for Human Consumption." *Journal of Agricultural Food Chemistry*, 1984; 32:173-175.

F

Feldman, F.A.; Johannes, C.B.; Araujo, A.B.; Mohr, B.A.; Longscope, C.; Mckinlay J.B. "Low dehydroepiandrosterone and ischemic heart disease in middle-aged men: prospective results from the Massachusetts Male Aging Study." *American Journal of Epemiology*, 2001; 153(1):79-89.

Filaire, E.; Duche, P.; Lac, G.; Robert, A. "Saliva cortisol, physical exercise and training: Influences of swimming and handball on cortisol concentrations in women." *European Journal of Applied Physiology*, 1996; 74: 274-278.

Filaire, E. and Lac, G. "Dehydroepiandrosterone(DHEA) rather than testosterone shows saliva androgen responses to exercise in elite female handball players." *International Journal of Sports Medicine*, 2000; 21:17-20.

Fishman, J. et al. " Increased estrogen-16-alpha-hydroxylase activity in women with breast cancer and endometrial cancer." *Journal of Steroidal Biochemistry*, April 1984; 20 (4B): 1077-81.

Fitzpatrick, Lorraine and Good, Andrew. "Micronized progesterone: Clinical indicationsand comparison with current treatments." *Fertility and Sterility*, September 1995; 72(3):389-97.

Flood, J.F.; Morley, J.E.; Roberts, E. "Memory-enhancing effects in male mice of pregnenolone and steroids metabolically derived from it." *Proceeds National Academy of Sciences USA*, March 1992; 89(5): 1567-71.

Folkard, S., Arendt, J., et al. "Can melatonin improve shift workers' tolerance of the night shift? Some preliminary findings." *Chronobiology International*, 1993; 10: 315-20.

Follingstad, A. "Estriol, the forgotten hormone." *The Journal of the American Medical Association*, 1978; 239 (1), 29-39.

Foidart, J., et al. "Estradiol and progesterone regulate the proliferation of human breast epithelial cells." *Fertility and Sterility*, May 1998; 69 (5): 963-68.

Formby, B., and Willey, T.S. "Progesterone inhibits growth and induces apoptosis in breast cancer cells: inverse effects on Bcl-2 and p53." *Annals of Clinical Laboratory Science*, November-December 1998; 28(6): 360-9.

Fortunati, N. "Sex hormone-binding globulin: Not only a transport protein." *Journal of Endocrine Investigation*, March 1999; 22(3):223-34.

Freeman, H.; Pincus, G.; Bachrach S., et al. "Therapeutic efficacy of delta 5 prenenolone in rheumatoid arthritis." *JAMA*, 1950; 143: 338-44.

G

Gajdos, Csaba, et al. "Breast cancer diagnosed during hormone replacement therapy." *Obstetrics and Gynecology*, April 2000; 95(4): 513-18.

Gambrell, R. Don, et al. " Decreased incidence of breast cancer in postmenopausal Estrogen-progensten users." *Obstetrics and Gynecology*, October 1983; 62(4):435-442.

George, M.S.; Guidotti, A.; Rubinow, D. et al. "CSF neuroactive steroids in affective disorders: Pregnenolone, progesterone and DBI." *Biological Psychiatry*, 1994; 35(10):775-80.

Gillson, G.R., and Zava, D.T. " 2003 Perspective on Hormone Replacement for Women: Picking up the pieces after the Women's Health Initiative Trial." *International Journal of Pharmaceutical Compounding*, 2003; 7(4): 250.

Gouras, G.K.; Xu, H.; Gross, R.S.; Greenfield, J.P.; Hai, B.; Wang, R.; Greengard, P. "Testosterone decreases neuronal secretion of Alzeheimer's beta-amyloid peptides." *Proceeds from the National Academy of Science USA*. February 2000;97(3): 1202-5.

H

Hansen, P.A.; Han, D.H.; Nolte, L.A.; Chen, H. Holloszy." Dhea protects against visceral obesity and muscle insulin resistance in rats fed a high fat diet." *American Journal of Physiology*, November, 1997; 273(5 Pt. 2):R1704-8.

Hargrove, Joel T., et al. "Absorption of oral progesterone is influenced by vehicle and particle size." *American Journal of Obstetrics and Gynecology*, 1989; 161(4): 948-51.

Heine, R.P.; McGregor, J.A.; Dullien, V.K. "Accuracy of salivary estriol testing compared to traditional risk factor assessment in predicting preterm birth." *American Journal of Obstetrics and Gynecology*, 1999; 180:S214-218.

Helzlsouer, Kathy, et al." Relationship of prediagnostic serum levels of dehydro-epiandrosterone and dehydroepiandrosterone sulfate to the risk of developing premenopausal breast cancer." *Cancer Research*, 1992;52:1-4.

Hennebold, J.D. and Daynes, R.A. "Regulation of macrophage dehydroepiandrosterone sulfate metabolism of inflammatory cytokines." *Endocrinology*, 1995;135:67-75.

J

Jenkins, T. "Male menopause: Myth or Monster?" *Vibrant Life*, 1995; 11(6): 12-15.

Johannes, C.B., et al. "Relation of dehydroepiandrosterone and dehydroepiandroste-rone sulfate with cardiovascular disease risk factors in women: Longitudinal Results from the Massachusetts Women's Health Study." *Journal of Clinical Epidemiology*, February 1999; 52(2): 95-103.

Johnson, Kate. "ERT halves testosterone levels, may warrant Tx." *Ob-Gyn News*, May 2000; 35(10): 18.

Jorgensen, Jens, et al. "Three years of growth hormone treatment in growth hormone-deficient adults: Near normalization of body composition and physical performance." *European Journal of Endocrinology*, 1994;130:224-8.

K

Kaiser, F. "Testosterone Therapy Shows Promise in Elderly Men." *Journal of American Geriatrics Society*, February 18, 1993.

Kall, M.A., et al. "Effects of dietary broccoli on human drug metabolizing activity." *Cancer*, March 1997; 114(1-2): 169-70.

Katznelson, L.; Finkelson, J.S.; Schoenfeld, D.A., et al." Increase in bone density and lean body mass during testosterone administration in men with acquired hypogonadism." *Journal of Clinical Endocrinology and Metabolism*. 1996; 81:4358-65.

Khan-Dawood, F.S.; Chloe, J.K.; Dawood, M.Y. "Salivary and plasma bound and "free" testosterone in men and women." *American Journal of Obstetrics and Gynecology*, 1984; 148: 441-445.

Kidd, Parris. "Phosphatidylserine." New Canaan, Conn.: Keats Publishing, 1998.

Kimonides, V.G.; Spillantini, M.G.; Sofroniew, M.V.; Fawcett, J.W.; Herbert, J.; "Dehydroepiandrosterone antagonizes the neurotoxic effects of Corticosterone and translocation of stress-activated protein kinase 3 in hippocampal primary cultures." *Neuroscience,* March 1999;89(2): 429-36.

Klatz, Ronald, and Goldman, Robert. "Stopping the Clock." New Canaan, Conn.: Keats Publishing, 1996.

Kudielka, B.M.; Schmidt-Reinwald, A.K.; Hellhammer, D.H.; Kirschbaum,-C. "Psychological and endocrine responses to psychosocial stress and dexamethanesone/ corticotrophin-releasing hormone in healthy postmenopausal women and young control: The impact of age and a two-week estradiol treatment." *Neuroendocrinology*, 1999;70: 422-430.

Kurzman, I.D.; Panciera, D.L.; Miller, J.B.; MacEwen, E.G. "The effect of dehydroepiandr-Osterone combined with a low-fat diet in spontaneously obese dogs: A Clinical Trial." *Obesity Research*, 1998; (6)1.

L

Lane, G., et al. "Dose-dependant effects of oral progesterone on the oestrogenised postmenopausal endometrium." *British Medical Journal*, 1983; 287: 1241-44.

Lee, John R., and Hopkins, Virginia. *What Your Doctor May Not Tell You About Menopause: The Breakthrough Book on Natural Progesterone.* New York: Warner Books, 1996.

Legros, John R. "Women's heart disease, heart attacks, and hormones." *The John R. Lee, Medical Letter,* August 1998; 1-3.

Legros, S., et al. "Premenstrual tension syndrome or premenstrual dysphoria." *Review Medical Liege*, April 1999; 54(4): 268-73.

Lemon, H. "Ostriol and prevention of breast cancer." *Lancet* 1, 1973; 802:546-547.

Lemon, H. "Estriol prevention of mammary carcinoma induced by 7,12-dimethyl- benzathracene and procarbazine." *Cancer Research*, 1975; 35: 1341-1353.

Lemon, H.M. "Clinical and experimental aspects of the anti-mammary carcinogenic activity of estriol." *Frontier Hormonal Research*, 1977; 5: 155-173.

Lemon, H. "Pathophysiologic considerations in the treatment of menopausal patients with oestrogens: The role of oestriol in the prevention of mammary cancer." *Acta Endocrinoligica*, 1980; 233: S17-27.

Lemon, H.M., et al. "Inhibition of radiogenic mammary carcinoma in rats by estriol by estriol or tamoxifen." *Cancer,* 1989; 63: 1685-92.

Leonetti, H. M.D.; Longo, S.; Anasti, J. M.D. "Transdermal Progesterone Cream for Vasomotor Symptoms and Postmenopausal Bone Loss." *Obstetrics and Gynecology*, January 1999; 94(2): 225-228.

Lissoni, P., et al. " Randomized study with the pineal hormone melatonin versus supportive care alone in advanced nonsmall cell lung cancer resistant to a first-line chemotherapy containing cisplatin." *Oncology*, 1992, 49:336-39.

Lu, Y.C.; Chatterton, R.T.; Vogelsong, K.M.; May, L.K. "Direct radioimmunoassay of progesterone in saliva." *Journal of Immunoassay*, 1997, 18: 149-163.

M

Manolagas, S.C. "Birth and death of bone cells: basic regulatory mechanisms and implications, for the pathogenesis and treatment of osteoporosis." *Endocrinology Review*, 2000; 21: 115-137.

Mauldin, Robert K. "New HRT approved." *Modern Medicine*, 1999, 67(7):55.

Michnovicz, J.J., and Bradlow, H.L. "Introduction of estradiol metabolism by dietary indole-3-carbinole in humans." *Journal of the National Cancer Institute,* June 1990, 82(11):947-49.

Mohr, P.E., et al. "Serum progesterone and prognosis in operable breast cancer," *British Journal,* June 1996, 73(12): 1552-55.

Monath, J.R. et al." Physiologic variations of serum testosterone with the normal range do not affect serum prostate specific antigen," *Urology,* 1995; 46(1):58-61.

Monteleone, P., et al. "Allopregnenolone concentrations and premenstrual syndrome." *European Journal of Endocrinology,* March 2000, 142(3):269-73.

Moon, Mary Ann. "HRT users more prone to mammography failures." *Ob-Gyn News* May 2000, 35(10): 15.

Morales, A. J., et al." Effects of replacement dose of dehydroepiandrosterone in men and women of advancing age." *Journal of Clinical Endocrinology and Metabolism,* 1994, 78(6) 1360-67.

Mortola, J. F. et al. "The effects of dehydroepiandrosterone on endocrinemetabolic parameters in postmenopausal women." *Journal of Clinical Endocrinology and Metabolism,* 1990, 71: 696-704.

Mosca, L. "The role of hormone replacement therapy in the prevention of Postmenopausal heart disease." *Archives of Internal Medicine,* 2000, 160: 2263-2272.

N

Nachtigall, Lila E. "Emerging delivery systems for estrogen replacement: Aspects of transdermal and oral delivery." *American Journal of Obstetrics and Gynecology,* 1995, 173(3): 993-97.

Nachtigall, M.J., et al.,"Incidence of breast cancer in a 22-year study of women receiving estrogen-progestin replacement therapy." *Obstetrics Gynecology* 1992, 80: 827-830.

Nafziger, Anne, et al. "Longitudinal changes in dehydroepiandrosterone concentrations in men and women." *Journal of Laboratory of Clinical Medicine,* 1992,131(4): 316-23.

Navarro, M.A.; Nolla, J.M.; Machuca, M.I.; Gonzalez, A.; Mateo, L.; Bonnin, R.M.; Roig-Escofet, D. "Salivary testosterone in postmenopausal women with rheumatoid arthritis." *The Journal of Rheumatology,* 1998, 25: 1059-1062.

O

Orentreich, N.; Brind J.L.; Rizer, R.L.; Vogelman, J.H. "Age changes and sex differences In serum dehydroepiandrosterone sulfate concentrations throughout adulthood." *Journal of clinical Endocrinology and Metabolism,* September 1984; 59(3): 551-5.

O'Rourke, M.T. and Ellison, P.T. "Salivary estradiol levels decrease with age in healthy regularly-cycling women." *Clinical Endocrinology,* 1986; 24:31-38.

P

Padwick, M.L., et al. " Absorption and metabolism of oral progesterone when administered twice daily." *Fertility and Sterility,* 1986; 46:402-07.

Petrie, K., et al. "A double-blind trial of melatonin as a treatment for jet lag in international cabin crew." *Biological Psychiatry,* 1993; 33: 526-30.

Pierpaoli, Walter. "Melatonin, the pineal gland and aging: A planetary and biological reality." In *The Science of Anti-aging Medicine* (Edited by Klatz and Goldman), Colorado Springs, American Academy of Anti-aging Medicine, 1996.

Pierpaoli, Walter, and Regelson, William. "The pineal control of aging. The effect of melatonin and pineal grafting on aging mice." *Proceedings of the National Academy of Sciences,* 1994; 91:787-91.

Plouffe, L., J. "Ovaries, androgens and the menopause: practical applications." *Seminars of Reproductive Endocrinology,* 1998; 16(2):117-120.

Plu-Bureau, G., et al. "Progestogen use and decreased risk of breast cancer in a cohort study of premenopausal women with benign breast disease." *British Journal of Cancer*, 1994; 70:270-77.

Powrie, Jake et al. "Growth hormone replacement therapy for growth hormone-deficient adults," *Drugs*, 1995; 49(5):656-63.

Prior, J.C. "Progesterone as a bone-trophic hormone." *Endocrine Reviews*, May 1990;11(2):386-98.

Q

Quissell, D. "Steroid hormone analysis in human saliva." *Annals of the New York Academy of Sciences*, 1993; 694: 143-145.

R

Raff, H.; Raff, J.L.; Findling, J.W. "Late-night salivary cortisol as a screening test for Cushing's Syndrome." *Journal of Clinical Endocrinology and Metabolism*, 1998; 83: 2681-2686.

Raz, Raul, and Stamm, Walter. "A controlled trial of intravaginal estriol in postmenopausal women with recurrent urinary tract infections." *The New England Journal of Medicine*, September 1993; 329(11):753-56.

Read, G.F. "Status report on measurement of salivary estrogens and androgens."*Annals of the New York Academy of Sciences*, 20 September 1993; 694:146-160.

Regelson, William, and Colman, Carol, *The Superhormone Promise: Nature's Antidote to Aging*. New York: Pocket Books, 1997.

Reiter, R.J. "The role of the neurohormone melatonin as a buffer against macro-molecular oxidative damage." *Neurochemistry International*, 1995;27:453-460.

Rosen, Thord, et al. "Consequences of growth hormone deficiency in adults and the benefits and risks of recombinant human growth hormone treatment, " *Hormone Research*, 1995; 43:93-99.

Rylance, P.B., et al. "Natural progesterone and antihypertensive action." *British Medical Journal*, January 5, 1985; 290: 13-14.

S

Sarrel, P.M. "Cardiovascular aspects of androgens in women." *Seminars of Reproductive Endocrinology*, 1998; 16(2): 121-8.

Schechter D. "Estrogen, progesterone and mood." *Journal of Gender-Specific Medicine*, 1999; (2):29-36.

Schwartz, E. M.D. *The Hormone Solution*. New York: Warner Books.

Seelig, Mildred. "Interrelationship of magnesium and estrogen in cardiovascular and bone disorders, eclampsia, and premenstrual syndrome." *Journal of the American College of Nutrition*, 1993; 12(4): 442-58.

Service, Robert F. "New role for estrogen in cancer?" *Science*, March 13, 1998; 279:1631-33.

Shaywitz, Sally et al. "Effects of estrogen on brain activation patterns in postmenopausal women during working memory tasks." *Journal of the American Medical Association*, 1999; 281: 1197-1202.

Sherwin, B.B. "The impact of different doses of estrogen and progestin on mood and sexual behavior in postmenopausal women." *Journal of Clinical Endocrinology and Metabolism*, February 1991; 72(2):336-43.

Shi-Zong B.; De-Ling, Y.; Xiu-Hai, R. et al. "Progesterone induces apoptosis and up-regulation of p53 expression in human ovarian carcinoma cell lines." *Cancer*, 1997; 79: 10.

Siegal, Sanford. *Is Your Thyroid Making You Fat?* New York: Warner Books, 2000.

Siller-Arenas et al. "Menopausal Hormone Replacement Therapy and Breast Cancer: A Meta-Analysis." *Obstetrics and Gynecology*, 1990; 79(2).

Stedman's Medical Dictionary. 27th ed. 2000.

Sternberg, T.H.; LeVan, P.; Wright, E.T. „The hydrating effects of pregnenolone acetate on the human skin." *Current Therapy Research*, 1961; 3(11): 469-71.

Suzuki, K. et al. "Endocrine environment of benign prostate hyperplasia: Prostate size and volume are correlated with serum estrogen concentration." *Scandinavian Journal of Urology and Nephrology*, 1995; 29: 65-68.

Swinkels, L.M.; Ross, H.A.; Smals, A.G.; Benraad, T.J. "Concentrations of total and free dehydroepiandrosterone in plasma and dehydroepiandrosterone in saliva of normal and hirsute women under basal conditions and during administration of dexamethasone/synthetic corticotrophin." *Clinical Chemistry*, 1990; 16:2042-2046.

T

Tan, D.X.; Chen, I.D.; Poeggeler, B.; Manchester, L.C.; Reitner, R.J."Melatonin: A potent, endogenous hydroxyl radical scavenger." *Endocrinology Journal* 1993; 1:57-60.

Tan, D.X.; Poeggeler, B.; Reiter, R. et al." The pineal hormone melatonin inhibits DNA-adduct formation induced by the chemical carcinogen safrole in vivo." *Cancer*, 1993; 70:65-71.

Taylor, Maida. "Alternatives to conventional hormone replacement therapy." *Comprehensive Therapy*, 1997; 23 (8): 514-32.

Tschop, M.; Behre, H.M.; Nieschlag, E.; Dressendorfer, R.A.; Strasburg, C.J. "A time-resolved fluorescence immunoassay for the measurement of testosterone in saliva: Monitoring of testosterone replacement therapy with testosterone buciclate." *Clinical Chemistry Laboratory Medicine*, 1998; 36: 223-230.

U

Ulrich, M. "Men who maunder about their fading virility should learn to grow old gracefully." *The Report Magazine*, 2001.

V

Vail, Jane. " 'Natural,' or ' Bioidentical' Hormone Replacement: What makes the difference? An interview with Christopher B. Cutter, M.D." *Inter-national Journal of Pharmaceutical Compounding*, 2003; 7(1).

VanVollenhovem, R. F., et al. "An open study of dehydroepiandrosterone in systemic lupus erythematosus." *Rheumatoid Arthritis*, 1994; 37: 1305-10.

Vermeulen, A.; Kaulman, J.M.; "Aging of the hypothalmo-pituitary testicular axis in men." *Hormonal Research* 43, no. 1-3, 1995; 25-28.

Vining, R.F.; McGingley, R.A.; Symons, R.G. "Hormones in saliva: mode of entry and consequent implications for clinical interpretation. *Clinical Chemistry* 1983; 29: 1752-1756.

Vining, R.F. and McGingley, R.A. "The measurement of hormones in saliva: possibilities and pitfalls." *Journal of Steroid Biochemistry*, 1987; (27): 1-3; 81-94.

W

Waddell, B.J. and Leary, P.C.O. "Distrubution and metabolism of topically applied progesterone in a rat model." *Journal of Steroid Biochemistry and Molecular Biology*, 2001; 80: 449-455.

Wagner, Janice. "Rationale for hormone replacement therapy in atherosclerosis prevention." *The Journal of Fertility*, March 2000; 45 (Supplement 1):73-80.

Wallis, Claudia. "The estrogen dilemma." *Time*, June 26, 1995; Cover article.

Wang, D.Y.; Fantl, V.E.; Habibollahi, F.; Clark, G.M.; Fentiman, I.S.; Hayward, J.L.; Bulbrook, R.D. "Salivary oestradiol and progesterone levels in premenopausal women with breast cancer." *European Journal of Cancer and Clinical Oncology*, 22 April 1986; (4): 427-33.

Wang, D.Y. and Knyba R.E. "Salivary progesterone: Relation to total and non-protein-bound blood levels." *Journal of Steroid Biochemistry*, 1985; 23:975-979.

Washburn, S.A. "Estradiol and Progesterone Effects on the Central Nervous System." *Menopausal Medicine*, 1997; 5(4):5-8.

Watts, N.B., et al. "Comparison of oral estrogens and estrogens plus androgen on bone mineral density, menopausal symptoms, and lipid-lipo-protein profiles in surgical menopause." *Obstertrics and Gynecology*, April 1995; 85 (4): 529-37.

Webb, C.M.; McNeill, J.G.; Hayward, C.S.; de Ziegler, D.; Collins, P.; "Effects of testosterone on coronary vasomotor regulation in men with coronary heart disease." *Circulation*, October 1999; 100(16):1690-6.

Wexler, Laura. "Studies of acute coronary syndromes in women-Lessons for everyone." *New England Journal of Medicine*, July 1999; 341(4): 275-6.

Willett, Walter, et al. "Postmenopausal estrogens-opposed, unopposed, or none of the above." *The Journal of the American Medical Association*, January 26, 2000; 283, (4): 534-5.

Women's Health Initiative. "Effects of Conjugated Equine Estrogen in Postmenopausal Women with Hysterectomy." *The Journal of the American Medical Association*, 2004; 291:1701-1712.

Worthman, C.M.; Stallings, J.F.; Hofman, L.F. "Sensitive salivary estradiol assay for monitoring ovarian function." *Clinical Chemistry*, 1990; 36:1769-1773.

Wren, B.; McFarland, K.; Edwards, L.; O'Shea, P.; Sufi, S. et al. "Effect of sequential transdermal progesterone cream on endometrium, bleeding pattern and plasma progesterone and salivary progesterone levels in postmenopausal women." *Climactric 3*, 2000; 155-160.

Wright, Jonathon V., and Morgenthaler, John. *Natural Hormone Replacement.* Petaluma Cal.: Smart Publication, 1997.

Wright, Jonathon V. "Comparative measurements of serum estriol, estradiol and E1 in non-pregnant, premenopausal women; A preliminary investigation. *Alternative Medicine Review*, 1999; (4): 266-270.

Y

Yaffe, K.; Lui, L.Y.; Grady, D.; Cauley, J.; Kramer, J.; Cummings, S. "Cognitive decline in women in relation to non-protein-bound estradiol concentractions." *Lancet*, 2000; 356(9231): 708-712.

Yang, R.; Bunting, S.; Gillet, N.; Clark, R.; Jin, H. "Growth hormone improve cardiac performance in experimental heart failure." *Circulation*, 1995;92(2):262-7.

Yen, S.S., et al. "Replacement of DHEA in aging men and women. Potential remedial effects."*Annals of the New York Academy of Sciences*, 1995; 774:128-42.

Young. D. "Common Misconceptions About Sex and Depression During Menopause: A Historical Perspective." *Female Patient* 17, 1993; 25-28.

Z

Zgliczynski, S. et al. "Effect of testosterone replacement therapy on lipids and lipoproteins in hypogonadal and elderly men." *Atherosclerosis*, March 1996; 121(1): 35-43.

Zussman, L. et al. "Sexual Response After Hysterctomyophorectomy: Recent Studies and Reconsideration of Psyschogenesis." *American Journal of Obstetrics and Gynecology*, 1981; 140 (7): 725-729.

INDEX

A

acne 10, 79, 119-120, 220, 289
acromegaly 102
ACTH 70, 200
adrenals 3, 25, 27, 107, 136, 149, 157, 187, 198, 201-202, 206, 208, 210
adrenocorticotropic 200
aldosterone 7, 198, 200
allergy 27, 201, 261, 263-264, 268-271, 273, 315
allicin 32
Alpha-Lipoic Acid 32, 220-221
Alzheimer's 83-84, 146-147
American Association of Pharmaceutical Scientists 240
American Family Physicians 166
American Journal of Cardiology 197
American Journal of Physiology 82, 324
amino acids 5, 95, 100, 230, 233-234, 296, 303
andropause 72, 106, 110, 141, 213, 283, 292
Androstendiol 85
Androstendione 85
Annals of Internal Medicine 197
Annals of New York Academy of Sciences 82
anti-aging process 251
antibiotics 193, 215
antidepressants 10, 164
antioxidants 29-32
anxiety 6, 23, 25, 34, 72, 112, 119, 137, 144, 147, 155, 160, 164-165, 268, 270, 302, 310
Archives of Dermatology 146
Archives of Internal Medicine 89, 328
arginine 100,164
aromatization 70, 112, 136, 141, 145, 158, 299
arteriosclerosis 73, 281, 283
arthritis xix, 28, 32, 89, 100, 278, 283, 293-294, 303, 323, 329, 333
Ashwaganda 32, 183

B

Baby Boomer 253
benign tumor 129, 145, 158
beta carotene xi, 220, 221
beta sistosterol 307
bioidentical hormone xi, 5, 13, 15-16, 18, 21, 37, 51-52, 57-58, 60, 63-64, 66, 302
biological age 10, 12-13, 17, 37, 287
Biological Trace Element Research 185
Biomedicina 146
black Cohosh 52, 302
blood pressure vii, 16, 32, 59, 102-103, 115, 150, 162-163, 174, 191, 198, 209, 298, 301
blood sugar 5, 26, 199, 201, 209, 257, 297
blood test 37, 39, 41, 102, 117, 182, 193, 271
body hair 115
bone density 99, 162, 306, 325
boron 32
bossiness 79, 119-120, 292
bound hormones 37-39, 44, 65
Bradlow 129, 319, 327
breast cancer 74, 126-131, 142-144, 157, 162-163, 185, 286, 299, 302, 307, 319, 321-324, 326, 328, 330, 334
breast pain 302
breathing 28, 35, 195-196, 199, 203-204, 259, 286
British Journal of Dermatology 216, 221

C

caffeine 171, 235, 236, 279
calcium 6-7, 98, 127, 171, 184, 267, 302, 306
cancer 16, 24, 28-29, 32, 54-56, 74-75, 82
capsules 64-65
carbos 27
carbs 19, 232, 245
cardiovascular disease 16, 23, 73, 76, 82, 104, 146, 191, 202, 283, 295, 297, 300-301, 318, 324
carpal tunnel syndrome 100-103
catabolic 9, 25, 35, 205
catalase 219-220, 232
cellulite 233, 235-236
Chaste tree berry 302

Chemical Research and Toxicology 146
cholesterol 85, 127, 144, 147, 159, 163, 180, 187, 223, 239, 282, 300, 303, 305
choline 63
Chondrocytes 97
chronological age 10, 13, 17
Chrysin 299-300
circadian rhythm 168
citrus extracts 289-290
Coenzyme Q10 231
collagen 23, 146-147, 214-216, 219, 221, 226, 228-229, 231, 233-234, 238, 250
constipation 21, 35, 192, 194, 263, 267, 303
Cordyceps Sinensis 28, 196, 279, 293
corpus luteum 148, 151
cortisol xi, 4, 7, 18-19, 25, 27, 38-39, 41-42, 44, 47, 65, 69-70, 81, 85-86, 136, 164,
169-170, 183, 198-204, 207-210, 213, 224, 245, 257, 290-291, 318, 330
cosmetics 217, 220, 238, 242
Curcumin 294, 303
cysts 24, 26, 127, 131, 148, 156-157, 162, 185, 289

D

deer antler extract 100-101, 305
delivery methods 58-66
dendrites 98
depression 5, 19, 56, 59, 71, 79, 86, 89-90, 98, 110-111, 113, 119, 132-133, 137,
146-147, 152, 155, 160, 164-168, 186, 200, 206, 263, 270-271, 290, 302, 335
DHEA xi, 7, 11, 16, 19, 24-25, 34, 38-39, 41, 44, 47, 61, 65, 69-82, 85, 90, 112, 136,
193, 201, 203-204, 207, 210, 213, 223-224, 226, 245, 287, 291-293, 319, 322,
324, 335
Diabetes xix, 27, 29, 61, 72, 75, 143-144, 188-189, 202, 210, 257, 266, 268, 270-271,
280, 295-297, 304
diamonds 51, 249
diet, diet plan xi, xx, 11, 13, 17-20, 27-28, 31, 82, 88, 102, 109, 130-131, 140, 153,
165, 178, 183, 186-187, 195-196, 201, 203, 214, 241, 245-246, 256-267, 269,
271, 273, 279, 303-305, 324, 326
DNA 4, 9, 29, 36, 53, 129, 219, 223, 276, 279, 296, 332
dong quai 302

Dr. Tai's Anti-aging Health Secrets
        adrenals 210
        delivery 66
        DHEA 81
        estrogen 145
        HGH 104
        hormones 16
        melatonin 177
        pregnenolone 90
        progesterone 165
        saliva testing 48
        skin 227
        skin care 253
        testosterone 120
        thyroid 196
dry skin 72, 104, 111, 119, 194, 220, 251, 288, 311

E

edginess 89-90
elastin 23, 214-215, 228-289, 243, 310
endocrinology 3, 54, 76, 79, 82, 88, 129, 131, 171, 204, 267, 301, 318-319, 321, 324-332
endometriosis 113, 123, 141, 143, 153, 299
energy, lack of 11, 20-21, 81, 119, 209, 253, 263, 268, 271, 283
environmental health perspective 223
enzymes 29, 59, 184-186, 232, 249-250, 279, 293-294, 303, 305-306, 311
epidermis 61, 158, 214-217, 230-231, 237, 239-240, 312
equine estrogen 55-56, 229, 335
erectile dysfunction 110, 112
estradiol 38, 41, 44, 47, 55, 65, 70, 85, 122, 126-129, 131, 145, 159, 181, 225-226, 300, 320, 323, 326-327, 329, 334-335
estriol 41, 44, 85, 126-132, 145, 225-226, 323-324, 326-327, 330, 335
estrone 41, 59, 85, 126-128, 130-131, 145, 226
evodia 293, 299, 300
exercise 13, 19-20, 28, 30-31, 35, 51, 95, 97-98, 171, 187-188, 195-196, 201, 207, 210, 259, 282, 305, 322
exfoliation 245, 247-250, 311
Experimental Molecular Medicine 229-230

F

fertility 5, 179, 320-323, 329, 334
fibroids 141, 143-144, 148, 156, 164, 185, 196, 299, 302
fibromyalgia 180, 200, 293, 295
follicle-stimulating hormone (FSH) 107, 122, 124, 134, 175
food allergies 261, 268-273, 315
Food and Drug Administration (FDA) 47, 56, 229, 239
Forgetfulness 89, 186
free hormones 37-39, 65, 77, 99, 117
free radicals 29, 33, 71, 214, 219, 221-223, 227, 292, 296, 305

G

GABA 291-292
genistein 222, 230, 302-303
gigantism 102
ginger 294, 303, 306-307
ginseng 230-231, 290-291, 305-306, 308
glucosamine sulfate 294, 303
glucose 29, 32, 41, 75-76, 93, 164, 200, 210, 263, 266, 297-298
glutamine, L-glutamine 33, 266
glutathione 171, 219-220, 231-232, 280, 296, 301
glycemic index 20, 26-27, 263, 279
GnRH 107, 134
goiter(s) 186, 192
green tea 33, 220, 260, 305-307

H

HDL cholesterol 119, 127-128, 147, 159, 164, 300-301, 305
headaches 34, 144, 149, 152, 155, 160, 261, 263, 267, 269-270, 290, 300, 303, 310
heart disease 16, 28-29, 32, 76, 126, 161, 170, 180, 188, 200, 210, 257
HGH xi, 23, 25, 61, 69, 93-105, 235
hormone replacement therapy 54-55, 57, 70, 90, 126, 143, 147, 181, 327-328
hormones, synthetic 12-14, 18, 51-56, 143, 146, 229
hot flashes 126, 128, 135, 137, 144, 146, 154, 160, 164, 229, 286-287, 302
huperzine A 291-292
hypertension 25, 32, 100, 104, 187, 202, 210, 257, 280, 301, 309-310
hyperthyroid 178, 182, 187-189, 192, 196
hypothalamus 7, 70, 107, 123-124, 134, 169, 184, 267, 304, 309
hypothyroid 16, 144, 178, 180, 182, 185-194, 196-197, 283
hysterectomy 136, 335

I

IGF-1 71, 82, 93, 95-102, 104, 233, 305
infertility   146, 200, 270, 283, 296
Infertility and Reproductive Medicine Clinics of North America 146
inositol-hexa-nicotinate 300
insulin 5, 8, 15, 25, 27, 73, 75-76, 82, 95-96, 101, 104, 144, 147, 183, 188, 198, 213,
        240, 263, 266, 297-298, 302, 304, 324
International Journal of Dermatology 225
International Journal of Obesity & Related Metabolic Disorders 267
iodide/iodine 178, 183, 185-187, 195-196, 258, 282
isoflavones 222, 302-303

J

Johns Hopkin's University 73

K

kefir xi
kukui nut oil 310-311

L

L-caffeine   235-236
L-carnitine   235-236
LDL cholesterol 127-128, 147, 180, 223, 300, 305
leydig cells 107
libido 21, 33, 56, 71-72, 81, 102-103, 109-112, 118-119, 136-137, 144-146, 163, 178,
        191, 196, 253, 290-291, 308
licorice 289-290, 301, 307, 311
linden 311
liposomes 63-64, 77, 101, 218, 224, 234, 239-243, 245, 249, 253, 310
lobelia 298
longevity 17, 24, 30, 33, 88, 147
luteinizing hormone 107, 122, 124, 134, 164, 171
lycopene 33, 220
lymphocytes 71
luteonizing phase 152, 155

M

magnesium 127, 266, 298, 303, 311, 331

marine collagen 331

melatonin xi, 4, 7, 19, 25, 41, 43, 136, 168, 169-170, 171-172, 174-176, 186, 193, 213, 223-224, 245, 319, 323, 327, 329, 331-332

memory and memory loss 6, 21, 24, 34-35, 53, 56, 71, 79, 83, 85, 87-90, 96, 98, 102, 109, 112, 114, 127, 137, 144, 146-147, 161, 181, 202, 278, 283, 291-292, 296, 320, 322, 331

menopause/perimenopause xi, 19, 55, 59, 106-107, 110-111, 113, 122, 125-128, 132, 134-140, 142, 145-147, 153-154, 160, 163, 170, 181, 200, 213, 222, 226, 283, 286, 288, 301-303, 322, 324, 326, 330, 334-335

menstrual cycle 5, 43, 123-125, 129, 134, 136, 144, 148, 150, 152, 155, 320

microdermabrasion 227, 249, 250, 311, 312

micro-encapsulations 224, 236, 241

migraines 24, 152, 268-270, 283, 303-304

monocytes 71

moisturizers 215, 217, 224, 227, 245, 250-252

mugwort 312

N

nausea 166, 190, 270

niacinamide 311

night sweats 110, 135, 137, 144, 146, 154, 229

norepinephrane 7, 109

nutrition xii, xvi, 19, 26, 64, 88, 200, 267, 296-297, 304, 307, 331

O

obesity 19, 24, 72, 143, 173, 181, 198, 210, 235, 256-257, 267-268, 270-271, 283, 297, 304, 324, 326

oily skin 79, 217, 247

olive oil xi, 28, 262

orgasmic response 112, 119, 308-309

osteoporosis 25, 29, 53, 79, 97-98, 109, 111, 137, 140, 144, 155, 158-159, 164, 200, 202, 209, 283, 292, 305-306, 327

ovarian cancer 143, 299, 302

ovarian cysts 127

ovulation 129, 134, 155, 191, 303

P

Panax ginseng 231, 290-291, 306, 308
pH 41, 128, 215, 227, 246-247, 289, 295
phosphatidylcholine 63, 66, 239
phosphatidylserine 325
photo-aging 234
phytoestrogen 223, 226, 229, 322
pineapple 311
pineal gland 168-169, 329
pinus 311
pituitary gland 7, 69, 95, 107, 123, 134, 170, 178, 184, 200
placebo 76, 221, 225, 281, 294
pleurotus 301
PMS 122, 125, 142-144, 148-152, 165, 190, 200, 302-303
poria 298
postpartum depression 132-133
pregnancy 8, 123, 127-128, 130, 132, 145, 149, 151, 155, 185, 226, 318
pregnenolone xi, 25, 69, 83-90, 180, 201, 213, 287, 291-293, 298, 322-323, 332
Premarin 55
prodew 310-311
progesterone xi, 5, 8, 11, 20, 23-24, 34, 40-41, 43-44, 47, 52, 54, 65, 80, 85, 123, 125,
131-132, 136, 138-139, 143-145, 147, 147-166, 196, 201, 203, 213, 245, 287,
300, 302-303, 319-324, 326-334
progestins 153, 162, 166
prostate 75, 101, 103, 111, 115, 141, 144-145, 157-158, 299, 306-308, 328, 332
puereria mirifica 222, 229, 230

Q

quercetin 295, 303

R

receptor sites 5, 12, 52-53, 95, 108, 127-129, 143, 157-158, 162, 230, 266, 297
red clover 52, 303
Retin-A 220-221
rheumatoid arthritis 89, 270, 293-294, 323, 329, 333
rhodiola-rosea 305, 310

S

salivary gland 38-39

saliva testing 37-48, 65, 77-78, 116, 210, 315

salicyclic acid 289

saw palmetto 118, 306, 308

secretagogues 100, 116, 309

sex drive xi, xii, 6, 22, 119, 181

sexuality 5, 112

SHGB (sex hormone-binding globulin) 39, 63-65, 108

side effects 51, 53-66, 90

sleep 5, 7, 18-19, 21, 30, 32, 43, 71, 73, 95, 102, 127, 136, 138, 144, 156, 160, 163, 168-177, 181, 188, 200-203, 209, 230, 238, 263, 280

smoking 18, 35, 62, 227, 232, 237

soybeans 304

steroid 5-6, 39, 65, 69, 82-83, 87-88, 148, 199, 224, 320, 322-323, 330, 333-334

stress 5, 7, 14-17, 19, 26-27, 32, 39, 42-43, 70-71, 77, 79, 81, 83, 85-87, 89-90, 112-113, 125, 164, 169-170, 172, 182-183, 198, 200-204, 209, 222, 231, 290-291, 296, 303, 310, 325-326

strokes 32-33, 56, 281, 301

sublingual 38, 58, 65-66, 100, 245

supplements xv, xxi, 13, 31, 34, 37, 51-52, 60, 65, 69, 100, 117-118, 158, 177, 192, 195, 199, 242, 245, 258, 265, 280, 289-312

sun exposure 219, 230, 237

sun protection factor (SPF) 227, 231-232, 244, 251-252

Syndrome X 297

synthetic hormones 12-13, 16, 18, 51-56, 143, 146, 229

T

T3 (triiodothyronine) 178-180, 182-187, 191

testes 5, 8, 69, 106-107, 122

testosterone xi, 7-8, 11, 20, 22-23, 34-35, 38-39, 41, 43-44, 47, 52, 55-56, 59, 61-62, 65, 69-72, 77, 80, 82, 104, 106-120, 136, 141, 149, 151, 157-158, 165, 170, 181, 183, 201, 210, 213, 223-224, 226, 233, 292, 300, 302, 308, 318-322, 324-325, 328-329, 333-336

thyroid xi, 3, 6-7, 22, 25, 136, 149, 162, 164, 178-197, 201, 203, 205, 213, 217, 243, 258, 332

toner 321

tribulus 293

tumors 74, 102, 129, 131, 142, 145, 148, 156-158, 227

U

unbound hormones 38-39, 65
urine testing 40-41
usnea extract 290
uterine bleeding 143
uterus 8, 123-124, 129, 136, 145, 147, 151, 153, 156, 159, 186, 290
UVA rays 231, 252
UVB rays 231, 252

V

vaginal dryness 128, 137, 144, 146
vitamin:
        A, 32, 183, 188, 220
        B, 169, 183, 188, 196
        C, 33, 183, 188, 216, 218-220
        E, 183, 188, 220
        K, 188

W

water retention 86, 100-101, 103-104, 144, 147, 150, 164, 187, 200, 209, 298, 302
weight gain 16, 56, 59, 110, 119, 124, 144, 186-187, 192, 194-195, 209, 242, 253, 267, 270, 286
weight loss 27, 70, 100, 191, 194, 256, 265, 267, 271, 304-305
white bean extract 305
white willow 295
wrinkles 104, 144, 172, 201, 212-213, 216, 219, 221, 226-227, 229-230, 234-235, 238, 242-245, 253, 285, 310, 312

Y

yams 56, 229

Z

zinc 28, 127, 164, 183, 197, 216